To Joe
From Jim Anderson.

(Now you're learning the <u>really</u>
important part of medicine!)

A METHOD OF PSYCHIATRY

A METHOD OF PSYCHIATRY

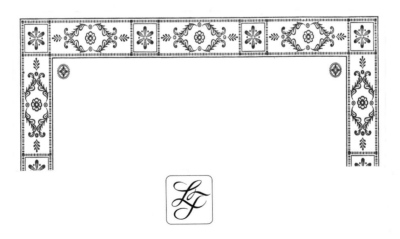

Lea & Febiger   1980   Philadelphia

Library of Congress Cataloging in Publication Data

University of Toronto. Dept. of Psychiatry.
  A method of psychiatry.

  Bibliography: p.
  Includes index.
  1. Psychiatry. I. Greben, Stanley E. II. Title.
[DNLM: 1. Mental disorders. 2. Physician-patient
relations. 3. Psychiatry—Methods. WM100 M592]
RC454.U54 1980   616.89   80-10348
ISBN 0-8121-0710-1

Published in Great Britain by Henry Kimpton Publishers, London

Printed in the United States of America

Print No.: 3   2   1

To the memory of
DR. ALDWYN B. STOKES,
Professor and Chairman,
Department of Psychiatry,
University of Toronto: 1947–1967

Preface

Faculty members of the Department of Psychiatry of the University of Toronto have prepared this text. We have done so because we have not found, among the many good and comprehensive textbooks available, one that reflects our particular method of teaching the basis of psychiatry.

This method is a broadly-based eclecticism which uses the contributions of many different points of view in the field of psychiatry. We emphasize the idea of the psychiatrist as a physician, a healer who uses the available knowledge of a given period to respond to the patient's suffering, with the awareness that the sources of suffering are ordinarily complex. These sources may range from the broadly sociological or even historical to the most narrowly identifiable somatic cause.

In the use of scientific knowledge the physician exercises a social role, but is not completely defined by it. The patient expects the physician to be sensitive to and aware of matters not usually covered in medical education, although sometimes now taught in the area called "Behavioral Science." At the same time, we expect that knowledge derived from rigorous investigation in the clinic, in the laboratory and in the community must occupy a central place in psychiatric practice.

Similarly, our approach takes into account that a patient is not simply defined by presenting oneself to a physician as a sufferer. The patient also has a social role that varies from society to society and from time to time.

The student should know about stressful situations in general, as well as the specific tensions and tasks of the various life stages, any of which may be pathogenic. He must also recognize the range of human needs—historical, sociological, economic, psychological and somatic—which may, when disrupted, generate suffering that becomes the concern of the physician.

Finally, as to our intended readership: This book is primarily presented for the medical student, and for all physicians who do not specialize in psychiatry. It is also hoped that it would be of value to members of other professions who handle these same patients, certainly including nurses, psychologists and social workers.

Acknowledgments

In 1973, Dr. Robin C. A. Hunter, the then Chairman of the Department of Psychiatry at the University of Toronto, invited Dr. Robert Pos to coordinate efforts towards producing student notes in psychiatry. This continued when Dr. Frederick H. Lowy became Chairman of the Department in 1974. A sub-committee consisting of Drs. Greben, Pos and Rakoff drafted the outline of this "Method of Psychiatry" which has been refined and amended by the Editorial Board.

We thank the Physicians of Ontario for the grant from The Physicians' Services Incorporated Foundation.

Contributors

J. Donald Atcheson, M.D.
  Professor, Department of Psychiatry
  University of Toronto
  Staff Psychiatrist, Clarke Institute of
    Psychiatry
  Toronto, Ontario, Canada

Joseph M. Berg, M.B., B.Ch.
  Professor, Department of Psychiatry
  University of Toronto
  Director of Genetic Services
  Surrey Place Centre
  Toronto, Ontario, Canada

David M. Berger, M.D.
  Associate Professor, Department of
    Psychiatry
  University of Toronto
  Staff Psychiatrist, Mount Sinai Hospital
  Toronto, Ontario, Canada

Alexander Bonkalo, M.D.
  Professor Emeritus, Department of
    Psychiatry
  University of Toronto
  Consultant, Clarke Institute of Psychiatry
  Toronto, Ontario, Canada

Gregory M. Brown, M.D., Ph.D.
  Professor and Chairman, Department of
    Neurosciences
  McMaster University
  Formerly Professor, Department of
    Psychiatry
  University of Toronto
  Staff Psychiatrist, McMaster University
    Medical Centre
  Formerly Head of Neuroendocrinology,
    Research Section, Clarke Institute of
    Psychiatry
  Toronto, Ontario, Canada

Paul M. Cameron, M.D.
  Associate Professor and Director of
    Postgraduate Education, Department of
    Psychiatry
  University of Toronto
  Staff Psychiatrist, Sunnybrook Medical
    Centre
  Toronto, Ontario, Canada

Clive G. Chamberlain, M.D.
  Associate Professor, Department of
    Psychiatry
  University of Toronto
  Chief Policy Adviser, Children's Services
    Division
  Ministry of Community and Social Services
    of Ontario
  Toronto, Ontario, Canada

Stanley J. J. Freeman, M.D.
  Professor, Department of Psychiatry
  University of Toronto
  Psychiatrist-in-Charge, Community
    Resources Section, Clarke Institute of
    Psychiatry
  Toronto, Ontario, Canada

Kurt Freund, M.D.
  Associate Professor, Department of
    Psychiatry
  University of Toronto
  Head of Research Section of Behavioural
    Sexology, Clarke Institute of Psychiatry
  Toronto, Ontario, Canada

Paul E. Garfinkel, M.D.
  Associate Professor, Department of
    Psychiatry
  University of Toronto
  Staff Psychiatrist, Clarke Institute of
    Psychiatry
  Toronto, Ontario, Canada

Stanley E. Greben, M.D.
Professor, Department of Psychiatry
University of Toronto
Psychiatrist-in-Chief, Mount Sinai Hospital
Toronto, Ontario, Canada

R. Ian Hector, M.D.
Associate Professor, Department of
Psychiatry
University of Toronto
Staff Psychiatrist, The Wellesley Hospital
Toronto, Ontario, Canada

Henry B. Kedward, M.B., Ch. B.
Professor, Department of Psychiatry
University of Toronto
Head, Research Section of Epidemiology,
Clarke Institute of Psychiatry
Toronto, Ontario, Canada

Edward Kingstone, M.D.
Professor, Department of Psychiatry and
Vice-Provost
University of Toronto
Staff Psychiatrist, Sunnybrook Medical
Centre
Toronto, Ontario, Canada

Stephen A. Kline, M.D.
Assistant Professor, Department of
Psychiatry, University of Toronto
Clinical Director, Dept. of Psychiatry,
Toronto Western Hospital
Toronto, Ontario, Canada

Sebastian K. Littmann, M.B., Ch.B.
Associate Professor, Department of
Psychiatry
University of Toronto
Psychiatrist-in-Charge, Outpatient Services,
Clarke Institute of Psychiatry
Toronto, Ontario, Canada

Frederick H. Lowy, M.D.
Professor and Chairman, Department of
Psychiatry
University of Toronto
Director and Psychiatrist-in-Chief, Clarke
Institute of Psychiatry
Toronto, Ontario, Canada

Marvin E. Miller, M.D.
Assistant Professor, Department of
Psychiatry
University of Toronto
Staff Psychiatrist, Mount Sinai Hospital
Toronto, Ontario, Canada

Harvey Moldofsky, M.D.
Professor, Department of Psychiatry
University of Toronto
Psychiatrist-in-Chief, Toronto Western
Hospital
Toronto, Ontario, Canada

Alistair Munro, M.B., Ch.B.
Professor, Department of Psychiatry
University of Toronto
Psychiatrist-in-Chief, Toronto General
Hospital
Toronto, Ontario, Canada

Emmanuel Persad, M.B. B.S.
Associate Professor, Department of
Psychiatry
University of Toronto
Chief, Affective Disorders Unit, Clarke
Institute of Psychiatry
Toronto, Ontario, Canada

Robert Pos, M.D., Ph.D.
Professor, Department of Psychiatry
University of Toronto
Director of Psychiatry, Owen Sound General
and Marine Hospital
Formerly Psychiatrist-in-Chief, Toronto
General Hospital
Toronto, Ontario, Canada

Quentin Rae-Grant, M.B., Ch.B.
Professor of Child Psychiatry and
Vice-Chairman, Department of
Psychiatry
University of Toronto
Psychiatrist-in-Chief, Hospital for Sick
Children
Toronto, Ontario, Canada

Vivian M. Rakoff, M.B. B.S.
Professor of Psychiatric Education,
Department of Psychiatry
University of Toronto
Psychiatrist-in-Chief, Sunnybrook Medical
Centre
Toronto, Ontario, Canada

Mary V. Seeman, M.D.
Associate Professor, Department of
Psychiatry
University of Toronto
Head, Active Treatment Clinic, Clarke
Institute of Psychiatry
Toronto, Ontario, Canada

Gerald Shugar, M.D.
  Associate Professor, Department of
    Psychiatry
  University of Toronto
  Chief, Adult Floor, Clarke Institute of
    Psychiatry
  Toronto, Ontario, Canada

Betty W. Steiner, M.B., Ch.B.
  Associate Professor, Department of
    Psychiatry
  University of Toronto
  Psychiatrist-in-Charge, Gender Identity
    Clinic, Clarke Institute of Psychiatry
  Toronto, Ontario, Canada

Paul D. Steinhauer, M.D.
  Professor, Department of Psychiatry
  University of Toronto
  Staff Psychiatrist, Hospital for Sick Children
  Toronto, Ontario, Canada

Richard P. Swinson, M.B., Ch.B.
  Associate Professor, Department of
    Psychiatry
  University of Toronto
  Staff Psychiatrist, Toronto General Hospital
  Toronto, Ontario, Canada

Graeme J. Taylor, M.B., Ch.B.
  Associate Professor, Department of
    Psychiatry
  University of Toronto
  Head, Psychiatric Consultation-Liaison
    Service, Mount Sinai Hospital
  Toronto, Ontario, Canada

George Voineskos, M.D.
  Associate Professor and Director of
    Undergraduate Education, Department
    of Psychiatry
  University of Toronto
  Chief, Primary Care Service, Clarke Institute
    of Psychiatry
  Toronto, Ontario, Canada

Gordon E. Warme, M.D.
  Associate Professor, Department of
    Psychiatry
  University of Toronto
  Chief, Child and Family Studies Centre,
    Clarke Institute of Psychiatry
  Toronto, Ontario, Canada

Donald A. Wasylenki, M.D.
  Assistant Professor, Dept. of Psychiatry
  University of Toronto
  Staff Psychiatrist, Clarke Institute of
    Psychiatry
  Toronto, Ontario, Canada

Contents

Chapter

1 The Patient and the Physician 1
   Vivian M. Rakoff, Robert Pos and Stanley E. Greben
2 Infancy and Childhood 9
   Paul D. Steinhauer
3 Adolescence and Young Adulthood 33
   Clive G. Chamberlain
4 Middle Age and Maturity (Old Age) 43
   Marvin E. Miller
5 Life Events and Illness 55
   Donald A. Wasylenki and Stanley J. J. Freeman
6 Biology, Behavior and Mental Functioning 71
   Alexander Bonkalo and Gregory M. Brown
7 Being with the Patient 77
   Stanley E. Greben
8 The Examination: History 81
   Sebastian K. Littmann and Gerald Shugar
9 The Examination: Mental State 91
   R. Ian Hector and Sebastian K. Littmann
10 The Examination: Physical and Special Investigations 101
   Paul M. Cameron
11 The Examination: Psychological Testing 107
   Gerald Shugar
12 The Examination: Formulation 113
   Paul M. Cameron and Stephen A. Kline
13 Common Psychiatric Disorders: Introduction 117
   David M. Berger
14 Anxiety and Anxiety Related Disorders 121
   David M. Berger
15 Dissociative Disorders and Depersonalization 131
   David M. Berger
16 Somatization, Conversion and Hypochondriasis 135
   David M. Berger
17 Psychosomatic Mechanisms 143
   Harvey Moldofsky
18 Psychosomatic Disorders 149
   Graeme J. Taylor

Chapter

19 Pain 157
    Robert Pos
20 Sleep Disorders 163
    Robert Pos
21 Affective Disorders 171
    Paul E. Garfinkel and Emmanuel Persad
22 Paranoid Disorders 185
    Alexander Bonkalo
23 Schizophrenic Disorders 189
    Henry B. Kedward and Mary V. Seeman
24 Personality Disorders 203
    J. Donald Atcheson and Gordon E. Warme
25 Disorders of Sexual Behavior 211
    Kurt Freund and Betty W. Steiner
26 Drug Use Disorders 221
    Richard P. Swinson
27 Organic Disorders (Intracerebral) 229
    Alexander Bonkalo and Alistair Munro
28 Organic Disorders (Extracerebral) 237
    Alistair Munro
29 Childhood and Adolescent Disorders 249
    Quentin Rae-Grant
30 Psychiatric Emergencies 267
    George Voineskos and Frederick H. Lowy
31 Suicide and Attempted Suicide 275
    George Voineskos and Frederick H. Lowy
32 Treatment: General 281
    Frederick H. Lowy
33 Treatment: Psychotherapy and Behavior Therapy 289
    Frederick H. Lowy and Robert Pos
34 Treatment: Somatic 297
    Edward Kingstone
35 Treatment: Hospital 319
    George Voineskos
36 Treatment: Social-Environmental 325
    George Voineskos
37 Difficult Challenges in Medical Practice 333
    Stanley E. Greben
38 Referral to the Psychiatrist 339
    Frederick H. Lowy
39 Mental Retardation 345
    Joseph M. Berg
A Short Glossary of Psychiatric Terms 355
Index 359

CHAPTER 1

The Patient and the Physician
Vivian M. Rakoff, Robert Pos and Stanley E. Greben

Although most physicians reject the idea that mind and body are separate, they often act as though the patient could be split into discrete entities. The specialization of medical practice encourages compartmentalizing of the patient.

Few patients have attended medical school, and they do not present themselves or their complaints to the physician in terms of his useful but somewhat arbitrary categories. Although the physician may find that breaking the patient up into systems is unavoidable, such an approach may prevent the perception of the patient as a whole. In psychiatric practice, for example, the patient who has a disorder that seems to be obviously psychological (because his emotions, perceptions and judgements may be disordered or because he is hallucinating or deluded) may in fact be suffering from metabolic, endocrinological, toxic, neoplastic, or infectious disease. Conversely, the patient whose signs and symptoms are obviously physical ones may, when he is examined, turn out to be sick because of emotional stress.

A number of studies have attempted to clarify the relationship between physical and emotional disorders. In the Stirling County Study (Leighton et al., 1963) and the Mid-Town Manhattan Study (Rennie et al., 1962) approximately 80% of the people studied had a psychological disorder of some kind. The Yale Medical Center Study (Duff and Hollingshead, 1968) showed that the percentage of people suffering from a psychological disorder was even greater in patients admitted to medical-surgical services. The Yale Study further showed that just before their illnesses became apparent, the patients studied had a significant increase in psychological symptoms compared with the general population. The work of Engel (1968) and of Schmale (1972) supports that observation. Engel and Schmale concluded that illness of any kind can be preceded by psychological distress that produces what they called the "giving up reaction," a response of despair and apathy. They estimated that the sequence, psychological stress—despair—illness, occurred in 70 to 80% of the patients.

In the Cornell Medical Project Study (Hinkle and Wolff, 1961) in which 3000 patients were observed for 20 years, it was found that illness was concentrated in 10% of the people studied. Those people appeared to have had more major and minor physical and psychological illnesses dur-

1

ing a given period. For some people that period lasted several years. It has been suggested that those patients were going through an "illness-prone phase of their lives" that could be related to the occurrence of severe psychological stress.

Koranyi (1978) has shown that psychiatric patients have more physical illnesses than people in general. In short, the link between physical and psychological suffering is important. Although this book concentrates on the psychological manifestations of disease, the relationship to physical disorders is not ignored or underplayed.

Both the patient and the physician may find the relationship between physical and psychological symptoms complex and bewildering. The patient may lack the ability to express his psychological suffering; and the physician, who is not aware of the many ways that psychological distress expresses itself, may miss the proper diagnosis or etiology of the disorder.

Eastwood (1971) and Goldberg and Blackwell (1970) studied the incidence of psychological illness in the practices of family physicians. Eastwood found that many patients in family practice clinics had psychological disorders. Usually the psychological disorders were minor, and were more common among women than among men. Eastwood's studies supported Hinkle's and Wolff's idea that both physical and psychological disorders tend to cluster in particular patients. The disorders are not distributed randomly.

Goldberg and Blackwell interviewed 533 patients of family physicians. They found that approximately 25% of the patients suffered from some form of psychological disorder. Not surprisingly the psychiatrists detected more psychological disorders than the family physicians did; nevertheless there was a high level of agreement between the psychiatrists and the family physicians, particularly in those cases in which the illnesses were clearly psychiatric. The criterion for considering

an illness a psychological one was that the patient concerned had few physical complaints or symptoms. Most important from the point of view of this book, Goldberg and Blackwell's study indicated that many patients who consult a physician for an apparently physical complaint suffer from "hidden psychiatric illness." A hidden psychological illness is generally not detected in the 10 to 15 minutes that the family physician usually spends with a patient. Patients with the hidden psychological illness formulated their complaints in purely physical terms—to the physician and to themselves. Since most of the patients did not consider themselves emotionally disturbed, the psychological nature of the illness was brought out only by direct questioning during the study.

Other studies have shown that although there may be a large amount of psychiatric morbidity in the general population, only a few people suffering from psychological disorders think that they should consult a physician. As Goldberg and Blackwell noted, the person may not realize that he is entitled to consult a physician for a disorder that is not clearly physical. They cite the sociologist Mechanic, who has stated that a person must consider himself ill in some way before he feels justified in consulting a physician. The physician who is aware of such an attitude can make certain that his patients feel free to discuss with him any psychological disorders.

THE PATIENT'S NEEDS

The physician must respond to various kinds of distress in the patient. The distress can be caused by a disruption of any part of the complex biological-social system that is necessary for well-being. Obviously, a healthy body is essential to well-being, and the physician is usually asked to restore health to the body. But the whole person extends beyond his body. He does so through his near and distant relationships that express and nurture important parts of his identity and are therefore relevant to his health and happiness.

A number of attempts have been made to classify and explain human needs and relationships. Maslow (1968) described such a hierarchy of needs. When the needs that are lowest in the hierarchy are satisfied, the next lowest needs press for satisfaction, and so on through the hierarchy. At the base Maslow places the physiological needs such as hunger and thirst. Then there is the need to feel physically and psychologically safe. Next, people need to feel that they belong to a community and experience love, and beyond that are the needs for esteem, for self-actualization, cognitive needs such as the thirst for knowledge, and finally aesthetic needs such as the desire for beauty.

All those needs affect happiness in ways that are relevant to medicine. Disruption of those needs may result in a host of disorders such as alcoholism, anxiety, and depression.

Human psychological integrity derives from many complex and interacting sources. If any of these is missing, distorted or disrupted it may result in suffering, ranging from minor distress to severe illness. "Systems theory" has tried to create an overall theory relating all these possible factors. It attempts to show how forces and events that seem remote from any particular person finally impinge on the simplest and most concrete parts of his life. For example: failure in industrial policy or world trading patterns can affect small towns in North America by producing economic difficulties. A particular factory making—let us say—gloves, has to discharge workers. An unemployed husband in a particular family already has doubts concerning his masculinity because of problems he had with learning difficulties at school, and troubles with his parents. The accumulation of distress produces depression which finally brings him to the doctor's office.

It is difficult to attribute one particular cause to his depression. Economic causes? But many workers who are laid off don't become depressed. Faulty infant rearing? Perhaps, but it didn't result in illness until there was an economic cause. A faulty educational system? Yes, but it only added to his problems at home. Some understanding of all these factors may be necessary to make sense of any particular case. At the very least it is desirable that the clinician should be aware of how complex the roots of psychological distress can be.

Under the umbrella of systems theory there are other sub-theories that help to understand the interrelationship of growth, development, and personal well-being: Psychoanalysis has provided a model for the importance of infantile relationships in establishing emotional health for the rest of the patient's life. Some recent concepts of ethology may clarify the genetic readiness for affection, close bonding to parents and the need for human intimacy, while learning theory explains how learning occurs within the context of these human needs and capabilities. And beyond the immediate and personally perceived processes, the disciplines of anthropology, sociology, and economics provide frameworks that make sense of the complex social needs of human beings.

THE PATIENT AND THE PHYSICIAN: WHO THEY ARE

Both patients and physicians operate within certain expectations of how they are to behave when the patient brings his suffering to the doctor's office. To a great extent the roles of patient and physician are defined by society.

THE PATIENT'S ROLE

Although sociologists and physicians have carefully studied the behavior of patients, they have not established that there is a predictable way that patients behave. Thus the models of patient behavior described in the following paragraphs are only diagrams. Still, they do explain much about the behavior that people exhibit when they consult a physician.

Patient behavior can vary from culture to culture; for example, in some cultures the model of how one may be sick is limited, and people in those cultures may use simple phrases such as, "I have a worm in my body" to describe different kinds of distress. Nevertheless, Talcott Parsons has been able to describe some common characteristics of the sick person: (1) The sick person is exempted by society from some or all of his normal responsibilities; (2) the sick person does not decide to become sick, and he does not decide to become better; but society expects him to want to get well as soon as possible; and (3) the sick person is expected by society to look for appropriate help (in Western society, from a physician or in a hospital) and to cooperate with that help toward the end of getting well.

A sick person, noticing signs of ill health, consults a physician. After the physician takes a history and examines the patient, he usually discusses with the patient the diagnosis, treatment, and prognosis. Ideally, the patient follows the physician's advice.

If the patient recovers, he abandons the sick role and resumes his normal life. But that is not always the case. Siegler and Osmond (and others) have examined the variations of the process, particularly as the variations affect the psychiatric patient, who is often an atypical patient.

The medical model of illness is the least complicated of the various models of illness. In the medical model the patient suffers from his illness without shame, and he behaves like a patient. In contrast, in the model of illness used in psychoanalysis, the question of sickness is avoided, and the person being treated is referred to not as the "patient" but as the "analysand."

The medical model ideally allows someone to be sick without feeling shame.

But there is also a moral model of illness that may affect the medical model; namely, the view that the patient is sick because he has been bad. Implicit in the moral model is the idea that if the patient strives for virtue, to be good, he will get better. The moral model implies that illness has a willful component. In many communities, the medical model (the "charitable model") is applied to physical illnesses but not to psychological illnesses. Since many patients who suffer from psychological illnesses also subscribe to the moral model of illness, they attribute physical causes to their illnesses; or they may believe that they themselves have caused their illnesses because they have been bad. A modern example of the moral model of illness is the "blaming" of parents for their children's psychological disorders. There may indeed be a causal relationship between the behavior of parents and psychological disorders in their children, but that relationship has often been discussed in tones that have been unjustifiably accusatory.

In the "impaired role" the illness is not a transient state that the patient enters and soon leaves. For the patient who assumes the impaired role, the illness extends over a long time, and that patient may be described as having not only an impairing illness but also an impaired life. The description fits the patient who is chronically ill.

Two other models of illness have been popular in recent years: (1) the social model, in which society is blamed for the patient's sickness and (2) a surprising model: the psychedelic model, in which through an inversion of the moral model the mentally ill person is considered to be more virtuous than the "bad people" in the surrounding society, who are masquerading as sane.

THE PHYSICIAN'S ROLE

The role of the physician, too, has undergone a number of changes. The obvious contemporary picture of the physician is that of the applied scientist that he has assumed over the centuries. It would be misguided to ignore the profound social benefits that have resulted from the emphasis that has been placed on the physician as applied scientist; but, most of the scientific knowledge that the modern physician uses is relatively new, whereas the role of physician is ancient. Until the Renaissance, most medical knowledge was speculative, folkloric, and unscientific (for example, the theory of humors, the fantasies about spirit possession, and impressionistic anatomy). The circulation of the blood was not demonstrated until the sixteenth century. The microscope did not exist until the seventeenth century. Until the middle of the nineteenth century the only effective medications were morphine and its derivatives and the botanical extracts that were effective principally in controlling the bowels. Digitalis was introduced only in the eighteenth century.

The medical advances of earlier centuries are minor ones compared with those of the nineteenth and twentieth centuries, when bacteriology, physiology, pathology, and biochemistry were established as sciences. And pharmacology, formerly confined to potions of doubtful efficacy, now includes a wide range of effective medicines.

Progress in medical science overtook progress in medical education. Until modern times medical training was based on the idea of medicine as a learned profession, and for hundreds of years medicine was taught in the university as one of the few alternatives to theology. For the most part, however, medical education took the form of an apprenticeship. In Britain there were (and still are) three routes to becoming a physician: (1) through the university, (2) through the professional guilds of the Royal College of Physicians, and (3) through the Apothecaries Hall.

In the United States, there were many routes to becoming a physician. Medical training sometimes took place in the university, but often it was unsupervised and not standardized. In 1911 the Flexner Report outlined a structure and standards for medical education in the United States. The report stated that the physician should be a physician-scientist. The Flexner Report was important, appropriate, and revolutionary. It established a science-oriented curriculum for the medical student.

Did the physician change the nature of his role when he became a scientist? To some extent, yes. When the physician became a scientist, he gave up the doubtful privilege of making decisions for the patient that were based solely on the physician's hierarchical authority, social license, and role as a magical healer. The change in role had negative as well as positive results. For one thing, the physician became somewhat depersonalized. In the effort to rationalize medical judgments and treatments, the relationship between the physician and the patient—formerly the essential curative element—was deemphasized.

The change in role also brought about medical triumphs. One has only to note how little fear there is today of random infection, the almost total disappearance of many childhood diseases, and the achievements of painless surgery. Yet the physician finds himself in a quandary that has been given much attention in the popular press. Before the breakthroughs of modern medicine, the physician seemed to command the respect of the layman. Ironically, before the physician became the physician-scientist, he could do little to cure his patients but he was held in great esteem by them. Now that there are rational therapies many patients feel as though a valuable part of the physician's identity was lost in the triumph of scientific medicine. The part of the physician's identity that was lost is the part that was split off from the physician's earlier priestly identity. In many cultures the magician-priest-healer is one person; at one time that was also true in the Western World. In ancient Greece, people who were sick went to the Temple of Aesculapius to be cured. The priests in ancient Greece were literate and knowledgeable, but it was not their literacy and knowledge that commanded the sufferer's respect and brought him to the Temple. The Greek priests also had a kind of authority that encouraged the ill person to entrust himself to their care.

The function of the physician is obviously different from that of the priest, particularly in the moral sphere. The priest administers to suffering within the context of moral judgement, whereas ideally the physician responds to suffering without making moral judgements. But like the priest, the physician has been placed outside the partisan causes of society, even to the point that in certain circumstances he is allowed—in fact, obligated—to treat enemy soldiers in time of war and to give medical direction to statesmen and even to royalty. Such authority has been called "Aesculapian authority."

Aesculapian authority makes it relatively easy for the patient to tell the physician things he would not ordinarily tell anyone else. It makes both physical and psychological exposure easier for the patients.

Some physicians can remain neutral more easily in regard to physical suffering, no matter how unpleasant or unesthetic that suffering may be, than in regard to psychological suffering. Some physicians feel uncomfortable in the presence of psychological pain. Their discomfort may arise from a belief that psychological pain is not a valid concern of the physician.

Some laymen also question whether the physician should treat psychological illnesses; and those who have an extremely "organic" view of the physician-scientist think that he should not. But, as we have said, patients do not always know the source of their illnesses, and physical illnesses may manifest themselves by psychological symptoms, and vice versa. In the past some illnesses that seemed to be entirely psychological have been shown to have an organic base. For example, G.P.I. (general paralysis of the insane) was considered a psychological disorder until it was shown to be related to tertiary syphilis. Until recently, many people were confined to mental hospitals for psychoses that were caused by myxedema; numerous pareses that derived from porphyria were diagnosed as hysterical; and it was not realized that islet-cell tumors of the pancreas could cause fugue-like states.

It has also been demonstrated that physical illnesses have emotional components. For example, asthma, peptic ulcer, and ulcerative colitis have been shown to be associated with intense anxiety.

Suppose that the physician were restricted to treating the body only. If that were the case, disorders that were apparently psychological would be excluded from the physician's care; and, conversely, physical disorders with emotional causes would be treated as though they had no psychological components—and so would possibly be mistreated.

The physician who does not treat both the physical and psychological manifestations of illnesses neglects important aspects of healing. Because physicians have followed a medical model that does not recognize a mind-body dichotomy, they have been able to ask the research questions that have led to the clarification of the genetic aspects of affective disorders (Winokur, 1973) and to knowledge of the biochemistry of those disorders. If physicians had not incorporated the new knowledge of human behavior into the medical curriculum, they would have excluded the medical student and the physician from a new "technology" that was not immediately applicable to the relief of suffering but that led to knowledge that was applicable to the relief of suffering. For example, before Bowlby (1952) and others demonstrated the importance of mother-child bonding and that children who are hospitalized often become depressed, hospitals restricted visiting on the pediatric wards. Now parents of hospitalized children are allowed to visit them freely. That change was based on the theory held by behavioral scientists that one's early years are important. That theory has altered the practice of pediatric medicine.

The physician fills a complex role that has a long history. He is a trusted confidant and adviser who in modern times works with the tools of modern science and modern technology. In his approach as a trained person to the patient as a person in need of help, the physician must maintain a comprehensive view of the patient. He must also remember that both he and the patient are real persons, not merely roles in a relationship.

REFERENCES

Bowlby, J. (1952): Maternal Care and Mental Health 2nd ed., Monograph Series No.2, World Health Organization, Geneva.

Duff, R.S., and Hollingshead, A.B. (1968): *Sickness and Society.* New York, Harper & Row.

Eastwood, M.R. (1971): Screening for psychiatric disorder. *Psychol. Med.* 1:197.

Engel, G.L. (1968): A life setting conducive to illness: the giving-up-given-up complex. *Arch. Int. Med.* 69:293.

Goldberg, D.P., Blackwell, B. (1970): Psychiatric illness in general practice: a detailed study using a new method of case identification. *Brit. Med. J.* 2:439.

Hinkle, L.E. (1961): Ecological observations of the relation of physical illness, mental illness, and the social environment. *Psychosom. Med.* 23:289.

Leighton, D.C., Harding, J.S., Macklin, D.B. et al. (1963): *The Character of Danger.* New York, Basic Books.

Maslow, A.H. (1968): *Toward a Psychology of Being.* New York, Van Nostrand.

Parsons, T. (1951): Social structure and dynamic process: the case of modern medical practice. In: *The Social System,* New York, Free Press.

Pos, R. (1963): *The Psyche-Soma Complex: Its Psychology and Logic.* Doctoral thesis. University of Utrecht.

Rennie, T.A.C., Srole, L., Michael, S.T., Langner, T.S., and Opler, M.K. (1962): *Mental Health in the Metropolis: The Midtown Manhattan Study.* New York, Blakiston (McGraw-Hill).

Schmale, A.H. (1972): Giving-up as a final common pathway to changes in health. *Adv. Psychosom. Med.* 8:20.

Srole, L., Langer, T.S., Michael, S.T., et al. (1962): *Mental Health in the Metropolis: The Midtown Manhattan Study.* New York, McGraw-Hill.

Winokur, G. (1973): Diagnostic and genetic aspects of affective illness. *Psychiat. Annals,* 3:6.

FURTHER READINGS

Koranyi, E.K. (1978): Morbidity and rate of undiagnosed physical illnesses in a psychiatric clinic population. *Arch. Gen. Psychiat.,* 36:414.

Eastwood, M.R. (1975): *The Relation Between Physical and Mental Illness.* Toronto, University of Toronto Press.

Mechanic, D. (1968): *Medical Sociology.* New York, The Free Press.

2

Infancy and Childhood*

Paul D. Steinhauer

One cannot begin to understand psychological problems in children without an adequate appreciation of normal development. All children at times show behavior which, were it to become sufficiently prolonged and pronounced, could be labelled pathological. Only a knowledge of the broad range and limits of the normal enables us to determine what is sufficiently pathological to merit our concern and to demand intervention. Many of the psychological disturbances of childhood either arise directly or have their roots in deviations from the normal developmental stream. When we do choose to intervene, we of course do so out of a concern for presenting symptoms. But perhaps more important we try to lessen or remove factors which, by their continuing presence, threaten to block or distort the ongoing developmental process.

An adequate understanding of child development is essential for the general psychiatrist and the child psychiatrist. The kind of adult one becomes is determined by the interplay between one's genetically determined biological endowment and the influences of the environment, especially those of the family. These environmental influences determine to a large extent the degree to which one's innate potential is realized or remains unfulfilled, the area in which conflicts and difficulties arise, the nature and extent of the psychological and behavioral defenses employed in response to these difficulties, and the resulting character structure, strengths, and vulnerabilities of the individual. How can one understand why the adult is as he is without an appreciation of how he came to be this way? How can one work responsibly with distressed adults without taking into account the predictable effects of the parental disturbance on children—effects which will vary according to the ages of the children?

GENERAL PRINCIPLES OF DEVELOPMENT

There is no single unitary theory of human development. A variety of theories have been advanced to explain different aspects of the developmental process. This chapter will first present and explore some general principles of development, and

*This chapter draws heavily upon material and clinical examples contained in Robson, B. and Minde, K. "Normal Child Development" in Steinhauer, P.D. and Rae-Grant, Q., eds. (1977), *Psychological Problems of the Child and His Family*, Toronto, Macmillan of Canada.

then it will examine the application of these basic principles to understanding children's development at different ages.

There are three major sets of concepts, each with its own associated theories, that require our attention. Let us examine these in turn.

Nature-Nurture Theories

Until recently, these theories have tended to stress either the influence of the genetic constitution (e.g. Kretschmer, 1925, Sheldon, 1949) or of the environment (e.g. Freud) while paying relatively little attention to the ongoing interaction between constitution and environment. Prior to the advent of psychoanalytic thinking in the early years of this century, the potential effect of the environment in modifying the basic constitution was largely unappreciated. More recently, largely in response to the increasing influence of psychoanalysis and, later, learning theory, the effect of environmental influence has been so emphasized that the importance of constitutional factors was frequently neglected.

It remained for Chess and her co-workers, Thomas and Birch, to establish a balance between the two. They selected and described nine basic variables which make it possible to define a child's basic temperament at any stage of his development. Then they demonstrated ways in which this basic temperament both influenced and was in turn influenced by the emotional and behavioral responses of the parents (Thomas, Chess, and Birch, 1968). Chess stressed that children do not respond passively to their environment; rather they play an active role in shaping environment and the ways in which it will respond to them. Parents, like children, have their own needs. The degree to which a particular infant either meets or frustrates these needs will do much to influence their response to and their enjoyment

of the child. In turn, this will affect the environment in which the child grows.

> Jamie, as an infant, was constantly fretful. A first child, he was a poor feeder, resisted a regular feeding schedule and, by screaming all night every night, he kept his family from having a good night's sleep for almost two years. Extremely active, he was always into things and strenuously resisted attempts to distract him. Consistently upset by new experiences, he was slow to adapt and frequently unhappy. Jamie's mother found herself at first feeling inadequate, then resentful and increasingly guilty as she began to reach the point of not wanting to have anything to do with Jamie. In contrast her younger son, Adam, was a delightful child, friendly, affectionate and adaptable. He fed easily and slept through the night within a few weeks. She soon found herself enjoying Adam as thoroughly as she resented Jamie who, in turn, became increasingly difficult in response to her rejection.

When one takes into account both the basic temperament of the child and the specific needs of the parents, one can see that in some cases parents and child may meet each other's needs while, in others, a mismatch may occur. The same child that would prove a delight to one set of parents may prove a source of severe and continuing disappointment to another couple with different needs and expectations. The cause of a mismatch may be related to the child's basic temperament (e.g. Chess' "difficult child") or to parental expectations (e.g. their wish for a child of the other sex, for one with a different temperament, etc.). In any event, the child's development will be continually molded by the ongoing interplay between constitutional traits and environmental forces.

The distinction between the effects of nature and those of nurture becomes less clear as our knowledge of the relationship between them increases. Intelligence, for example, was once considered genetically determined. Over the last two decades, however, the influence of the environment on the level and even on the potential level of intellectual functioning has become abundantly clear. At the same time, other conditions once thought to result from environmental influences, such as early infantile autism, have been related to previously unrecognized biological factors.

Development as an Integrated Process

Development proceeds simultaneously across a number of related fronts. Thus development occurs concurrently in the biological, cognitive, language, emotional and social areas, with advances in one sphere being synchronized with progress in the others. For example, a child will not have developed to the point where he can experience separation anxiety until emotionally his cognitive development allows him to achieve object permanence. Similarly the gradual attainment of independence (a process termed "individuation" by Mahler), and an essential step in emotional development, is dependent on biological maturation: the achievement of locomotion, the ability to feed and care for oneself, ongoing language development, all of which allow for a greater control over the self and mastery over the environment. When this has been attained the child is freed to function more independently than before.

Continuous-discontinuous Theories

Some learning theorists hold that development occurs on a continuing basis. They argue that the child is exposed to a constant bombardment of experiences (i.e. stimuli) to which he is bound to respond by making simple connections. They perceive learning as the cumulative result of these connections constantly recurring in response to new experiences. Development is thus thought to be the result of a continuous process of learning rather than as a series of specific phases, each with its own particular age-related tasks or challenges.

Other major developmental theories, such as Freud's psychoanalytic theory and the cognitive theory of Piaget are *epigenetic* theories (Flavell, 1963). They hold that development proceeds not continuously, but in an orderly though step-like manner through a predictable series of stages. Such stages result from the nearly simultaneous occurrence of a group of behaviors which normally develop about the same time. For example, it is invariably just a short time after the child learns to distinguish between strange and familiar faces that he first begins to show anxiety when exposed to strangers. Epigenetic theories hold that the successful completion of one stage is a prerequisite for success in the next but, as Keniston has pointed out, they do not imply that development is like an escalator that carries one surely and effortlessly to its eventual conclusion (Keniston, 1974). There may be problems on the way. Blocks and distortions may occur at any level, causing either temporary or permanent developmental arrest. Thus many individuals never successfully complete their development to achieve their genetic potential. Examples might include the lasting cognitive deficits common to children raised in the inner city; the blighted social and educational aspirations of ghetto blacks or Indian children; the common failure to achieve adult morality or mature heterosexuality in psychoanalytic terms. Particularly important is the failure of over fifty per cent of all adults to master the capacity for abstract thinking that Piaget terms formal operations, although this highest level of cognitive functioning is commonly achieved during adolescence.

Each potential advance, at least at the emotional and social level, presents the individual with a series of choices which are not always conscious. In order to progress developmentally he must set aside the comforts, coping mechanisms, and defenses that, in the past, may have been the bulwark of his sense of security. Dare he risk this, or should he stay with the familiar and the comfortable, avoiding the challenge of the new and unknown and the anxiety that comes with pushing beyond past limitations? These periods of development at advanced and heightened vulnerability are termed developmental crises by Erikson and Lidz. They present the individual with an opportunity either for further growth and the achievement of mastery or, if the challenge is not met by backing away from it, the anxiety generated by it. And if old inadequate defenses are used there is a rise of location (block) or falling back (regression).

No discussion of epigenetic theories of development is complete without some mention of the concept of the *critical stage*. This implies that certain developmental tasks are necessarily linked to specific developmental stages. Biological (primarily neurological) maturation frequently sets a lower limit to these stages. For example, no amount of training will teach a child to talk before age six months or to read before three years, although attempts to do so may play a major part in emotional development and the subsequent acquisition of language. But while there is little doubt that lower limits for the appearance of various developmentally linked phenomena exist, the evidence is less clear on whether there are upper limits beyond which are many areas of development in which second chances may occur, allowing a child to achieve success at a later stage in an area failed at an earlier time. An example would be the boy who was socially unsuccessful in middle childhood because of a lack of the basic athletic skills which are so important to boys of this age. This may have been aggravated by an insufficient mastery over his own feelings that resulted in his frequently bursting into tears of frustration and rage when things didn't go as he wished. That same boy, by mid-adolescence, might have developed a much better control over his own feelings.

With his good looks, his intelligence and his charm he will have attained an attractiveness to girls which in turn would win him new respect and status in the eyes of his peers. Thus the social success and confidence denied him in middle-childhood might be successfully achieved at a later developmental stage.

However, it is generally believed that there are some developmental areas in which a major set-back at an earlier stage of development cannot entirely be compensated for by advances made in response to later developmental opportunities. For example, it appears that a prolonged period of emotional privation (grossly inadequate, inconsistent parenting) and deprivation in the first year or two of life may result in permanent damage to the capacity for basic trust and the potential for intimacy that cannot entirely be overcome by subsequent exposure to even an optimal environment. Similarly there is considerable doubt as to whether the potential for full cognitive development can survive two or three years of consistently minimal stimulation, no matter how intensive or prolonged the subsequent attempts at remediation. While clinical impressions seem to support the concept of a critical stage for at least some major basic developmental functions, there is not enough convincing evidence that is true for the entire process of development.

From the above, it should be clear that child development is a complex process. How does one begin to integrate and make sense of so many different, and at times conflicting, theoretical attempts to explain its progress? Generally speaking, it is agreed that no single developmental theory is enough, in itself, to explain all developmental phenomena. Some aspects of development, such as cell growth and socialization, occur continuously, while others, such as capacity for symbolic and increasingly abstract thought, develop in stages. Because of the frequency with which individuals may have a chance to revise or make up at a later stage for deficits or distortions resulting from blocks or deviations at an earlier one, it is difficult to predict with accuracy the final outcome of a child's development. Only severe and persistent pathological interactions between a child and his environment, whether because of a severe defect in or damage to the child's integrative mechanisms (e.g. severe brain damage, early infantile autism) or an extremely abnormal environmental situation (e.g. severe and persistent parental neglect), can be expected to produce predictable and lasting deficits.

BASIC DEVELOPMENT PARAMETERS

Biological Development

All aspects of development are predicated upon the continuing growth and maturation of the body, particularly that of the central nervous, musculoskeletal and endocrine systems. The readiness to learn, and thus the accessibility to environmental influences including training, are highly contingent upon biological maturation. No amount of training or stimulation prior to the achievement of the necessary maturation will allow for the achievement of coordination and control over motor skills, bowel and bladder control, cognitive, language or emotional development. It is the state of biological maturation that sets the lower limit for the acquisition of a number of related functions that we term a developmental stage. Gesell's pioneer work in correlating developmental skills with maturation levels is reflected in tables at the end of this chapter.

Biological development affects, and is affected by, the environment in which development occurs. There is considerable evidence that a failure to meet the minimal need for external stimulation may have the effect of impeding physical as well as emotional growth. The association of failure to thrive with severe environmental deprivation is supported by Spitz's studies on hospitalism and important animal studies relating brain development to the presence or absence of adequate stimulation.

The expression of genetic factors through the basic constitution also represents an important biological contribution to ongoing development. There are numerous studies which relate maternal responsiveness to the innate activity level of the neonate (Levy, 1958; Yarrow, 1968). Earlier in this chapter there has already been some discussion of ways in which a child's basic temperament will affect the quality and intensity of his relationship with his mother. Table 1 summarizes nine basic temperamental variables or traits which Chess et al. see as providing the biological basis for the constitution. These basic traits may be altered by experience, but nevertheless will affect to a major degree how a child will be perceived by others and, thus, the nature of the environment which will play so crucial a role in his ongoing development.

Cognitive Development

Cognitive development refers to the development of the intellectual processes. It allows the child first to conceptualize what is perceived, next to represent these perceptions in symbolic terms, then to organize these perceptions into groups, and eventually to think at an increasingly abstract level. This, in time, allows the child to think in terms of ideas and concepts, which he can then integrate to construct some sort of world view.

The major theories of cognitive development are epigenetic, in that they suggest that while the rate of cognitive development may vary, the development sequence remains constant. For example, a prerequisite for learning to name and group objects is the acquisition of the concept of object permanence. This is just one of many possible illustrations of the way that cognitive development proceeds in a step-like man-

TABLE 1   BASIC TEMPERAMENTAL TRAITS

1. ACTIVITY LEVEL	Describes the level, tempo, and frequency of motor behavior, ranging from hypoactive to hyperactive.
2. RHYTHMICITY	Describes the rhythmicity of repetitive biological functions such as sleeping and waking, eating and appetite, bowel and bladder functioning. Ranges from regular (establishment of pattern) to irregular (failure to establish even a partial pattern).
3. APPROACH AND WITHDRAWAL	Describes the child's initial reaction to any new stimulus, be it food, people, places, or procedures.
4. ADAPTABILITY	Describes the child's sequences of responses to a new or altered situation; deals with the ease or difficulty with which the initial response can be modified by parents or others.
5. INTENSITY OF REACTION	Describes energy content of the response, irrespective of its direction, ranging from mild to intense in either a positive or negative sense.
6. THRESHOLD OF RESPONSIVENESS	Refers to the level (quantity) of extrinsic stimulation required to produce a discernible response, regardless of the nature or quality of the stimulus.
7. QUALITY OF MOOD	Describes the amount of pleasant, joyful or friendly as opposed to unpleasant, crying, unfriendly behavior.
8. DISTRACTIBILITY	Refers to the effectiveness of external environmental stimuli in interfering with, or in altering the direction of, the ongoing behavior.
9. ATTENTION SPAN AND PERSISTENCE	By attention span is meant the length of time a particular activity is pursued. By persistence is meant the child's continuing with an activity in spite of obstacles either external (e.g. environmental interferences) or internal (e.g. limitation of ability related to the activity).

Data from *Behavioral Individuality in Early Childhood* by Alexander Thomas et al. New York University Press, 1963.

ner, with concepts already assimilated at an earlier stage paving the way for later advances. The progression typical of cognitive development will be discussed in more detail later in the chapter.

Emotional Development

In discussing emotional development, we are considering intrapsychic development as inferred through its derivatives in the child's interpersonal behavior. Traditional psychoanalytic theory held that the infant is acutely aware of strong biological needs because of the bodily tension or dis-

comfort he experiences when these remain unsatisfied. It pictured the neonate's perceptual and cognitive processes as so immature that the infant is, initially, incapable of the awareness of a world outside of himself. He only "knows" that when he cries, milk (or whatever is needed for comfort) comes, and presumably assumes that his cry makes it come. This leads to a rude awakening when, as a result of the advance of cognitive development, he reaches the point of recognizing that not only does he depend on someone out there to supply his comforts and relieve his tensions, but that the someone—the primary caretaker, usually the mother —has the power either to provide or to withhold the needed gratification. Traditional psychoanalytic theory pictures this recognition, suddenly achieved, as leading to the first primitive distinction between self and other (Ferenczi, 1916; Freud, 1961). More recently Fairbairn and other object relations theorists have seen the infant, even at birth, as having some ability both to perceive and to influence the environment (Fairbairn, 1952). Instead of a sudden breaking through of awareness, they postulate a gradually developing recognition of the difference between self and other. Whether this distinction comes about suddenly or gradually, however, its perception strips the child of any illusions that he is all-powerful or omnipotent, forcing him to face the fact that he is helpless and dependent on his primary caretaker for his comfort and, ultimately, for his very survival. From this point, continued security presumably depends on his ability to succeed in controlling the source of his comforts and in subordinating her to his will.

This series of hypotheses attempts to explain the earliest stage of emotional development, which occurs as the child first begins to distinguish between self and others and then starts to come to terms with the implications of this distinction, including the inevitable conflict between his biological (instinctual) needs and the frustrating influences of the environment. As he gets older, increasingly the mother demands that he accept the frustration and discomfort that come from containing or modifying urgent instinctual demands for immediate and total gratification. He is expected to adapt to a schedule for eating and sleeping and, as he gets older, is increasingly pressured towards some degree of cleanliness and obedience in order to retain the approval and avoid the displeasure of the caretaker(s) to whom he has become attached. The process of attachment will be discussed later in more detail, but at this point it is introduced to show how the young child is caught between the conflicting claims of his basic instinctual drives demanding release and satisfaction, and equally strong but frequently incompatible social drives which demand that these powerful biological demands be modified or contained in order to protect his relationship with his primary caretaker. As he grows older and begins to identify with the parents, their standards of good and bad or right and wrong will increasingly become his. At first, it is as if he had within him an echo of their voices. Later, as this inner representative becomes integrated within his own personality, he shuns misbehaving both to avoid offending others and to escape the censure of what he is increasingly aware of as his developing conscience.

Thus by this time the child's instinctual drives are opposed both by environmental restrictions (pressure from parents and others) and, increasingly, by the growing inner voice of conscience. This inevitable clash generates anxiety within the child, who then develops a series of defense mechanisms which he uses to contain the anxiety generated in this basic conflict. The normal child develops defenses sufficient to keep him relatively free of anxiety and to allow continuing growth without significantly restricting the scope or enjoyment of his life and without distorting the structure of his developing personality. In other children, the defenses developed may prove inadequate to the task, so that the child constantly fears lest his instinctual drives, escaping from their precarious controls, expose him to the threat of punishment or rejection. In still other children, the use of defense mechanisms in response to this threat is so excessive or inappropriate that the child's behavior and personality are dominated by these abnormal manifestations of defense which we see as symptoms.

Superimposed on this basic struggle and as the growing child moves toward emotional maturity, are a number of major tasks to be negotiated. The child must achieve a stable and integrated self-concept and adequate self-esteem; he must develop healthy attitudes toward authority; he must gradually but successfully negotiate the process of individuation in order to achieve emotional independence and to be free to relate intimately to others; psychosexual development must proceed, allowing the adoption of an appropriate gender identity and healthy attitudes toward his own sexuality. The process by which these are achieved will be discussed in more detail later in the chapter.

Personal/Social Development

From the start, there is a major overlap between development in the emotional and in the personal/social spheres. We have seen how the origins of emotional development lie in the young child's struggle to contain his instinctual demands in response to the pressures of his family environment and, especially, the primary caretaker. With an increasing number of infants and children having much of their primary care provided not within the family but in day-care, the question of how emotional development is affected by attachment to a number of primary caretakers is one increasingly being explored. In any event, by middle childhood, the child who is now attending school is exposed to a number of models and to pressure from a variety of extra-familial figures (in particular teachers and admired members of his peer group). Increasingly their influence will compete with and, during adolescence, may often contradict and supplant that of the parents in shaping the values, behavior and attitudes of the child.

Thus some ability to renounce or modify some of his basic needs and to deal acceptably with the resulting tension and frustration is an essential part of learning to live successfully within the family, the peer group and, eventually, society at large. The hope is that within broad limits this will be achieved in a manner that affords the child reasonable satisfaction while helping him develop adequate adaptability, while avoiding the extremes of alienation from the self (i.e. over-conformity and over-socialization) or from society (asocial or antisocial personality).

Language Development

While language development might well be considered as just one of the specialized aspects of cognitive development, it will be followed separately. This is partly because of the key role that the use of language plays in the continuing emotional, social and cognitive evolution of the child, but also because of the way that Gesell and others have demonstrated how language usage can be used as an indicator of the level of biological and cognitive functioning (Knobloch and Pasamanick, 1974).

THE PROCESS OF NORMAL DEVELOPMENT

Development can be described as the result of the various interlocking forces which create change in each of the basic developmental parameters previously defined. Through their constant interaction, these forces continually influence their mutual progression. For this reason, development in all areas should be surveyed in any assessment of possible emotional and intellectual deviations in either children or adults. To assist the reader, Table 2 at the end of this chapter will illustrate the level of achievement and the synchronized progress along each developmental parameter at each of a number of commonly defined age-related stages. First, though, let us describe some of the main features of development in each of these key areas as it proceeds. To illustrate its progress in concrete terms, we will follow the development of two normal, healthy but very different eleven-year-old boys. Beginning by introducing them as they are now, we will return to them following the discussion of each chronologic stage, observing how each boy appeared at that level and how each of their personalities took shape as development proceeded.

William, called Bill by everyone, has a mass of dark brown, curly hair, a pleasant, round face and a sturdy frame. Bill is in Grade Six, an average student who prefers gym and math. He is the goalie for the second-string school team, and plays league hockey on the team for which his father is assistant coach. Bill has six really close buddies but no one special friend. All the guys say Bill is okay. He has never gotten into any real trouble, but recently he was caught with three other boys climbing on the roof of the recreation center after Scouts. His dad seemed quite angry and hit him, but that was the last heard of the incident. Over the past year Bill has taken an increasing interest in his appearance. He now insists on accompanying his mother on shopping trips to select carefully his jeans, T-shirts and jean jackets. All Bill's friends are dressed practically identically. They kid one another about girls, and their interest in rock music is second only to their enthusiasm for hockey and football.

Kristian, called Krissie since birth by his mother, is also in Grade Six. Krissie is a tall, lean, pale, blond boy. A bright, attentive student, he is well-liked by his teachers, performing better than his classmates. Krissie and his best friend, Peter, are inseparable. They build models of cars, trains, trucks and airplanes. Although they feel it is babyish, they even "play" with their car collections at times. Krissie enjoys reading, particularly science fiction, and reads at a grade 10 or 11 level. Krissie is considered by everyone to be very artistic and creative. He has a good imagination. His art teacher at school has been especially encouraging, although this embarrasses Krissie who rather shyly avoids praise. He thinks such accomplishments are sissy, but he is proud of his ability in electronics. He just finished building a radio, and would like to be a space pilot.

Prior to Birth

The birth of their first child plunges the married couple into a new developmental stage. Before, they were a couple; now they are a family. Being a parent is not easy. Parenthood presents many pressures which may not be recognized, let alone reported to a physician. It may cause strain on a marriage, psychological stress for either or both parents and dissatisfaction and resentment of the child who has complicated their lives.

The stage is set for the development of a given child twenty to thirty years previously. This is because the attitudes and patterns we employ as parents are significantly influenced by the parenting we received as children. Our own parents serve as our role models and, even if we consciously repudiate their values and techniques in the upbringing of our own children, there is a frequent tendency, especially under pressure, to revert and to repeat the type of parenting we experienced. Parenting is a major task, yet one in which we receive little formal advance preparation. Unless she has had the experience of feeling cared for, it will be difficult for the new mother to provide this for her infant, especially should the child prove frustrating and difficult in spite of her best efforts. Unless the father is sufficiently identified with his own father or a father surrogate, he will find it hard to take a paternal role, though he must also be sufficiently identified with the baby to tolerate crying, sleepless nights, and repeated demands without excessively resenting the time and attention his wife now has to share with the newcomer. Should the baby in any way fail to meet the parents' needs or expectations, by being physically deformed or mentally handicapped, by having a congenital illness, or even by not having the sex or the temperament on which the parents were set, the resulting disappointment may place both child and marriage seriously at risk.

The experience in utero may have major and lasting effects not just on the condition of the infant at birth but on the whole course of subsequent development.

Syphilis and gonorrhea, toxoplasmosis and viral infections (especially rubella) during the first trimester have been clearly associated with serious congenital defects in the developing fetus. Incompatibility of maternal and fetal blood types used to be a major source not only of intrauterine death but also of kernicterus which was commonly complicated by cerebral palsy. Maternal drug-taking during pregnancy has been implicated in a whole range of complications and handicaps, including: the effects of steroids administered early in pregnancy on the differential development of the sexual organs; the interference of thalidomide with the normal development of the limbs; the effects of barbiturates and opiates on the condition of the infant in the neonatal period; the association of maternal smoking with a lower birth weight and an increased incidence of prematurity.

Knobloch and Pasamanick (1974) have focused attention on a whole continuum of reproductive casualty which they describe as an acquired vulnerability leading to results which vary with the severity of the intrauterine or perinatal insult. Results may range from severe (miscarriage, intrauterine death or stillbirth) through moderate (cerebral palsy or epilepsy) to minimal (vulnerability to learning and behavior disorders). On reviewing their work later, the authors noted that social class was probably the key factor responsible for this differential variability, as general hygiene and nutrition during pregnancy, the frequency and quality of medical care during pregnancy and delivery, and the circumstances of the delivery itself statistically undermined the prospects and increased the risk of complications for the child born to a mother in the lowest socioeconomic groups.

The First Year of Life

The normal infant, at birth, seems to function neurologically at an extremely primitive level with only basic reflexes and systems necessary for survival and for the maintenance of physiological homeostasis such as breathing, sucking and swallowing, grasping, circulatory and temperature control, all relatively well developed. The sensory system, however, remains incomplete, with sensory impulses registering at the thalamic level rather than in the cerebral cortex. Further development and differentiation of the sensory system requires adequate external stimulation, possibly within a critical period, if development is not to be permanently impaired. Riesen's demonstration of irreversible atrophy in up to 90 per cent of the retinal cells of chimpanzees reared in total darkness, and the irreversible loss of sight in one eye in children with severe strabismus left uncorrected for six years support this hypothesis.

As important as environmental stimulation is, it should not be imagined that even the newborn infant merely responds passively to the ministrations of the parents. Despite their apparent helplessness at birth, infants have available to them an innate repertoire of available behaviors. These include clinging, crying, sucking and following with the eyes. A differential following in response to the mother's voice and a pre-smile grimace have been demonstrated within ten hours of birth. By as early as two weeks, infants may show differential smiling, and precursors of social smiling are often present well before two months. All these behaviors will play an important role in shaping maternal responsiveness, a process that will be discussed later in the chapter.

Over the course of the first year, the infant gradually gains control over his body. Control over the eyes is achieved in the first quarter, over the head and arms in the second quarter, over the trunk and hands in the third, and over the forefinger and thumb in the fourth. The ongoing process of biological maturation prepares the child to begin developing the motor skills that are essential for independent functioning.

These include: achieving the control over his hands and arms which will allow him to begin exploring his world; acquiring control over his legs which will allow him to become independently mobile, thus expanding the field of his explorations; an increasing elaboration of and control over his cognitive apparatus and functioning.

Cognitive development during the first year proceeds from the sensory-motor level present at birth. As maturation proceeds, the infant passes from a stage of reflex activity (e.g. the involuntary grasping of an object placed in the hand) through one of voluntary repetition of reflex activities (such as repeatedly thrusting the thumb or fist in the mouth, removing it and reinserting it) to one of deliberate placing of the thumb in the mouth. True convergence of the two eyes on an object in the field of vision, essential for fixation and depth perception, first occurs at about seven or eight weeks. Some time around ten weeks of age, the infant can be shown to be capable of storing the memory of a stimulus. He gradually begins to recognize that pushing an object changes its position, thus providing a different view. When he reaches the point where he learns to associate these different visual perspectives with the same object, he is ready to grasp the concept of object permanence.

Object permanence is an essential prerequisite for further cognitive, emotional and social development. Usually developed gradually sometime during the first year, it becomes possible only when the child can develop and retain a memory trace of an object removed from his line of vision. By this stage, if the child sees a favorite toy hidden, he will uncover it and regain it with delight, although if the task is complicated by first hiding and then shifting the toy without the child's knowledge, he will continue to search for it in the original hiding place. It is not until between 18 and 24 months that the child will overcome the added complexity of this maneuver to continue the search beyond the original hiding place until the toy is recovered.

The achievement of object permanence has important implications on the child's relationship with his mother. By a year of age, if his mother leaves the room and the child is free to follow, he is usually not distressed; presumably he recognizes that she still exists beyond the doorway, so that he has only to follow to find her. Toward the middle of the second year, however, he is likely to be distressed at her leaving. With his increased awareness and understanding, he now seems to comprehend that his mother, though just outside the door, might at any moment move away again. He therefore feels the need to follow her, to maintain some visual or auditory trace of her lest she move to a more distant area of what his increasingly sophisticated memory map tells him lies beyond the door. These general developmental sequences are in no way rigid and can be drastically modified by changes in the particular situations such as interesting distractions, past experiences with other adults, etc.

Kagan (1962) has hypothesized that much early intellectual development occurs when the child develops a particular cognitive set (i.e. a way of organizing what is perceived) which he then attempts to match with sets which he observes in the outside world to form a single gestalt. For example, if the face he sees outside does not correspond with his internal concept of face, he does not smile. This, naturally, has its effects on ongoing social development. At anywhere from two weeks to two months the infant begins to smile in response to the human voice. Soon he smiles noticeably more in response to the mother (or other primary caretaker) than to others. As his visual discrimination and his ability to recognize his surroundings increase, he becomes noticeably more comfortable in her company than in that of strangers. Some time after six months, he will begin to "make strange," hiding his face in his mother's shoulder or staring impassively when a stranger approaches.

In his language development, the infant of two months cries frequently but does little cooing or babbling. Cooing and squealing increase during the second and third months, apparently independently of environmental factors. After the third month, however, these vowel-dominated sounds increasingly occur in response either to being stimulated or to the sound of his own voice. New sounds begin to be produced, resulting more from continuing neuromuscular maturation and postural changes than from imitation. By six months, babbling consisting of an increasing number of one-syllable repetitions has replaced cooing as the dominant mode of expression. The babbling is typically interspersed with consonants, and by the end of the first year the words "mama" and "dada" have entered the vocabulary of the child who, by this stage, gives definite evidence of understanding common words and simple commands.

> Krissie, at a year, was especially shy with strangers. From about eight months of age, he had been able to pull himself up and move about in his walker. By a year, he was tall, already wearing an 18-month size. His mother had been the only one to look after him except for an occasional babysitter in the evening. His family took vacations together at the cottage. Krissie's father, a town planner, was busy at work or making repairs and improvements to the house. He never considered it his role to participate in the direct care of his son. Krissie had two quite severe colds during his first year, and his mother often worried about his becoming ill. When he was distressed, his mother seemed to be the only one who could comfort him.
>
> Bill at a year, was already a sturdy child. Less tall than Krissie, he had trouble standing or walking, but that did not stop him from creeping about and getting into things or trying to get up the stairs when no one was looking. His parents considered his behavior a great joke. Bill could say a great many things with words and was very clear in his wants. Like Krissie's father, Bill's dad was not much involved with his early care, but he began to enjoy playing as soon as Bill was old

> enough to toss about, laugh with and play peek-a-boo. Bill was frequently cared for overnight by both sets of grandparents from an early age, becoming happily excited if a visit to his "Bopa's" was suggested. He could be comforted by his mother, father or grandparents, although he had a slight preference for his mother.

In the area of emotional development, the crucial advance during the first year is that of the bonding which gradually develops between infant and mother referred to as *attachment*. Contrary to popular belief, attachment between mother and child is by no means inevitably present at birth. It develops gradually over a period of time as a result of ongoing exposure and mutual interaction. Anything that interferes with this ongoing interaction in the first days and weeks of life, such as prematurity or serious illness which keeps mother or infant in hospital and away from the other for weeks at a time, may interfere with a successful bonding, thus increasing the risk that a satisfactory attachment wil not occur.

If attachment is not universally present at birth, how then does it come about? In addition to the mother's usual attitudes of caring and protectiveness derived from an instinct towards the preservation of the species and from the personal pleasure that many but by no means all mothers feel at having given birth to a healthy child, the infant through his behavior does much either to assist or to impede the attachment process. Many of his instinctual behaviors such as crying, sucking, clinging, smiling, and stroking play an active part in keeping the mother close and in encouraging maternal involvement. But the closeness that develops between mother and child only becomes a mutual attachment at about eight months of age, the stage at which cognitive development has reached the point where, concurrent with or slightly after the development of stranger anxiety, the child recognizes the primary caretaker, usually the mother, as more important than any other adult for his comfort and security. Once it has become mutual, attachment makes it hard for either mother or child to endure a separation from the other. One might equate the development of attachment with the growth of love, and future relationships and the capacity to love will to some extent be determined by the quality and strength of this early attachment. Attachment behavior intensifies, typically reaching a peak at eighteen months, and then declining over the next two to three years as the child becomes increasingly self-reliant and independent.

Severe neglect and failure to develop a successful attachment are generally associated with a broad range of severe and lasting cognitive, emotional and social deficits, which may include a virtual disruption of development and a blighting of the capacity for social relationships. Some children who are removed from homes in which they are suffering severe neglect and privation and placed in families who provide adequate security and stimulation, show marked developmental gains. Bowlby was a pioneer in studying the persistent and irreversible effects of separation from the primary caretaker. Subsequent work of Rutter and Bowlby has questioned whether it is the separation itself that is so damaging or primarily the quality of care preceding and following the separation that governs the response. Though much remains to be learned in this area, it appears that the consequences of separation for a given child will depend on the degree of privation to which he has been exposed previously, the duration of the separation, the age at which the separation occurs (with children between the ages of one and four years being particularly vulnerable), and the adequacy and prompt availability of a suitable alternative. The work of Spitz (1945, 1946) and Goldfarb (1955) as well as that of Bowlby stress the irreversibility of the damage done, though a study by Skeels (1966) strongly argues for reversibility.

Ages One to Three

Frequently called the "toddler" years, this period is one in which locomotor controls and skills are perfected, allowing the child more freedom, greater independence and an expanding environment. By fifteen months he can crawl, climb stairs, and frequently walk on his own. Running away from parents and other games related to his new-found mastery over his body become a source of pleasure and delight as well as a means of reinforcing his attachment to parents. By this age, he is generally given the run of the house and by three years he runs easily, jumps with some control and negotiates stairs alone with alternate feet. By this stage fine motor control has improved sufficiently that he can hold a crayon and scribble "letters" or pictures of his own, thus demonstrating the first signs of his potential creativity.

Intellectually, the toddler who is in what Piaget has termed the preoperational period deals with his world through play, beginning by ordering and grouping objects. He may, for example, line up all his toy animals, placing them in the farmyard in contrast with the toy people whom he placed in or near the house. The most striking development during the second year usually occurs in the area of language. At eighteen months, the average child, despite a vocabulary of between three and fifty words including a few set phrases (e.g. thank you), is not yet spontaneously combining words to form phrases. Both vocabulary and understanding progress rapidly, however, and by his second birthday the child is combining words to form two-word phrases and, increasingly, using language as a way of communicating his wants to others. Much of his vocabulary develops out of his ordering and grouping, as he uses language to group objects together to form categories and then to define the nature of categories. Pigs, cows and horses all fall into the category of animals and animals go in barns, in farmyards, or in trucks, but not in houses or cars. While constantly adding to his vocabulary, this sort of play also provides a way of organizing and understanding the world around him.

The toddler also develops a sense of himself through language. He learns his name, and begins to group himself into certain categories, each for its own specific meanings and rules for behavior derived primarily from his family but also from teachers, peers and other representatives of his culture. For example, he learns that he is Johnny, and a member of the Smith family, unlike Janie next door, who belongs to the Brown family. He is a boy while she is a girl. He learns quite a bit about boys, about what they are and what is expected of them. What specifically he learns (that is the way that his role as a boy is defined for him) will reflect the definition and attitudes of what is considered boyish in his particular family and their social circle. For example, he learns that when he grows up, he may become a daddy or a husband, but will never be a wife or mother. He learns that boys don't wear dresses (unless in special situations, when they are dressing up and pretending to be girls). He will learn a whole list of "do's" and "don'ts" that his particular family associates with being a boy: certain toys (e.g. dolls), activities (e.g. skipping), games (e.g. playing school) or attitudes (e.g. timidity, noncompetitiveness, sensitivity) may evoke their criticism while others (e.g. playing cars, climbing trees, playing ball, toughness, and bravery) may be encouraged. At some point often around age three, he will become aware that boys, like men, have penises which allow them to urinate standing up, unlike girls. Thus a whole series of language-linked concepts help him develop a sense of himself, but this can only come when cognitive and language development allow him to grasp the concept of categories and the characteristics of each.

Emotional development passes through three important phases during this period, well described by Margaret Mahler (1976).

As his motor skills and use of language increase, he is able to venture forth and do more things for himself, thus becoming somewhat less dependent on his mother. He may develop a strong sense of himself as a separate person, becoming fiercely independent in his behavior; during the "terrible two's," it is quite normal for him to assert his independence by refusing to cooperate with parents around routines, dressing or toilet training. But while initially the child takes great pleasure in asserting himself as someone separate from his mother, there routinely occurs approximately between fifteen and eighteen months a phase of *rapprochement*. During this stage, attachment bonding hits a peak as the child returns to an intensified closeness with the parents. Often whiny, demanding and more babyish, the child at this stage is extremely vulnerable to separation anxiety if the parents leave, even to go out for the evening. Shortly, however, this anxiety recedes and again the child, usually with the support and approval of the parents, begins to show signs of more independent and self-sufficient behavior.

At this time, many parents notice their child becoming intensely attached to a special blanket or toy that seems to be essential for his ongoing security. While often dragged and taken everywhere, it seems especially necessary when he goes to sleep or faces unfamiliar situations. It has been suggested that something about this object, its shape, texture or gestalt, reminds the child of the safe, secure world of the early part of his first year, before he realized that he needed someone outside himself to ensure his continuing security. The blanket seems to serve as if he had a part of his mother, and all the security she represents, available to him at all times. Such an object—Linus's blanket is possibly the best contemporary example—is often termed a *transitional object*, in that it provides security while the child steps forth from the safety of the relationship with his mother and experiments with less certain and at times anxiety-provoking relationships with other people, sometimes termed "object relationships."

This is also a stage where the child begins to differentiate his wants and needs from those of the parents. As the parents gradually begin to introduce limits and controls the child may struggle against them although usually, by three years of age, the child is prepared to submit to the will of the parents. In this, probably the earliest stage of moral development, the child does as the parents say, not because he wants to or in order to be good, but to avoid the loss of love or parental anger that he fears will follow should he disobey. Toilet training is one situation typical of the potential conflict of wills inherent in this stage. The child, who has reached the point where he has both the capacity for delaying evacuation and the ability to recognize and signal the imminent event sufficiently in advance, is expected to hold in his stool and place it in the appropriate place at the proper time. This may make great sense to his mother, but rarely does so for the toddler, who often experiences mild discomfort while holding in, which is sometimes associated with some anxiety when placed on the toilet. If the mother, for any of a variety of reasons, tries to force the child to train before he is ready or prepared to do so, an intense power struggle may result leading to withholding at times complicated by constipation and pain for the child and a severe strain on the mother-child relationship. Usually, however, training is completed within a few weeks when the child is ready and soiling rarely persists beyond age three in the normal child.

This is also the age when some children create an imaginary playmate. Often larger than life, this playmate serves to protect the child, his master, against monsters or the dark while, at the same time, helping the child who feels constantly hemmed in by rules and adult authority feel that he is no longer lowest in the family pecking order. This is an age when children are almost constantly involved in play. Play serves much more than just a recreational function: it helps drain off energy; it allows the child to practise new skills; it serves as a way of mastering anxiety about feared situations; it makes it possible for the child to behave like parents or other adults, fantasied or real, whom he sees himself as being like, thus providing him an opportunity to become and feel that he is like the role model.

Bill, who according to his parents had always had a mind of his own, certainly began to show this at about a year. His father announced proudly that Bill had never walked, but that once he got the idea at around 14 months he always ran. Bill's father played baseball with some friends every Sunday. Bill loved to go with his mother to watch, chanting "play ball" over and over. Bill was into everything at home, emptying drawers and cupboards. At 18 months, toilet training was tried for the first time with no success. Bill had the idea; he would smile and say "put poopy in potty" but he never performed. At 26 months, however, he learned within a week. As a special treat, Bill loved to stay with his grandparents for the weekend. But when his parents went away on vacation and left Bill, then 20 months, with his grandparents for two weeks, he became withdrawn and played quietly by himself on the floor— not the usual Bill at all. When his parents returned, he acted as if they had never been away, but for three days after behaved very badly. At two, Bill's favorite word was "no" and he wanted only trucks for presents at his birthday party.

Krissie was quite sickly in his second year. His mother was constantly on the phone to the doctor. An early walker, he was able to go up and down stairs well by 16 months, but although he was able to do a number of things for himself he preferred to have his mother do them for him. He did enjoy the mastery of certain skills. He was quick at manipulating toys, working with plasticine, Playdoh and crayons. His mother, a sculptress, was proud of his primitive creative abilities, spending long hours helping him make things. Krissie's father also enjoyed his son's creative ability, but even though Krissie wanted to join him, he felt it was too dangerous for Krissie to be around where he himself was building.

The Preschool Years, Ages Three to Six

Improved muscle coordination allows the development of further motor skills during the preschool years. The child learns to hop, skip, throw a ball, becoming expert in riding a tricycle and, late in the period, possibly even a small bicycle. Improved observational skills and eye-hand co-ordination allow him to draw first a circle and later a square. By the end of this period he is capable of drawing a person with six parts.

Meanwhile, the child continues to explore his physical world, expanding his cognitive development by grouping and naming objects. Much of the learning occurs through action-linked concepts: apples are eaten, books are read, shovels are for clearing snow, etc. Each of these objects, however, is also included in other groupings. An apple, for example, is a food and also a fruit; as it begins with the letter "A" it is an "A-word," but it also has a shape and a red color that can be painted or crayoned. Thus the original action-linked concept is extended by a series of associated images, thus leading to the acquisition of new words. During this period the vocabulary which by age three consists of about a thousand words, expands at the rate of 50 new words each month.

By age three, about 80 per cent of the child's verbalizations can be understood even by strangers. Although he still makes errors, in general his grammatical constructions compare in complexity with those of colloquial adult speech, and by age four his grasp of language has advanced to the point where his speech differs from that of adults more in style than through the number of errors. By about four years, the child begins using complete sentences of up to eight words which are complex in their organization and notable for the increased use of relational words such as personal pronouns. By this time the child has mastered vocal inflections, and can use language to negotiate with the environment and to instruct himself.

Toward the end of this stage, the child increasingly begins to enter the community, learning to cross roads safely and to find his own way to school and home. By now he can dress and undress himself completely, usually by age six tying his own shoelaces. During this period, children become aware of their peers and spend an increasing amount of time playing with them. At first, they are not really able to play together, but rather interact with each other as they play or follow a parallel symbolic theme. By age six, however, they are capable of playing simple games by rules without adult supervision.

Until well into the preschool years, children regulate their behavior in response to environmental controls, but by about five they are beginning to develop a set of internalized standards or conscience on their own. Thus their actions are increasingly controlled not by the fear or shame of getting caught but by a growing personal sense of right and wrong. Their system of values develops as they increasingly decide what they want to be like and how they want to be seen by others. Heavily influenced by parental expectations, they take pride in activities they know that parents admire, and play out long and complicated fantasies on these themes.

Psychoanalysts refer to this as the oedipal period, as they see it as characterized by the child's developing a sexual interest in the parents, particularly the parent of the opposite sex. Determined partly by the strength of innate biological drives and partly by dynamic alignments within the family environment, this attraction and the guilt and anxiety resulting from it are normally resolved by identification with the same-sexed parent along with the relinquishing of the opposite-sexed parent in favor of extra-parental interests and activities. Failure to successfully achieve this resolution is seen by psychoanalysts as the nuclear conflict in psychoneurosis, and as a decisive influence in adult sexuality.

As the child continues to align himself with parental expectations, he increasingly begins to see himself and to behave in a manner appropriate to his biological sex. The attitudes of one generation regarding what is sexually appropriate are passed on to the next. Children increasingly learn to avoid acting in ways they associate specifically with the other sex. They begin to imitate, not always consciously, the parent of the same sex who serves as a role model, while the opposite-sexed parent, under normal circumstances, allows and encourages this identification.

During the preschool years, children not infrequently experience severe anxiety, possibly related to the at times stringent demands of their newly developed conscience, to increasingly demanding environmental expectations and to the need to be like the parent of the same sex. This anxiety may lead to transitory and intense but usually normal fears which may take the form of nightmares, night terrors, transient phobias, fear of the dark or monsters, fear of bodily harm, or bedwetting.

> Krissie made a friend of a little girl down the street. Although she was about five months younger and shorter by a head, she tended to dominate their play. At first, Krissie could not tolerate his mother leaving him at her house to play. Later he became willing to stay and play with her for short periods. When he started nursery school, Krissie had to have his mother stay with him for about the first month. Later he enjoyed all the activities, particularly the group singing. He had a series of repeated colds, and was absent more than he was there. As his mother still worried about his health, she kept him away from children on the street if they seemed to have colds. At five, Krissie still had difficulty sharing his toys with the neighborhood children. A faster runner than the others, he loved riding his two-wheeler with training wheels. He would act sullen and angry if his mother worried over him, but he looked forward to being with his father on weekends and helping him build a new porch.

> When Bill was three and a half, his new baby brother was born. At first Bill was pleased because he had wanted a brother.

> Later he came to resent the time his parents spent with the baby. At this point, his speech became less clear and he reverted to baby talk and wetting his bed. On their physician's advice the parents, particularly his father, spent more time with Bill and soon he was his old self again. Bill was always covered with bruises from falls, not that he was clumsy, but because at four and a half he was rather aggressive and trying everything. His father built a rink in the backyard, so Bill could skate sloppily by four and fairly well at five. Bill didn't go to nursery school or junior kindergarten, but looked forward to half-day kindergarten. After two weeks' supervision, he walked to the school three blocks away by himself. He enjoyed playing with boys his own age, but at times would leave them to do something on his own. He tended to play by the rules, waiting for outside authority to step in to settle a dispute.

Middle Childhood, Ages Six to Eleven

This period, extending from the end of the infantile period (about six) until just prior to the resurgence of sexual and aggressive drives that initiates adolescence, is one in which the child's attention and energies are focussed primarily on continuing socialization and on his adjustment to the external world, including school. Often an easier, less stressful period for both parents and children, it is one in which the strong drives and inner conflicts of the earlier years often seem to lose some of their urgency. Psychoanalysts have termed this the stage of *latency,* as they see it as providing a biologically-determined breathing space between the psychological conflicts of the preceding oedipal period and the subsequent physiologically increased stresses and conflicts of preadolescence.

Others (e.g. Chess et al.) prefer the term "middle childhood", as their observations refute the regular existence of a period of significantly reduced intrapsychic turmoil during these years. They suggest rather that with entry into school and the emphasis on continued socialization, the focus of development shifts as the child increasingly begins to compare himself to his peer group. Competition with peers in every conceivable area, intelligence, strength, athletic ability, social acceptance, and material possessions may be acute, and the child's self-image, no longer merely a reflection of his parents' perception of him, increasingly takes into account the judgments of peers and teachers as well. Children, though they may at times deny it, are keenly aware of acceptance or rejection by peers and of their place in the pecking order. These inevitable social stresses lead in turn to intrapsychic conflict as the child struggles to deal with his fear of rejection. This he can do either by withdrawal or by retaliation. Should he tend toward withdrawal, he can do so physically by not participating in activities or by avoiding volunteering answers in class for fear of disapproval or rejection. He may rationalize this withdrawal, implying that he has no interest in being involved though he really does, or he may forget or steer entirely clear of threatening or stressful situations. Since mastering the basic academic skills which are being taught at this time requires accepting the possibility of being wrong, the child who is solidly committed to avoiding any risks is likely to develop learning difficulties, which in turn will further undermine his self-confidence and self-esteem.

Other children attack anxiety-rich situations head on, attempting to overcome them. If successful, their success and the resulting confidence will reinforce their pattern of direct confrontation of problems, but failure, especially repeated failure, may compound the difficulties and further undermine the child's confidence in himself and in his abilities. Should he react to lack of success by clowning around or acting up in class, the reaction to his behavior may compound the damage to his self-concept and, if continued, may alienate him from the school and its goals. Thus throughout middle childhood, repeated experiences in school with friends and in the home result in changes and elaboration in the child's self-image and, with it, in his sense of self-esteem.

Most children, particularly girls, look forward to beginning school, although social and cultural factors will do much to influence a child's attitude and adjustment to school. While entry into school is geared increasingly over the years towards cognitive development, it can be seen from the above that school has an impact on the total personality and on the psychological and social adjustment of the child. While school achievement is obviously influenced by basic intelligence, other equally important determinants of academic success include motivation, work habits, creativity both innate and cultivated, cultural opportunities in and outside the home, and family encouragement and support for the value of school. Most middle- and upper-class families support education, but many lower class children enter school lacking many of the experiences, facts, concepts and skills possessed by their middle-class peers and valued by their middle-class teachers. Teachers often react against the action-oriented behavior and the attitudes and values lower-class children need for survival on the streets of the inner city. Their parents, who frequently mistrust the school system, frequently do little to motivate their children to persevere in the face of these initial disadvantages, and instead of presenting a model encouraging academic achievement frequently give at least tacit support to their child's growing alienation from the school.

During these years, the child's thought patterns gradually shift from the concrete ordering and grouping of objects that Piaget terms the period of *concrete operations* to a stage where he begins to understand concepts that allow him to start working with ideas with less need for specific objects to serve as visual props. However, true abstract reasoning or what Piaget terms *formal operations*, that is the ability

TABLE 2 AGE AND DEVELOPMENTAL CORRESPONDENCES*

At End Of:	Biological:	Language:	Cognitive:
2 months	Develops eye & head control —looks at rattle in hand. —chin and chest held up. Real binocular color vision.	Impassive face—considerable crying.	Basic reflexes: sucking, grasping, tracking objects in field of vision.
6 months	Vision: depth perception. Sits bending forward, uses hands for support, bears weight when put in standing position but cannot yet stand without holding on. Reaches and grasps toy —transfers toy from hand to hand.	When talked to smiles, squeals and coos. Consonants begin to be interspersed with vowel-like cooing. Cooing changes to babbling resembling one syllable utterances.	Coordination of basic reflexes, e.g. can look at toy, reach for it, grasp it, mouth it. Grasps for rattle, but if hidden forgets it: —unable to retrieve rattle if even partly hidden from view —significance: part is not yet indicative of the whole
8–9 months	Sits well; pulls self to feet at railing. Plays with 2 toys; picks up pellet with thumb and index finger.	Reduplication (more continuous repetitions). Utterances can signal emphasis and emotion.	Recognizes top and bottom of baby bottle as belonging to same object: —if presented with bottom will rotate bottle to get nipple.
15 months	Crawling, climbing stairs; walks alone. Toddler builds tower with two cubes, puts six cubes into cup. Imitates vertical stroke.	Says Dada, Mama; a vocabulary of 3–20 words. Responds to "Give it to me", "Show me your eyes." Little ability to join words into spontaneous phrases. Pronoun "I" and "mine" understood.	Object permanence: —hidden object will be retrieved by the child. —significance: object has permanence, independent of child's immediate ability to perceive it. —not until 18–24 months will child be able to find an object first hidden, then removed to new hiding place.

*Reprinted with permission from Robson, B. and Minde, K. (1977): Normal Child Development in Steinhauer, P.D. and Rae-Grant, O., eds, In *Psychological Problems of the Child and His Family*. Toronto. Macmillan of Canada.

TABLE 2   AGE AND DEVELOPMENTAL CORRESPONDENCES (Cont'd)

At End Of:	Biological:	Language:	Cognitive:
3 years	Runs, rides tricycle, goes up and down stairs alone with alternating feet, tip-toes, jumps 12 inches, stands on one foot momentarily. Builds tower of 6–7 cubes. Imitates circular scribble, imitates "+" and "0".	Vocabulary 1,000 words; 80% of utterances intelligible, even to strangers. Grammatical complexity roughly that of colloquial adult language. Gives full name and sex.	True symbolic play. —continues exploration of world. —objects seen as entities and named. —child begins to group objects together, naming the whole group.
6 years	Hops on one foot, stands on alternate feet with eyes closed for 10 seconds, jumps 12 inches high, landing on toes; can throw a ball. Imitates ◆ (age 6) ▲ (age 7)	Language well established: deviations from adult norm tend to be more in style than grammar. Can name values of coins. Can name all colors. Can give description of pictures.	Builds on objects to form concepts, and on concepts to form classes of concepts. —continues grouping, re-grouping, naming and exploring.
8–10 years	Can tap either foot on floor, and right or left finger on table at the same time, maintaining rhythm for 20 seconds. By age 10, good fine motor control. Can balance on board, standing with arms out in front, palms down, eyes open.	Good understanding of general language and its rules —knows plural of man is men —gives 3 rhyming words for "map" or "cat" within 30 seconds. By age 10–11, can express self in abstract concepts, e.g. —can name 10 wild animals in one minute.	By age 9, can group objects in 2 categories simultaneously, e.g. a bead is both red and wooden: this is still a building process of reflexes and groupings. True abstract reasoning (i.e. the ability to go beyond the concrete and envision changes without visual processes) does not occur until adolescence.

TABLE 2   AGE AND DEVELOPMENTAL CORRESPONDENCES (Cont'd)

Personal-Social:	*Psychological:*
Number of feedings reduces from 7–8 to 5–6. Spontaneous reflex smiling (12 hours). Unselected social smile at human voice (14 days). Smiles at face in motion (5 weeks). Smiles at face with some detail, e.g. eyebrows and eyes (2 months).	Primary caretaker's bond to the child forming: caretaker responsive to child's needs. Infant aware of this responsiveness: develops sense of predictability of his surroundings—begins to develop sense of security. Infant biased toward the familiar from birth—settles into routine of home. Begins to differentiate between primary caregivers and strangers.
Smiles selectively to mother's face Plays with feet. "Teething"	Begins to distinguish between himself and others; with discriminatory vision, able to distinguish visually faces and people. Able to differentiate primary caregivers well; reacts with more pronounced apprehension and withdrawal to those who are unfamiliar: "makes strange".
Taking fine solids and rusks; feeds self crackers. Smiles only to whole familiar face.	Links good things (warmth, food) with the familiar: links security with caretakers. Has developed special *attachment bonding* with significant adults: anxious or disturbed when separated from them.
Toilet regulated during day. Carries and hugs doll. Assists and co-operates in dressing.	Demonstrates a sense of self separate from mother: begins to individuate, i.e. do things adults used to do for him; seems to enjoy separateness. *Rapprochement Phase* (15–18 months): —returns to close, intense relationship with primary caretaker —appears more vulnerable to separation than previously —attachment bonding at its peak. *Transitional Object*: behaves as if favorite toy or security blanket can protect from harm; object appears a substitute for contact with primary caretaker.

TABLE 2   AGE AND DEVELOPMENTAL CORRESPONDENCES (Cont'd)

Personal-Social	Psychological:
Puts doll to bed, feeds self well, puts on socks, unbuttons, asks for toilet during day, begins to want to play with peers. Interested in difference between boys and girls.	Parents expect some obedience and socialization —child establishes "self" by opposing will of parents: the "terrible two's". By age 3, child subjects his will to wishes of parents —often experiences anger at having to give up own wishes —fear of punishment, imaginary dangers and monsters common: fears physical injury through play —may defend against these dangers via imaginary playmate or animal, who, while ferocious and larger than life, is subject to child's whims.
Ties shoelaces. Walks to school by self, crosses road at lights safely, plays co-operatively with peers. Can play simple game by rules without adult supervision.	Acceptance of parents' morals and wishes. Child "identifies" with parent of same sex, taking on that parent's values, sex-role behavior: conscience and value system develop. Child increasingly behaves as if controlled and regulated by own internal standards and ideals: not as influenced by external punishment or reward.
Uses knife at table, combs and brushes hair. Catches a baseball, plays complicated games by rules.	School involves: —accepting rules and regulations —adapting to others —competing with others —possibility of defeat, ridicule, humiliation —persisting at task even if unpleasant until it is complete. Child's self-image and self-esteem are cemented by sense of own accomplishments and feedback from others.

to think and to understand changes in terms of concept with no need for concrete examples to serve as props, is not achieved until well into adolescence.

During these years, the process of moral development and gender-identity formation, begun earlier on the basis of identification, continue. The influence of the initial role models, the parents, may find increasing competition with the values and attitudes of the peer group. Especially toward the end of these years when children begin to develop moral standards which reflect their own values, there may be much preoccupation with what is right or wrong in others' behavior. The growing ability to think in abstract terms increasingly allows them to consider moral issues in a general or abstract way. This preoccupation with good and evil spills over into their fantasy life. Their imagination, continuing strong, elaborates on themes of universal good and bad, as fairy tales and monsters are replaced by police and gangsters or Kung-Fu. The search for values and for a clearly defined sense of oneself as a unique individual will not be completed during middle childhood, but will be among the major tasks remaining to be achieved during the continuing development that will occur during the adolescent years.

Bill had no trouble entering school, but he seemed more anxious before he got on the hockey team. When the team lost a game he tended to be sullen and angry, but he very rarely talked back to either of his parents. His teachers thought he could probably do better than average at his studies. Bill himself, although not afraid of success, preferred to be one of the boys than to stand apart by seeming outstanding. His father admired this in Bill; although he would, at one time, have wanted his son to be a star, he was pleased to see that Bill had friends, was well-liked and played fairly. He was not terribly concerned about Bill's school work, rarely inquiring if he had any homework. He considered that Bill's responsibility.

Kris, who insisted everyone stop calling him Krissie, was pleased by his progress in school as were his parents. Always margi-

nally ahead of his classmates, he could read and write at home before he went to Grade 1. Although quick to grasp concepts, Kris always preferred not to compete openly with other students. Learning for him has been more a personal challenge, not unlike his parents' striving for individuality.

His mother is now a nationally-known sculptress. Kris, who still enjoys working with his father, is getting to be almost as good a skier as he. They often kid one another about their ability. Kris is very close with his friend, Peter, with whom he shares everything. They have been friends since nursery school, their interests having grown together as they matured.

REFERENCES

Erikson, E. (1959): "Growth and Crises of the Healthy Personality." *Psychol. Issues.*, 1:50.

Fairbairn, W.R.D. (1952): *Psychoanalytic Studies of the Personality.* London, Routledge.

Ferenczi, S. (1916): Stages in the development of the sense of reality. In *Contributions to Psychoanalysis.* Boston, R. C. Badger.

Flavell, J.H. (1963): *The Developmental Psychology of Jean Piaget.* New York, Van Nostrand, Reinhold.

Freud, S. (1961): The ego and the id. In *The Standard Edition of the Complete Psychological Works of Sigmund Freud.* Volume 19. London, Hogarth Press.

Goldfarb, W. (1955): Emotional and intellectual consequences of deprivation in infancy: A re-evaluation. In *Psychopathology of Childhood.* Edited by P. H. Hoch and J. Zubin. New York, Grune and Stratton.

Kagan, J. and Moss, H.A. (1962): *Birth to Maturity.* New York, J. Wiley.

Keniston, K. (1974): Youth and its ideology. In *American Handbook of Psychiatry.* 2d ed. Edited by S. Arieti. Vol. 1. New York, Basic Books.

Klaus, M.H., Jerauld, R., and Kreger, N.C., et al. (1972): Maternal attachment: importance of the first post-partum days. *N. Engl. J. Med.* 286:460.

Knobloch, H. and Pasamanick, B. (1974): *Gesell and Amatrude's Developmental Diagnoses.* 3d ed. Hagerstown, Harper and Row.

Kretschmer, E. (1925): *Physique and Character.* First ed. New York, Harcourt, Brace.

Levy, D.M. (1958): *Behavioral Analysis: Analysis of Clinical Observations of Behavior as Applied to Mother-Newborn Relationships.* Springfield, Ill., Charles C Thomas.

Lidz, T. (1974): The life cycle: introduction. *American Handbook of Psychiatry.* 2d ed. Edited by S. Arieti. Vol. 1. New York, Basic Books.

Mahler, M.S., Pine, F., and Bergman, A. (1975): *The Psychological Birth of the Human Infant.* New York, Basic Books.

Sheldon, W.H. (1949): *Varieties of Delinquent Youth*. New York, Harper.

Skeels, H.M. (1966): Adult status of children with contrasting early life experiences: a follow-up study. In *Monograph Soc. Res. Child Dev. 31*:1.

Spitz, R.A. (1945): Hospitalism: an inquiry into the genesis of psychiatric conditions in early childhood. *Psychoanlyt. Stud. Child. 1*:53.

Spitz, R.A. (1946): Hospitalism: a follow-up report on investigation described in volume 1, 1945. *Psychoanlyt. Stud. Child. 2*:113.

Thomas, A., Chess, S., and Birch, H.G. (1968): *Temperament and Behavior Disorders in Children*. New York, New York University Press.

Yarrow, M.R., Campbell, J.D., and Burton, R.V. (1968): *Child Rearing: An Enquiry into Research and Methods*. California, Jossey-Bass.

FURTHER READINGS

Bowlby, J. (1969): *Attachment and Loss. Vol 1: Attachment*. New York, Basic Books.

The classic textbook on attachment theory.

Erikson, E. H. (1959): Identity and the life cycle. *Psychol Issues. 1:1.*

The classic volume, describing Erikson's developmental theory.

Flavell, J.H. (1963): *The Developmental Psychology of Jean Piaget*. New York, Van Nostrand, Reinhold.

A very concise summary of Piaget's theoretical concepts. Fairly hard reading.

Fraiberg, S. (1959): *The Magic Years*. New York, Scribner's.

A psychoanalytic approach and a beautifully descriptive book of the early pre-school years.

Kagan, J. and Moss, H.A. (1962): *Birth to Maturity*. New York, J. Wiley

A classic volume introducing modern concepts of cognitive development.

Mahler, M.S., Pine, F., and Bergman, A. (1975): *The Psychological Birth of the Human Infant*. New York, Basic Books.

The text of Mahler's theory of development from the symbiotic phase through separation-individuation, rapprochement, and beginning of later separation, with complete research data.

Thomas, A. and Chess, S. (1977): *Temperament and Development*. New York, Brunner and Mazel.

Arising from the 20-Year New York Longitudinal Study, this book shows the significance of temperament as it interacts with the environment, for normal and deviant psychological development.

Weiner, I. B. and Elkind, D. (1972): *Child Development: A Core Approach*. New York, J. Wiley.

A concise but comprehensive and well written introduction to the basic facts and issues in child development. Presents and integrates a number of major theoretical approaches, and provides an annotated bibliography at the end of each chapter.

3

Adolescence and Young Adulthood

Clive G. Chamberlain

Adolescence is best defined as a development process: It begins as a clearly recognizable sequence of biological changes, but the definition of its termination, the end of adolescence, is not only largely determined by social and cultural factors but also depends on the view of particular authors. Some restrict the term adolescence to the process of puberty and the period immediately following it, while others include a much longer phase ending with social and financial independence. This may have the result that in the developed world and, in particular among prosperous social classes, individuals may see themselves and be seen by others as adolescent until they are in their thirties.

In the sense that each life phase has a particular task, it is the task of adolescence to make the transition from childhood to adulthood: to achieve the capacity "to love and to work." It involves abandoning the safe plateau of late middle childhood for more complex and sophisticated levels of personality functioning. This has to include the integration and mastery of gradually increasing sexual and aggressive drives and the final development of intellectual capacity and talents. It is during this period that most individuals first experience an essential separateness from all others: the adolescent often experiences loneliness and an ill-defined nostalgia which can be thought of as the entry to the necessary adult capacity to suffer and endure. There is a paradox in this phase: while the adolescent encounters loneliness for the first time, he also faces the strong need for others, as a truly social being.

The approach taken in this chapter will be first, to discuss the biological, cognitive, psychological, and social aspects of adolescence and then, next, to look in somewhat more detail into the substages of this developmental phase. We will conclude with a short discussion of some clinical and conceptual problem areas.

ASPECTS OF DEVELOPMENT

There is great normal variation in the beginning and the pace of the biological changes during adolescence. However, the developmental *sequence*, the phases of change and growth, is highly consistent in both sexes.

Biological Development

Morphologically in boys, pubescence is signalled some time between the age of 10 and 13½ by testicular and scrotal enlargement followed usually within three months or so by the growth of pigmented pubic hair, at first straight, then becoming more curled as it darkens, coarsens and spreads. About a year after the first evidence of testicular growth, the average boy experiences a dramatic acceleration in the rate of skeletal and muscular growth. This coincides with the onset of increase in the size of the penis, which has lagged behind scrotal growth. Approximately two years after the first sign of scrotal enlargement, the average boy will have achieved his peak skeletal and muscular growth rate. Ejaculation becomes possible at about this time. See Figure 1.

Morphological changes for girls begin earlier than in boys. Characteristically, the height-growth spurt, early breast development (areolar enlargement and "budding") and pubic hair growth, all begin more or less simultaneously, between the 8th and 13th year. As with boys the growth rate peaks about one year later and this coincides with fairly advanced breast development. Menarche occurs at about age 13 (normal range from ages 10 to 16½). See Figure 2.

The enormous variation noted above may create considerable problems for some youngsters, even while they are physiologically normal. Because of an early or late development they may feel themselves to be oddities. Of course, considerable change may occur within a relatively short period of time. Yet, merely being ahead of one's peers or behind them by several months can engender acutely uncomfortable degrees of self-consciousness. The morphological and physiological changes force the youngsters to modify their perception of their own body and the way they relate to their own body: they must learn to accommodate to the new person they see in the mirror. They must also

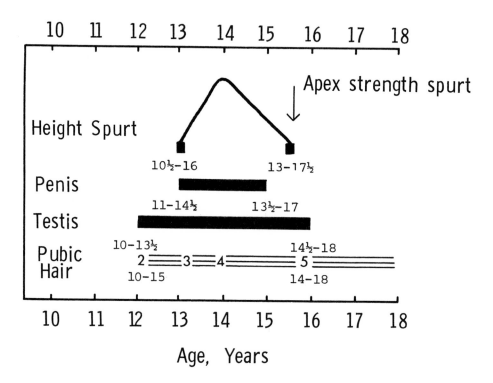

FIG. 1.

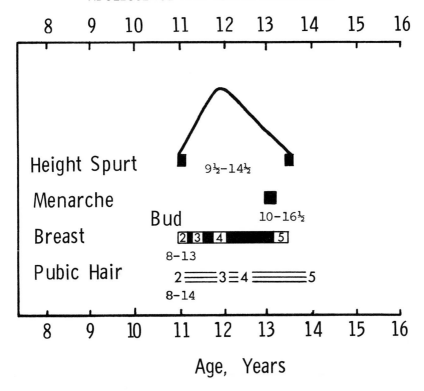

FIG. 2.

Cognitive Development

accommodate to changes in how they are perceived and treated by others, especially by adults and peers of the opposite sex. Because self-perception often lags behind the way others see them, adolescents may be confused about the meaning of the behavior of other people towards them and they are constantly open to considerable embarrassment.

While morphological development is more accessible to direct observation, there is good reason to believe that the variation, so obvious in this sphere of development, is paralleled in the cognitive-psychological and social dimensions.

Cognitive Development

Between the ages of seven and eleven, the child achieves a considerable sense of order in his surrounding world of objects and events. But the categories in which he

classifies experience are rather limited. His ability to generalize, to move from the particular to the general, to abstract, remains limited. He is still locked up in the concrete and immediately contemporary facts of the surrounding world. Because he is so limited by immediate, tangible data he has but a limited capacity to imagine alternative kinds of experience, or ways of responding. Intellectual activities or operations are not yet abstract events in their own right which can be reflected upon and manipulated. This stage, preceding adolescence, has been labeled the stage of "concrete operations" by Piaget.

Around age ten to twelve, however, i.e. at the stage of early adolescence with its rapid physiological changes, a shift to a higher level of intellectual functioning also takes place: the development of the capacity for formal operations which Piaget called the "crowning achievement" of intellectual development. The young adolescent acquires the capacity to imagine complex alternate situations and possibilities, to hypothesize, to test "simulation models." Thus the power of prediction and, consequently choice, is vastly extended. This includes, of course, his own and others' social roles. For the first time, the adolescent can "look at himself," i.e. he can treat himself as an object seen "from the outside," and he becomes able to imagine how another person might experience a given situation and react to it. He develops a capacity for empathy—to feel and perceive the world from the point of view of others.

While the development of concrete operations is a universal process across cultures and social strata, there appears to be less universal consistency in the development of formal operations. The level of intellectual and emotional sophistication relates to the demands and expectations of the family and social environment. A high level of demand stimulates the development of the adolescent in this regard. The development of formal operations does not progress as a uniformly advancing front. There are advances with temporary regressions, while islets of more primitive functioning may remain amidst general progress and may indeed persist throughout life.

Psychological Development

This includes emotional development, e.g. the integration and acceptance and the appropriate expression of intensified sexual and aggressive drives; the changes in ways of relating to others and to oneself. Equally important is the development of the sense of relationship to society, its history, and to dominant systems of myth and belief.

Erikson stressed that adolescence has a major, phase-specific task: the consolidation of a personal sense of identity. During this time the individual is preoccupied with such questions as "Who am I?" "What are my values?" "What is my style?" "What are my talents and eccentricities?" In short, he must exercise choice and engage in self-definition across a wide range of experience and behavior. If successful, there results some coherence and consistency in attitudes, values and behavior patterns. Obviously, physiological maturation and cognitive development are preconditions.

Anna Freud has also contributed considerably to our understanding of the psychological aspects of adolescent development. She focused on the challenge of having to establish within oneself a new equilibrium between intensifying sexual-aggressive drives, and new social demands for their control and appropriate expression. The tension between these forces in the life of the adolescent generates a state of inner turbulence, which may have little overt behavioral expression. She pointed to the development of 'phase specific' ego defense mechanisms for dealing with unpleasant emotions, such as asceticism and intellectualization. The first refers to a prudish, anti-sensual defensive posture often taken by the young adolescent who feels threatened by sexual opportunity, but who is still uncomfortably dependent on his parents and for whom sexual activity may still retain some incestuous meaning. Intellectualization, of course, is fostered by the newly acquired level of cognitive functioning.

Anna Freud was also preoccupied with the resolution of the conflict between infantile attachment to parents and independence. She suggested that adolescents characteristically shift the object of their dependency before the intensity of the dependency relationship itself is altered. In other words, they still need to be closely attached to some supportive people other than their parents. The peer group may become a substitute, or they may shift their dependency to intellectual ideas or socially oriented ideologies. So that there is a period of relative "ideological" vulnerability in early, normal adolescence, resulting from the search for something or someone to depend on other than one's parents. This often involves reaching out and becoming dependent on others, partly perhaps to salvage self-esteem but also to conduct the struggle for independence with respect to the family unit.

Social Development

The human needs for personal meaning and identity clearly involve the need to see oneself as part of the group, of society, of the surrounding world which carries more permanence or significance than the isolated individual. In other words, personal identity is felt and conceived of within a social context. This need for social belonging and social meaning may be expressed in many different forms and may be explored in the strangest of directions.

Returning to Erikson: once the individual has achieved some sense of personal identity, it is the next task of the emerging adult to prepare for and seek intimacy in relationships. At an ethical level this involves sensitivity to others and regard for another individual who is seen as someone with personal rights, feelings, and idiosyncrasies and not as a stereotype or an interchangeable member of a category. As always with any developmental process, failures at any level of development have a limiting effect on the potential for development in subsequent stages and may lead to an accumulating deficit. Thus an adolescent emerging into young adulthood with a precarious and conflicting sense of who he or she is will find the demands of an intimate relationship overwhelming if the tasks of adolescence have not been achieved. And new adult intimacy would be all too reminiscent of the earlier version—that of the parent-child relationship.

STAGES OF DEVELOPMENT

Preadolescence

Before puberty, small amounts of androgen and estrogen are produced, probably by the adrenals, in both boys and girls. The level of these substances begins to rise in both sexes between the ages of seven and ten.

Children in the year or two just prior to pubescence will, for the most part, have reached a considerable level of physical, psychological and social skills. These permit them far greater senses of personal competence, self-assurance and independence than were previously possible. Children of this age appear to have a sense of wholeness or completeness; they are predictable, usually happy, and easy to live with.

Early Adolescence

In girls pubescence begins with a dramatic increase in estrogen production and a much smaller increase in production of testosterone. With boys, of course, it is just the reverse. As already indicated, the variance in time of onset is immense and the physiological aspect of the developmental process spans about four years.

The age at which puberty begins may have psychological consequences. For example, there is a tendency for boys who are late in reaching puberty to be less confident and assertive, but more talkative and attention-seeking. This may be related to the fact that early puberty often goes along with a well-developed muscular physique. High value is often placed on physical and athletic prowess by adolescent boys. On the other hand, girls on the average mature two years earlier than boys. If the onset of puberty is very early, they may become quite self-conscious and make efforts to conceal the evidence of their maturation. Because of all these variations there is no general, clear-cut relationship between the time of onset of puberty and attitudes towards self.

In the earliest phase of adolescence, group activity tends to be mainly with the same sex, in spite of the frequent attempts by adults to promote early heterosexual socializing. Both sexes experience heightened body awareness demonstrated by the capacity to spend enormous amounts of time before a mirror. The preoccupation with appearance is sometimes the subject of much amusement to younger and older siblings. This increased preoccupation with their bodies is probably necessary for adolescents to accommodate to very rapid changes without losing their sense of who they are. Girls become concerned about their weight, acne, their menses (do others know they are having a period?) and their breast development. Similarly, boys are concerned about developing muscularity and height, genital size and the growth of pubic, axillary, and facial hair.

There are few youngsters who, at this stage, do not have moments of exquisite self-consciousness and concern for the way others perceive them. Particularly poignant are the difficulties of youngsters who bring to this stage already existing stigmata or disability. A boy who has compensated very well for a physical handicap may suddenly during early adolescence feel himself alienated and despised by his peer group. He may seem to lose all the self-assurance that was so painstakingly developed in earlier years. For all children this is a time when partially resolved developmental problems from earlier periods may re-emerge. Typical examples: temporary heightened dependency on parents may often alternate with rebellion, or, a regressive intolerance of group activity in favor of one-to-one relationships.

This is a time of much interest in sexuality as evidenced by conversation, themes in humor, and sexual activity. Most surveys on the subject indicate that the overwhelming majority of boys and a sizable minority of girls begin to masturbate, more or less regularly, shortly after the onset of puberty. This continues until it is supplemented or substituted by sexual involvement with other persons. Once thought, both by the general public and professionals, to be not only sinful but dangerously unhealthy, masturbation is now regarded by most as healthy and normal. It is important, however, to note that some youngsters find themselves in an intense conflict around masturbation: masturbation may in such cases become the central issue over which the struggle for developing self-control rages. Without such a struggle, a significant degree of adult maturity is probably not possible. One must, therefore, be cautious about the way in which reassurances are given, lest the wish to be one's own master be mistaken for anxiety about normality.

During early adolescence youngsters tend to remain home-centered. Increasingly oppositional behavior may occur. If so, it usually is in direct proportion to the intensity of the dependency upon the parents. To use a cosmic metaphor it is as if they must somehow find the energy to achieve escape velocity from the parental gravitational pull. However, children who have already achieved a high degree of self-assurance and independence usually proceed through this stage with little turbulence.

Both boys and girls begin to seek transitional dependency relationships to replace some of their dependency on their parents. "Crushes" and "hero-worship" are vital ingredients in the important activity of separating from parents. By passing through a series of identifications the adolescent extends and consolidates personal identity. There are nuances to "crush" and "hero-worship" relationships that are important to note in understanding and helping early adolescents. It is a characteristic of such relationships that they possess a somewhat transparently disguised erotic component. The purpose of the relationship for the youngster is to serve as a way-station on the road to decreasing dependency, and increased erotic and intimate attachment to appropriate others. The object of such a transitional attachment is rarely perceived clearly and is expected to live up to some very demanding and unrealistic expectations, or at least not disappoint them. The impact of such flattery upon the person chosen can be seductive. Gentle interest is the response which best suits the needs of the young adolescent, but it may not always be evoked, particularly if the person to whom the adolescent becomes attached is lonely or finds the flattery all too welcome. Just as a bored, disinterested response would be hurtful to self-esteem, a response seeking intimacy and closeness may well produce panic or confusion.

In counselling youngsters of this age, it should be remembered that they need some assurance from the adult that an appropriate distance will be respected and that the responsibility for maintaining this will not be the young person's alone. It is worth remembering that so long as the young person is seeking such "transitional relationships" there is an implicit demand for some parenting involving limit-setting and advice. When this is no longer required to the same degree, the stage is set for mid-adolescence where the center of social gravity shifts from the family to the community and especially to the peer group.

Mid-Adolescence

When this stage begins, physiological changes of adolescence are well advanced, although as yet incomplete.

Whereas in early adolescence preoccupation with self took a decidedly bodily form, attention now shifts to personality, life style, attitudes, beliefs, ideas. The early turbulence and awkwardness appear only infrequently. Whereas in early adolescence transient periods of ambiguity in sexual orientation frequently occur, for example as manifested by homosexual play, in mid-adolescence gender identity and sexual orientation consolidate rapidly. Explicit sexual explorations often begin at this time, although there is great variation.

As the first tentative interests in the opposite sex are expressed, peer group standards begin to dominate and independence from parents and parent figures ripens and extends. As form and coherence begin to characterize personality structure, Erikson's notion of identity becomes important in the psychological life of the young.

In the intellectual sphere this is a time when ideologies begin to fascinate and make strong claims for commitment. Ideas are passionately held and rapidly discarded, as the emerging person tastes the whole smorgasbord of ideas and points of view in the general culture. An aspect of the pace at which these processes occur is the intolerance of ambiguity and uncertainty that is a characteristic of this substage of adolescence. The heroes of adolescence tend to be figures identified with action, and proceeding from a "black and white" point of view. It is at this time that religious or quasi-religious organizations with these characteristics begin to exert their appeal. There may be intense concern with such philosophical themes as the "meaning of life" or with personal and political values.

Psychotherapy with the early adolescent often demands the use of activity or play therapy as with younger children. However, one has to begin accommodating the emerging formal cognitive operations of the youngsters. But mid-adolescents enjoy discussions and become amenable to conventional verbal psychotherapies. They are less frightened by growing sexual and aggressive drives. Their advanced maturity in interpersonal functioning permits them to engage in conscious therapeutic alliances. Viewing the young patient as an independent person makes it possible to deal with attempts to seek parenting from the therapist as transference behavior rather than age-appropriate behavior.

Late Adolescence and Young Adulthood

This is the stage in which the promise of the capacity to love and to work must be made good.

In the sphere of human relationships the ideal of achieving a capacity for intimacy (the I—Thou relationship of Buber) is most significant. To achieve this, others must be recognized as having their own reality and feelings. There is not only one's own personal reality, but also the reality of others. Just as Piaget's young child "discovers" that the same object looks different to two observers in different locations—the older adolescent rediscovers the same principle at the interpersonal level. It is this shift that makes mature love possible.

In addition to personal relationships, the adolescent must acquire the ability to work. Ideally this involves not only the ready mobilization of energies and the application of skills which had their major growth in latency, but also the harnessing of these to a sense of direction and purpose, acquired chiefly during the period of adolescence. One is reminded of the perhaps apocryphal story attributed to Christopher Wren, who, on an inspection tour of the site of St. Paul's Cathedral, asked one workman what he was doing. "Digging a hole" he was told. On encountering another to whom he put the same question, a very different answer explained the same activity: "Building a cathedral."

Perhaps because this stage of life demands actual performance in both spheres—love and work—rather than some expectations for the future, it is a time of great stress. Of course, pubescence is also a phase of particular stress and turbulence as pointed out by romantic theorists and some serious students of personality. But one should be particularly aware of the unbending demands for performance which occur for the first time in one's life, during adolescence. The protection of parents is diminished and one knows that one is responsible for oneself and one's performance, a fact which characterizes emerging adulthood. Failures at this stage are no longer readily forgiven and consequences of poor judgement have become less reversible.

It is at this stage that the incidence of serious psychic decompensation, psychosis, and the first indications of mood disorders become significant. The etiology of such disorders is far from clearly established, yet the coincidence of life stress and emerging psychopathology is unlikely to be entirely coincidental.

SOME CLINICAL AND CONCEPTUAL PROBLEM AREAS

Much theorizing about early childhood has been dominated by the false dichotomy of "nature versus nurture." A similar issue tends to affect thinking about adolescence. The polarities here are the individual versus the group; or, personal consciousness versus community and culture. Obviously, just as in childhood, it is not a question of either one or the other. However, there is some support for the view that adolescence, especially mid-adolescence and late adolescence, is to a significant extent a social artifact: characteristics of individuals at this stage are those of adults at any age who are forced by circumstance to accept a dependent role. Perhaps, such a perspective helps to explain the variation seen in this stage of life amongst different social classes and societies.

However, it is, in general, much more difficult to be sure about the interrelation of two sets of variables, for example, biological and psychological ones, as one moves away from childhood. For example, the intrinsic (biological) development of Piaget's perceptual object constancy, is clearly a precondition for the development of separation anxiety. Certain psychological developments can only occur on the basis of certain biological developments. This mode of thought, involving particular and specific links, becomes much more difficult to maintain when one tries to account for the branching out of various "styles" or patterns of personality development in adolescence. In adolescence multiple social and cultural variables begin to interlock with internal necessities, and theorizing about the adolescent does not easily accommodate simple polarities.

Another troublesome issue in thinking about adolescent personality and adolescent psychopathology has been the confusion between genuine illness or disorder and normal turbulence. There existed (especially during the 1960's) a tendency among some clinicians to regard with optimism serious psychiatric symptoms which would be regarded as ominous at any other stage of life. Thus, adolescents were often described as suffering from emotional turbulence and, consequently, behavioral turbulence could also be viewed as "normal." "Acting out" was perceived as some kind of self-cure or therapeutic catharsis, or, at least an age-appropriate defensive strategy. The next step in this kind of theorizing led to the development of treatment approaches which encouraged free expression while playing down the essential development of self-control. Not only did a particular forbidden impulse or wish become appropriate, but its behavioral expression was

to be encouraged as well. While this therapeutic approach may have counteracted the development of self-control, with others it began supporting nonintervention altogether. For, if most, if not all adolescent upheaval was normal and underlying impulses and wishes appropriate, intervention seemed futile: it was thought that most youngsters with upheaval and symptoms would "grow out of it."

Accumulating evidence tends not to support such views. Studies of "normal" adolescent populations reveal a developmental stage which is essentially continuous. Upheavals are more subjectively experienced than overtly expressed in action. Long term follow-up studies of symptomatic adolescents confirm the impression that normal adolescent behavior resembles psychopathology only in romantic fiction. Prolonged early adolescent antisocial behavior, far from being "sowing wild oats" or healthy rebellion, is all too often the harbinger of serious disability. Just as we sometimes admire the appearance of wit in the schizophrenic, there is a risk that the self-defeating and compulsive misbehavior of some young patients can be taken for healthy emancipation. It is particularly important to pay attention to severe manifestations of psychiatric symptomatology such as hallucinations or delusions: they suggest serious illness and are not simply signs of turbulence.

This chapter has attempted to develop an overview of the significant themes in the second major "cycle" of life. Beginning with a well-balanced and "complete" organism, the pre-adolescent child, we have traced the vicissitudes of a process beginning with the disequilibrium imposed by a changed self arising out of increased instinctual drive, and a changed world brought about through new powers of cognition. The cycle ends as it began: the organism, again well-balanced, is more complete and ready once more to encounter new challenge.

FURTHER READINGS

Group for the Advancement of Psychiatry, Committee on Adolescence (1968): *Normal Adolescence: Its Dynamics and Impact.* New York, C. Scribner's.

Feinstein, S.C., Giovacchini, P.L., and Miller, A.A. (1971): *Adolescent Psychiatry, Vol. I.* New York, Basic Books.

Holmes, D.J. (1964): *The Adolescent in Psychotherapy.* Boston, Little, Brown.

Offer, D. (1973): *The Psychological World of the Teenager.* New York, Basic Books.

Robins, L.N. (1966): *Deviant Children Grown Up: A Sociological and Psychiatric Study of Sociopathic Personality.* Baltimore, Williams & Wilkins.

CHAPTER 4

Middle Age and Maturity (Old Age)
Marvin E. Miller

A person enters middle life about the age of 40. By common agreement it is considered that the middle age span lasts about 20 to 25 years, so that 65 becomes the threshold of old age.

At the onset of middle age the concept of "aging" becomes a meaningful one. It is true that we are "aging" throughout life and that it begins at birth. But the essence of aging as decline rather than growth and development makes itself apparent during the middle years and gathers momentum as the individual approaches death.

The aging process takes place according to a variety of "profiles." Some age gracefully and in concert with their chronology, whereas others show a tendency to be old before their time in both appearance and behavior. Yet others remain active, alert and engaged in life well into their 90's.

In general there are many things as yet unknown about the aging process, but it appears that senescence with its accumulation of losses is part of the normal life cycle and is not a pathological entity.

THE AGING PROCESS—GENERAL CONSIDERATIONS

When considering the aging process one must remember that the person is both a physical and psychological being. The aging process manifests itself in both aspects; it is essential for the doctor's approach to the older individual that he keep in mind their constant interplay.

PHYSICAL CHANGES

The functioning of the mind depends on an intact cerebral cortex. As the individual ages, neuronal degeneration and necrosis take place continuously, so that gradually a significant depletion of neuronal tissue occurs. And since neuronal tissue cannot regenerate, tissue loss is absolute. There is however a significant reserve of functional capacity in the cerebral cortex that compensates effectively for the depletion for a long time, and the "functional neuronal mass" continues to allow acceptable mental functioning as the individual ages. However, as time goes on there will be some slowing in mentation, some minor degree of memory difficulty and perhaps some minimal problem of orientation. This will be the state of affairs in the senescent individual. However, in the presence of a disease process such as Alzheimer's disease, the changes in mental functioning will be more profound. There will be a decrease in brain weight with evidence of

43

cerebral atrophy and ventricular enlargement on radiological evidence. These latter changes represent a pathological entity in contrast to the former process with its expected loss of neuronal mass as part of normal aging.

Theories of Aging

Intracellular Theories

Cell loss is thought to occur as a result of random events which may take place over many years. These events lead to mutations in cell structure and eventually cell necrosis. In general, longevity in an aging animal is inversely proportional to the rate at which the animal develops mutations. Thus dogs live about six times longer than mice and develop mutations at about one sixth the rate. Radiation, for example, may produce a mutative effect. According to Busse and Pfeiffer (1977) "the exposure of a living organism to repeated small doses of ionizing radiation or to a larger sublethal dose, appreciably reduces the life span of the organism. Radiated animals and aging animals both show an increase in the number of somatic cell mutations."

Others consider that cellular degeneration results from a biologic clock mechanism linked to genetic programming which controls the aging process that becomes increasingly apparent as neuronal deterioration and other somatic cell changes occur in time.

Another theory postulates a "wear and tear" mechanism that results in cell degeneration which appears to be also time related and results in obsolescence of the cellular tissue.

Curtis (1966) in his "composite" theory of aging suggests that a series of changes initiates the degenerative diseases which are increasingly probable in the aging individual. As an individual becomes older he develops at different rates most of the degenerative diseases. The changes take place in the somatic cells, and these changes cause these cells and their prog-

eny to function to the detriment of the organism. Mutation is an important step in the detrimental change, but the extent of the change cannot be explained as the result of a single mutation.

Finally, some have postulated that alterations occur in the structure of the molecule leading to defective enzymes which in turn lead to abnormal metabolic processes. This is the so-called "error theory," a more specific variant of theories concerning chromosomal aberrations.

Extracellular Theories

The aging process affects the connective tissue of the body in a way which reduces its elasticity and results in more fibrous, rigid connective tissue strands. It is thought that the collagen in connective tissue is altered by way of a cross linkage between polypeptide strands in the collagen molecule. As time passes there is a switching of the ester bonds from within the polypeptide strands to between the individual collagen molecules. This cross linking between the strands alters the structure of the collagen, particularly affecting its elasticity. The connective tissue is thereby altered in its quality, and crowding may occur which hastens the eventual degeneration of the somatic cells.

Walford (1964) has posited an immuno-protein theory. He points out that in time the individual develops mutant protein and in response to the changed protein immune reactions may bring about a change in various anatomical structures which may in turn lead to age-related diseases, for example, arteriosclerosis, cancer or maturity onset diabetes.

The life span of members of any one species tends to be fairly uniform. There appears to be a time clock for each species which governs genetic material regulating the phases of the life cycle. In this connection the brain is the only organ whose size is correlated with potential life span in several species. The cephalization index is the ratio between the weight of the brain and the body, and seems to be correlated with longevity in the case of mammals and birds. Roughly,the greater the brain mass governing a unit of body mass, the more long-lived is the species.

AGING AND SOCIETY

The older individual is often rejected from the community on the basis of economic issues. The older person no longer capable of making a contribution to the group may, in his need, threaten the resources of a poor community and disturb its homeostatic balance.

Among the Hopi and the Crow Indians as well as the Bushmen of South Africa, for instance, it was customary to lead the aged person to a hut specially built for the purpose, away from the village, and to abandon him there leaving only a little food and water. The Inuit persuaded the old to lie in the snow and wait for death; or left them to die on an ice floe when the tribe was out fishing. Sometimes they shut them into an igloo to die of cold. Among the semi-nomadic African Hottentots older members of the tribe were usually highly esteemed. They actively participated in important tribal rituals, presiding over all rites of passage and particularly the initiation of adolescent boys. However even in this community when dementia was well established, the older person was hoisted onto the back of an ox and escorted to a remote hut. There he was left to die (Simone de Beauvoir, 1972).

Where there is a greater margin of economic security in a particular society, there tends to be a greater tolerance for the existence of the infirm aged. Yet this tolerance is a relative matter, and although there is no overt death-dealing blow or abandonment in a remote hut there are, nevertheless, many subtle rejections which pervade the social and economic systems. It is a commonplace that many old people in the Western world live in a situation of poverty because of the disparity between their meagre incomes and the cost of living during an inflationary period.

Another aspect of the social experience of the older person may be understood in terms of "disengagement theory." Some old people withdraw from close relationships as they age. Similarly people with whom they previously had involvements withdraw reciprocally from the old so that a state of mutual isolation develops. It has been proposed that this mutual withdrawal may be an adaptive mechanism which serves a healthy purpose for some old people. It results in a state of relative well-being in spite of the fact that they are not actively engaged with others. In a sense the disengagement theory supports schizoid behavior, seeing it as appropriate for some older individuals. It allows for solitude wherein the old person may gradually come to terms with the final stage of life.

There have been some who have proposed that "life review" activity of the old is an adaptive mechanism which bolsters self-esteem so vulnerable at this time in life. In the process of reminiscing old people set in order highlights of their lives, and by so doing give a retrospective structure and meaning to their existence.

On the other hand there are those who maintain that activity and involvement with the environment are essential to maintain effective functioning in old age. It is felt that isolation may lead to stagnation of physical and mental activity and result in disease processes which can affect both body and mind. The "need to exercise" concept is an important determinant of health throughout life including the health of the aged. It appears that both activity and disengagement are relevant to the phenomenon of aging.

AGING AND CREATIVITY

We tend to view the life cycle as having an ascendance followed by a decline. This decline has generally been thought to occur somewhere in early adulthood after a peak period in sexual activity and creative output. Elliot Jacques (1965) suggests that there is an efflorescence of creativity which emerges from the artist or scientist in an almost tempestuous way early in adult life. He contrasts this with the creative output of persons in middle life and old age where a slower and more deliberate shaping of the creative product, much as a sculptor shapes his medium, is more common. The younger person's productivity may relate more directly to unconscious psychological process, whereas the creativity of the older person emerges from a "cooler crucible" and the required effort is related more to neutralized energies that have been modified by experience. There are many instances of persons in middle and old age who have produced significant work: Titian, Michelangelo, Goethe, Sibelius, Churchill and Freud are examples of creative artists, scientists and statesmen who have made outstanding contributions long after they passed their mid-life period. The so called period of decline, then, is not necessarily synonymous with deterioration, decrepitude and despair.

AGING AND THE MEDICAL PROFESSION

The population of older people in our society has been increasing significantly since the turn of the century. Since that time there has been an increase in the numbers of people age 65 and over from approximately 4% to approximately 9% at the present time. A projection of population figures suggests that this will increase by about 2% by 1990. The sheer weight of numbers of the old in our society will put an increasing demand on services from medical professionals.

The old have not been particularly attractive to medical personnel, and have often suffered indignities and rejection in the context of being a patient. For many years a climate of therapeutic nihilism prevailed. It was thought that chronologic age was synonymous with irreversible disease and that efforts to deal with disease processes (not only symptoms) were futile. Older people were often only treated in a palliative way, and proper assessment required to lead to meaningful diagnoses was not performed.

This state of affairs has shifted in recent years and there is a climate of greater therapeutic optimism than was formerly the case. Practitioners both in physical and psychological medicine are becoming increasingly interested in the variety of health problems that beset the older individual. For example the use of psychotherapy with the old has in recent years become more common. We know that older people can "learn" as long as they have not entered a state of dementia due to marked diminution in the "functional neuronal mass" and that they may potentially benefit from psychotherapeutic intervention.

THE DEVELOPMENTAL POINT OF VIEW

The individual who successfully manages to deal with the intrapsychic and interpersonal problems that occur in earlier life is better able to confront the crises of the latter half of life. The shifting facets of life experiences repeatedly offer potential for change, and old age, too, is a time of potential development of the person in the same way as earlier periods of life.

By the time the person has lived about 40 years a wealth of experience has accrued. As Erikson proposes, the best use of this accumulated experience for the next 20 years is to impart something of it to others. The middle aged have gained knowledge in the management of life's problems, and in general, by occupying positions of advantage and power are able to offer help both to the young as well as to the old. At the same time the men and women of this age group are required to face and deal with that "change of life" referred to as the climacteric in which both psychological and physical involution processes occur.

The middle aged person is on the one

hand an acknowledged "expert" in living, but has yet to develop an "expertise" in the process of decline (involution) as it relates to physical, psychological and psychosocial functioning. The involution experience in another sense is preparatory to the final stage of life during which what has gone on before must be accepted and worked through as the person prepares to face death.

During the decade of the 40's and for the first half of the 50's men and women are in the first throes of what we might call "manifest aging." Physically, there are significant changes that reveal the inevitable alterations in appearance and body functioning. The graying of hair, the appearance of facial wrinkles, major deterioration of dentition, musculo-skeletal problems and a tendency to paunchiness are the outward manifestations of the aging process. Within, there is a diminution of physical strength, vigor and perhaps stamina. The feeling of self-satisfaction that comes in moving the body effectively, with ease, and with a sense of mastery, begins to be threatened. For many people this can result in reduced self-esteem. Yet, the ensuing anxiety can become either a stimulus for adaptation to the changes or may result in symptom formation. The concept of adaptation helps one to understand that the periods of aging (both middle and old) have a developmental aspect. Where adaptation occurs to changing circumstance, there is implied an addition to the repertoire of behavior skills the individual has come to master.

Furthermore, the developmental point of view underscores the notion of continuing psychological work on the problem of autonomy. The pursuit of separation-individuation is a lifelong process. Along the way a number of age-related crises are encountered, each of which requires resolution. The outcome of these struggles can lead to: further development in the individual's growth; a lack of movement forward or backward (stasis); or, a regression to an earlier stage of development. This process begins early in the first year of life and proceeds in an accelerating fashion during early childhood. The process is still operative during adolescence when the question of identity or sense of self is being worked out. Similarly at the time of retirement, when energies are required to be redirected into activities which serve to reaffirm feelings of worth and sense of self, the process continues. And finally, as Erikson's concept of "ego integrity" in old age states, the task is relevant to the older person facing death. Clarity about who one is, and who one has been, is actively sought by the autonomously developing individual.

THE RETIREMENT EXPERIENCE

The relationship that a person has to his or her work serves as a model for exploring adaptive potential in the mid-life period. A man whose sense of worth has been significantly linked to the idea of himself as a worker is required, at the time of retirement, to shift ground and redirect his energies toward new enterprises which will allow him to find continuing satisfaction. And the new-found interests may tend to buoy up his sagging self-esteem and may ward off a depressive illness. A fall in self-esteem tends to result in feelings of inferiority as a consequence of not living up to one's ideals. Following this collapse in self-esteem, a depressive illness may occur. It is postulated that an individual may continue to weather the "slings and arrows" of many life crises without falling victim to an abandonment of ideals as long as he continues to be dedicated to a task consistent with past standards. When this "performance" is no longer possible, as occurs with retirement or the loss of one's job because of an arbitrary corporate decision, the unprepared person is hard pressed to mobilize sources of self-approval necessary to negotiate the transition. A similar situation occurs in the case of the woman whose adult life has been dedicated to the task of childbearing.

In middle age, early or late, when the grown children leave home, a void is left in her life that was previously filled by the gratifying experiences of the maternal role. In her case, too, the potential for psychological decompensation exists if she has not previously diversified.

To limit one's experience, to put "all of the eggs in one basket," is likely to lead to difficulties during middle and old age since these are characteristically times of life that inevitably rob one of many healthy narcissistic satisfactions.

SEXUALITY AND AGING

The subject of sexuality and aging has been conspicuously absent from the literature until about twenty years ago. In recent times, constricting attitudes have given way to more open and tolerant considerations of human sexual behavior (an openness and tolerance that may be more apparent than real), and we are beginning to get a better picture of the alterations in sexual activity as they affect aging people.

The phenomenon of the climacteric (menopause) was briefly mentioned earlier. It was thought that this time in life had inevitably to be difficult for women as they began to experience the involutional processes associated with the endocrine changes that lead to a cessation of the menses and fertility. Traditionally this has been conceived of as a time of emotional upheaval for the woman who, having experienced the menopause, feels her femininity seriously compromised. Yet a recent study has revealed that many menopausal women accept their "change of life" and experience few debilitating symptoms. Neugarten (1968) studied a sample of well-educated, upper-middle class women. The study used questionnaires to assess conscious attitudes and brief interview surveys were also conducted. The fact that many of these women indicated they were not unduly distressed by their menopausal experience affirms that it is not universally debilitating. On the other hand it is well known that many women are less successful in their adaptation and may experience a variety of physical and psychological symptoms. It is a time when irritability and depressive symptoms are manifest. Yet it can also be a time when the woman may begin to demonstrate an assertiveness in her behavior which was not previously apparent. Some authors have suggested that there may be a reversal of traditional male/female behavior vis-a-vis assertiveness during the involutional period and that one tends to see more aggressivity in women and more passivity and compliance in men than was the case earlier in life. Apart from mild to moderate debilitating symptoms the individual, during the climacteric, may tend to develop a full-blown psychological illness which can be either acute or chronic, self-limiting, or one requiring therapeutic intervention. At times such illness can form the nucleus of an altered life style, which may persist to the end of life. A prolonged and chronic depressive state beginning in the involutional period and sometimes associated with paranoid trends, may in some cases be intractable.

The work of Kinsey and his associates in the late 1940's is helpful in considering, more specifically, the matter of sexuality and aging. He observed that in men there is a decline in frequency of ejaculations from youth to old age. He pointed out that in youth there occurred approximately 4 ejaculations per week which then declined to 1.8 at age 50 and subsequently 1.3 at age 60 and 0.9 at age 70.

Masters and Johnson (1966) studied 133 men above the age of 60 (52 of whom were older than 70). In the same study 54 women age 60 and over (17 were 70 and over) were interviewed. They concluded that although male sexual responsiveness decreased with age, men with a high sexual output in younger years are likely to continue to be sexually active in old age. For women, they agree with Kinsey that a large proportion of women after menopause show a sex drive which is related to sexual habits established in earlier years.

A longitudinal study at the Duke University Department of Gerontological Research has been proceeding since 1954. A cohort of 254 people (age range 60 to 94) has been followed every three years to assess changes in their sexual interest and their sexual activity. It has been noted that what happens to sexual interests is not necessarily paralleled by what occurs in sexual activity. The study reveals that both sexual interest and activity are not rare in persons beyond the age of 60. It also demonstrated that patterns of sexual interest and activity differ substantially for men and women of the same age. Ten years after the study began they found that for 80% of men in the study there had not been a significant decrease in their *sexual interest* when their health, intellectual status, and social functioning were unimpaired. By contrast, although 70% of this group had been *sexually active* at the beginning of the study, only 25% remained so ten years later. Thus although sexual interest remained high, sexual activity dipped significantly.

With women they observed that only about 33% reported sexual interest at the beginning of the study, and ten years later, there was little change in the number remaining interested. With regard to sexual activity, only about 20% were active at the beginning of the study and ten years later approximately the same percentage of women reported they were still sexually active. The researchers reported some surprise at the fact that far fewer women than men were still sexually interested and active at this time in their lives. They wondered whether the differences represented a cultural or biological double standard, but they also considered that women might tend to be less open about revealing their sexual interest and activity in such a study.

When it is recalled that the term "sexuality" may have the broad meaning of multi-varied satisfaction-seeking in relation to different erogenous zones, it may be appreciated that the possibility of continuing sexual satisfaction is a reality for the old. In spite of the many and varied physical infirmities that affect very old people, the experiences of touching and being touched (skin eroticism); kissing and being kissed (oral eroticism); and mutual genital stimulation continue to afford a degree of sexual pleasure. However, it has been noted that cultural stereotypes of sexually driven old men ("dirty old men") and old women ("the aging whore") have unfortunately inhibited the normal expression of sexual longings in the broadest sense among many old people in their 70's and 80's.

Similarly it is not unusual to find that the children of older people may reject or mock the need for sexual satisfaction in the older person. Similar disapproving attitudes towards sexual behavior in the old can be seen in members of the helping professions. When it is remembered that sexuality in older people is a normal part of human behavior, it becomes apparent that responses of ridicule or outright condemnation are inappropriate and irrational.

The normal decline in male potency cited by Kinsey can be further increased by both physical and psychological problems. There are some neurological syndromes as well as diabetic problems that impair erectile potency. Prostatic surgery may result in this problem and diseases affecting more distant organ systems, e.g. arthritic problems and cardiovascular difficulties, may similarly compromise sexual functioning.

But, most commonly it is anxiety concerning failure and/or fear of damage to an already compromised organ, e.g. post-myocardial infarction, that may lead to sexual impotence. Some people give up sex following myocardial infarction because of the belief that it will endanger their lives. A resumption of sexual activity following the necessary period of recuperation after the infarction (roughly 8 to 14 weeks) may be encouraged in most patients. The doctor can play an important role in reminding such a patient that sexual activity following his illness is an important aspect of his overall functioning and quality of life, and the physician should give support to its resumption as soon as it is considered safe to do so.

In the woman, problems with dyspareunia* may follow on the development of senile vaginitis which results in a significant decrease in vaginal lubrication. A woman whose sexual interest has been minimal throughout her adolescent and early adult life may find in this physiological change a rationalization for her longstanding reluctance to engage in intercourse. But, for the woman whose sexual interest has been relatively free of conflict throughout her adult life, the menopausal and post-menopausal changes may provide a stimulus to join with her partner in finding an acceptable adjustment through alternate ways of satisfying the needs for sexual intimacy.

Sexual partners who have been together for many years may require, as the aging process affects them both, to continually enliven their sexual experience if boredom is not to set in. Again, it will be an indication of successful adaptation to the aging process if both partners can individually, and in relationship to each other, seek and find new and mutually satisfying sexual experiences.

THE "MIDDLE" GENERATION

The mid-life man and woman are in the middle of the generation stream. On the one hand vis-a-vis younger people they are the experienced "norm-bearers" of the mainstream societal structure. They are in a position to impart information and attitudes they have acquired in the course of their own development. It is in this sense

that Erikson speaks of the essential task of this stage of life as "generativity versus stagnation." It relates to the development of the middle aged individual in terms of his function in the broadest sense as a "teacher." The middle aged are in the position of being able to consolidate from their past the lessons of many experiences and tasks (obligatory and self-gratifying) that have been traversed. Patterns of thinking, feeling and behavior have become well established in a characteristic mode for that individual. A certain rigidity may be noted in the behavioral trends of the middle aged person. At the same time new events are continuously becoming part of that person's life. We have already spoken of some such events, for example the endocrine shift of the climacteric. Still other events that herald the manifest progress of the aging process appear. Intellectual and cognitive functioning begins to show subtle changes which are often more likely to be demonstrated on finely-tuned psychological tests, than may be apparent in the every day functioning. Such alterations are more related to psychomotor aspects, e.g. the speed of accomplishing the task rather than in terms of the accuracy of the task performed. In general, verbal skills tend to be relatively well preserved, whereas performance skills tend to show some degree of deterioration.

The use of the Wechsler Adult Intelligence Scale (WAIS) demonstrates that the use of verbal skills required in the portion of the test measuring information, comprehension, arithmetic, similarities, digit span, and vocabulary is maintained relatively well in spite of the aging process. On the other hand performance tests such as digit symbol, picture completion, block design, picture arrangement and object assembly are not handled as efficiently by the older subjects.

The commonly held stereotype concerning the old person and his rigidity finds expression in the metaphor about "the old dog" and "new tricks." Researchers who

* dyspareunia — the occurence of pain in the sexual act.

have looked into the question of new learning in older people have demonstrated that older individuals with average I.Q. do better at more slowly paced (or self-paced) tasks than at more rapidly paced situations (Eisdorfer, 1977). New learning can indeed take place, but frequently the older person resists responding to the stimuli of new tasks and fails to express the appropriate responsiveness essential to mastering the new task. Learning may not take place as a result of fear of failure rather than significantly altered cognitive ability.

While mid-life individuals struggle with gradually developing "losses" they are still in the throes of interpersonal relationships with younger and older people, family and others. The "gains" they have made through living are offered as help to the younger members of the family who may challenge the teaching of the parents as anachronistic or insensitive. At the time that fathers and mothers in the three generation family are faced with the striving for independence on the part of adolescent children, they may be required to shift position and offer support and empathy to aging parents. Ideally it requires that the parents must have worked through the attainment of their own separateness and individuality. If this has happened satisfactorily, they will be able to tolerate the struggles of the adolescent child, and the dependent needs of the older generation.

THE LAST STAGE—OLD AGE

In old age, as we have seen, the aging process acquires a more definitive character. The intimations of aging that are manifest in the mid-life span become unmistakable as the individual moves from the decade 65 to 75, to 75 to 85. When we consider the "old-old" in contrast to the "young-old" of middle age, we note that there are many more losses and the relative strengths and achievements of the middle aged individual have given way to a process of decline. The task with which the

person is now concerned is that of achieving some state of equanimity in facing his own death.

The modes of adaptation of individuals to growing old are variable. There are the successful agers who continue to express in the way they live an affirmation of their individual life cycle. They remain interested and involved with people and events of the real world, and they will experience a continued zest and feeling of self-regard as they participate in social experiences with others, or solitary pursuits such as hobbies or studies. For a few, the creative process remains alive, and significant products of their creativity result. In general these people are able to harness their energies in individually and socially meaningful ways (sublimations) and thereby achieve a degree of satisfaction in a way that is relatively free of conflict. They are people who can be considered to have successfully dealt with the crises and problems of earlier periods in their lives and so have developed internal strategies for facing the stresses of old age.

Only 5% of the population aged 65 and over live in institutions such as nursing homes, homes for the aged, or chronic care hospitals. That is to say 95% of elderly people live in the community in relative states of health or illness. A large number of these people have psychiatric problems of a degree which merit a thorough-going assessment and therapeutic intervention where indicated. The holistic approach to psychiatric problems of the aged is important inasmuch as physical illness along with psychological problems frequently co-exist and a confident understanding of the interaction of these factors is important. For example, confusional states can be related to both transient cerebral ischemic episodes and the effect of a dysfunction in more distant organ systems (cardiovascular, endocrine, genital, urinary, or liver). An older person receiving diuretics may have delirium because of electrolyte shifts. Anxiety states and paranoid and depressive syndromes sometimes accompany Parkinsonism that frequently affects the elderly. Similarly, paranoid ideation as well as affective disturbances related to cerebrovascular disease or cellular degeneration are not uncommon features of that not uncommon condition of old age—"brain failure."

Significantly, these symptomatic concomitants of brain failure (confusional behavior, thought disorder or affective disturbances) can frequently be successfully treated and the psychopathology diminished in intensity.

It is vitally important to know that depressive illnesses are the commonest of the psychiatric syndromes seen in the elderly. A proper diagnostic assessment of the patient must be made in order to distinguish between organic dementias and depressive illnesses which may resemble an organic dementing process. The cognitive difficulties of the organically impaired patient (memory and orientation impairment) may be present in an essentially depressed patient, but with careful examination it can be determined that the difficulty is more apparent than real and is probably related to concentration difficulties rather than to some essential dysfunction of cognitive abilities.

This brief reference to some aspects of the psychopathology of the aged is made in order to highlight another fact, namely that psychiatric problems of the elderly can often be successfully treated using psychological and physical means. The treatment of psychiatric illness in the elderly is now an active part of medical psychiatric practice. With the advent of the major tranquilizers it became possible to relieve the distress of affective disorders (e.g. agitation, anxiety, depression) in many patients of all age groups. The older patient could now be offered specific treatment for a depressive illness, and in many cases one could expect a complete remission. Similarly, psychopharmacologic treatment might be offered to the old person suffering from chronic brain syndrome (brain failure) due to cellular or cerebrovascular pathology where the syndrome is characterized by an important degree of mood and/or behavioral pathology. So that even if the therapeutic efforts cannot bring about a significant reversal of the cognitive impairment (memory and orientation disturbance) they may normalize the mood and behavioral disturbance.

In general, one must be particularly cautious, when using drug treatment in the elderly, not to produce side effects which are worse than the illness for which the patient is being treated. Problems surrounding the ingestion, absorption, assimilation, distribution, metabolism (detoxification) and excretion of drugs are frequent in the population we are discussing. Therefore the approach must be cautious and informed. This is not to say that the doctor should be unduly timid in prescribing appropriate types and dosages of drugs. Nonetheless in the lower range of efficacy, the elderly patient may do quite well on a total daily dose of 75 mg of a tricyclic antidepressant, whereas a younger patient may require at least twice the amount for effective therapeutic action. In general, older patients tend to be over-medicated and it behooves the doctor to rule out the iatrogenic effects of individual drugs or drug-drug interactions in the case of older patients who present with confusional states. Neurological complications of the extrapyramidal type are often encountered. Tardive dyskinesia, which is characterized by involuntary movements of the tongue, mouth and facial musculature as well as limb and trunk muscles, is a syndrome which may occur after the patient has been on neuroleptic medication for some time. It can be a persistent and distressing complication of therapy and at this time there is no effective way of treating it, although smaller dosages of medication may prevent some dyskinesias from appearing. Low dosages to begin with are recommended. Individual and group psychotherapy is frequently helpful.

Electroconvulsive therapy is a safe and effective treatment for some cases of intractable depression and should be considered in the elderly where pharmacological methods are ineffective and perhaps more dangerous. For example, certain tricyclic antidepressants may produce life-threatening ventricular tachyarrhythmias.

Lastly, a fact that is sometimes forgotten about aging individuals is that they are still thinking and feeling human beings. The doctor's therapeutic efficacy is put to the test in dealing with the old patient. Although there are many occasions in which an illness has been reversed and a cure obtained with appropriate therapy, we must frequently be satisfied with small gains as we engage with the older person in our role as physicians. The doctor's therapeutic presence, even when he is not always objectively effective as a healer of specific diseases, means to the older person that he (the patient) is perceived as worthy.

REFERENCES

Busse, E.W. and Pfeiffer, E. (1977): *Behavior and Adaptation in Late Life*. 2nd ed. Boston, Little, Brown.

Curtis, H.J. (1966): A composite theory of aging. *Gerontologist*, 6:143.

de Beauvoir. S. (1972): *Old Age*. (London) Andre Deutsch.

Eisdorfer, C. (1977): Intelligence and cognition in the aged. In *Behavior and Adaptation in Late Life*. Edited by E.W. Busse and E. Pfeiffer. Boston, Little, Brown.

Jacques, E. (1965): Death and the mid-life crisis. *Int. J. Psychoanal*. 46:502.

Neugarten, B. (1968): *Middle Age and Aging: A Reader in Social Psychology*. Chicago, University of Chicago Press.

Walford, R.L. (1964): The immunological theory of aging. *Gerontologist*, 4:195.

Group For the Advancement of Psychiatry: Report #59—*Psychiatry and the Aged: An Introductory Approach*.

FURTHER READINGS

Bromley, D.B. (1974): *The Psychology of Human Aging*. Rev. ed. London, Penguin Books.
  A consideration in depth of the developmental processes related to the aging experience is provided. Cognitive functioning and psychosocial adaptations are well explored.

Pitt, B. (1974): *Psychogeriatrics: an Introduction to the Psychiatry of Old Age*. Edinburgh, Churchill Livingstone.
  A paperback edition is available of this neatly compiled compendium of clinical experiences. Psychiatric syndromes are well described and there is a helpful treatment of the psychosocial, community psychiatry aspects of the aging process.

Stotsky, B.A. (1968): *The Elderly Patient: Mental Patients in Nursing Homes*. New York, Grune and Stratton.
  A paperback encompassing both psychosocial and psychiatric problems of the aged including a point of view that concerns itself with the mental hygiene of aging.

Verwoerdt, A. (1976): *Clinical Geropsychiatry*. Baltimore, Williams & Wilkins.
  An excellent concise, up-to-date and informed overview of the psychiatry of old people. Recommended to the student who wishes to obtain a solid grounding in the biologic-psychologic-psychosocial parameter of geriatric problems.

CHAPTER 5

Life Events and Illness

Donald Wasylenki and Stanley J. J. Freeman

In 1907 a physician who had observed the effects of a severe earthquake on the people of Messina, Italy, described a clinical syndrome that he labeled earthquake neurosis. He noted that the syndrome "was produced immediately, that in general its duration was brief, as in acute illnesses, and that the symptoms disappeared without leaving any trace" (Dohrenwend, 1973).

People have known for centuries that trauma can induce physical and psychological symptoms. However, only during the last 40 years have investigators studied that phenomenon systematically. The concepts of stress and crisis are contemporary formulations that relate disruption of the environment to dysfunction of the individual.

Many of the ideas discussed in this chapter have their roots in the tradition established by Adolph Meyer (Leif, 1948) the outstanding figure in the early development of American clinical psychiatry. Meyer's emphasis on the relationship of biological, psychological, and social phenomena to health and disease provided the basis for modern psychiatric history taking. He prescribed the careful study of events in the patient's life as a pathway to understanding the patient's dysfunction. He urged the physician to concern himself with the continuing interaction between the patient and his life events. Meyer developed what he called a life chart, which reflected his interest in the significant events in the patient's life: "changes of habitat, of school entrance, graduations, or changes, or failures; the various jobs; the dates of possibly important births and deaths in the family, and other fundamentally important environmental incidents." Meyer's work gave birth to crisis theory and the study of the impact of life events. The following terms, used throughout the chapter, require definition:

Life event is any change in a person's social setting requiring change in ongoing life adjustment. The life event may be ordinary or extraordinary; examples of life events are bereavement, marriage, and loss of one's job. A life event usually requires that the person involved make some kind of change.

A *crisis* is a state of temporary disequilibrium that is precipitated by a life event. Disequilibrium refers to disruption of the steady state pattern when a person responds to an internal or external change. Caplan (Darbonne, 1967) defined crisis more descriptively:

> Crisis is a state provoked when a person faces an obstacle to important life goals that is, for a time, insurmountable through the utilization of customary methods of problem solving. A period of disorganization ensues, a period of upset, during which many different abortive attempts at solution are made. Eventually some kind of adaptation is achieved which may or may not be in the best interest of that person and his fellows.

Stress has been defined as "the organism's response to stressful conditions or stressors, consisting of a pattern of physiological and psychological reactions, both immediate and delayed." (Rabkin, 1976). That definition sounds like the definition of crisis. In this chapter, the term stress is used to describe the state of internal arousal in a person who is responding to a life event, whereas the term crisis is used to describe a broader process of disruption, disequilibrium and/or regression that is both experienced by the person and observable to others.

Social support is information that leads a person to believe that he is cared for, loved, esteemed, and considered a member of a group whose members are obligated to one another (Cobb, 1976). The quality of that "emotional feedback" and the task-oriented assistance provided by a person's social network, particularly during a crisis, establishes his degree of social support (Caplan, 1974).

Coping and adaptation are often used as synonyms. Adaptation, however, is a broader term than coping. It describes the continuing interaction that maintains an equilibrium between a person and his environment. Adaptation ranges from the simplest ways of dealing with minor problems and frustrations to the most complex strategies for managing disruptions. It is a process that develops in time, and it may at any point be either progressive or regressive. Coping, a category of adaptation, refers to adaptation under difficult conditions. When a person has a problem that brings about a drastic change, or that challenges his accustomed ways of behaving, or that requires him to change, or that makes him feel uncomfortable, then coping becomes necessary.

This chapter is written from a psychosocial perspective. It discusses how life events, including public disasters, private occurrences and cumulative changes precipitate stress. It then discusses the development of the crisis state and the relationship of stress and crisis to physical and psychological dysfunction and illness. Finally, the chapter discusses how social supports, coping, and adaptation are buffers against the potentially harmful effects of changes in one's environment.

REACTIONS TO DISASTER

A disaster can be defined as a catastrophic alteration of the environment. The study of the psychiatric aspects of disasters demonstrates that disasters can induce symptoms. The symptoms may be physical or psychological, or both and short term or long term or both.

In 1954 a rural section of Arkansas was hit by a severe tornado. Ninety percent of the survivors who were interviewed reported that they had "some form of acute, emotional, physiological, or psychosomatic after-effect." The most common after-effects were nervousness, excitability, or hypersensitivity (59%) and sleeplessness or poor sleep (46%).

In 1972 several communities in the Buffalo Creek Valley in West Virginia were destroyed by a tidal wave. The flood killed 125 people and left 4,000 people homeless. Ninety percent of the survivors had neurotic reactions to the trauma. Two years after the disaster those reactions were still present. A "Buffalo Creek Syndrome" was described; its symptoms were severe anxiety, nightmares and other sleep disturbances, obsessive ruminations and phobias about wind, rain, and water, and grief over the death of relatives and friends, and over the loss of possessions. The grief evolved into an apathetic, depressed state. The syndrome was thought to have arisen from both the immediate experience of the catastrophe and the destruction of communities. Underlying the symptoms were unresolved feelings of grief, "survivor shame," and impotent rage. The coping mechanisms the survivors used to master their overwhelming feelings —apathy, severe restriction of activity, and limitation of emotional expression—were disabling and caused some long-lasting character changes in the survivors. The persistence of those changes challenged the earlier belief that post-disaster symptoms subside quickly and easily.

From studies of the disasters in Arkansas and Buffalo Creek Valley—and of other public disasters—four characteristics of disaster reactions have emerged:

(1) The event must be catastrophic.
(2) In the immediate disaster period, personal factors are not significant.
(3) Almost 100% of the survivors have post-disaster symptoms.
(4) Some survivors have lasting neurotic, psychotic, or psychosomatic symptoms.

Trying to conceptualize reactions to disaster as a process, Tyhurst (1970) described three overlapping phases:

(1) During the *impact phase* of a disaster, about 75% of the survivors are stunned and bewildered. The psychological manifestations of their fear are inhibited, and their behavior is automatic.
(2) During the *recoil phase* of a disaster, the survivors have a gradual return of awareness, recall, and emotional expression. They feel dependent, and they have a desire to ventilate their feelings.
(3) In the *post-traumatic phase*, the survivors become fully aware of what the disaster has meant. Their reactions in that phase include anxiety and depression.

The reports of reactions to various disasters support Tyhurst's observations. Diagnosis of psychological disorders in the immediate post-disaster period is often complicated by physical injuries, especially those of the central nervous system, or by alcohol or drug intoxication, various deprivation states, and the failure of some survivors to take prescribed medications.

Edwards (1976) described some specific reactions to disaster. Anger may be seen in individual survivors; or the anger may be collective and organized, resulting in the scapegoating of other groups. When many people have died in a disaster, the survivors may feel guilty for having survived. When the disaster is life threatening and escape is believed to be possible for only a short time (as in a ship's sinking), panic often occurs, and the panic is often contagious.

Chodoff (1970) considered the experience of the Jews and others in the Nazi concentration camps the most severe example of psychic traumatization by a catastrophe. The survivors' immediate response to internment had been the familiar shock-apathy-depression triad described above. A long-term "survivor syndrome" was found in nearly every person studied. It included severe anxiety, sleep disturbance, depression, and guilt, including survivor guilt. Rakoff (Epstein, 1977) studied the children of people who had survived the Nazi concentration camps. An unusually high percentage of those children had sought psychiatric help as adolescents. Their problems seemed to stem from their parents' exaggerated concern for them. It may be that the parents expected the children to provide meaning to the parents' lives.

The long-term effects of disasters have not yet been studied systematically. Much of the evidence in this chapter is based on clinical observation.

"PRIVATE" LIFE EVENTS

Most individual crises are ones of private life, such as the death of a relative, marital disruption, or an economic problem. In line with Meyer's view, certain stressful private life events are associated with an increase in morbidity and mortality.

In 1944 Lindemann gave the now classic description of acute grief—in Boston families that were suddenly bereaved as a result of the Coconut Grove nightclub fire. Lindemann listed five reactions of the bereaved that pointed to the presence of grief: physical distress, preoccupation with the image of the dead person, guilt, hostility, and loss of patterns of conduct. Lindemann also described what he called the "grief work," a necessary reaction in the bereaved person to loss that results in the bereaved person's "emancipation from the bondage to the deceased, readjustment to the environment in which the deceased is missing, and the formation of new relationships." Lindemann listed the following as manifestations of "inadequate grief" (that is, signs that the bereaved person had not completed his grief work): anniversary reactions, overactivity without a sense of purpose or a sense of the loss, acquisition of symptoms of the dead person, psychosomatic illnesses, furious hostility, altered relationships, blunted emotions, loss of patterns of social interaction, detrimental activities, and agitated depression.

Lindemann showed also how a therapist could help a bereaved person overcome any resistance to doing grief work—any tendency to "avoid both the intense distress connected with the grief experience and the necessary expression of emotions."

Lindemann's pioneering work affected the development of crisis theory. Adjustment to change has often been viewed as adjustment to loss and the emotional reactions to change have been viewed as similar to grief. Much of crisis intervention work is similar to grief counseling.

Many private life events have significant sequelae. Leaving one's job has been associated with changes in the person's serum levels of norepinephrine, creatinine, uric acid, and cholesterol. More people who had been laid off work had peptic ulcers than did the people in the control group in a carefully done prospective study (Cobb, 1976).

Weiss (Caplan, Killilea, 1976) described severe cognitive and emotional problems in people he studied who had recently been separated from their spouses. Those people reported the following reactions to the separation: obsessive review of past events, anger, guilt and related emotions, uncertainty regarding the self, a tendency to make false starts, impulsiveness, self-doubt, and lack of self-confidence. Weiss observed also that people who were not prepared for their negative reactions were more vulnerable to them than were people who expected to have negative reactions.

As mentioned, many of the private life events that have been studied involved losses. Parkes (1972) described reactions common to the loss of a limb, the loss of a home, and the loss of a spouse.

In Parkes's view and terminology, any significant change in a person's life space (the world external to him) is accompanied by a change in his assumptive world (the world as he sees it). Changes that involve a person's assumptive world require him to give up some beliefs he holds about the world and thus bring him varying degrees of grief.

CUMULATIVE EFFECTS OF LIFE EVENTS

Several groups of investigators studied whether the effects of life events are cumulative. Their studies indicated that people who have had a number of life events are prone to physical and psychologic disorders and to accidents.

To measure the amount of change in a person's life over a given period, Holmes and Rahe (1967) developed a device they called the Social Readjustment Rating Scale. The scale listed 43 life events; each event was assigned a value of from 1 to 100. Not all the events were negative in the conventional sense. Many were "socially desirable," that is, they were consistent with ideals of achievement. The point of the scale was that each event, positive or negative, called for some adjustment by the person experiencing it. The scale emphasized change, whether the change was desirable or undesirable.

In early studies, Rahe and his associates (Rabkin, 1976) showed that people who had fewer than 150 life change units (LCU's) for a given year had good health for the following year and that 70% of the people who had more than 300 LCU's for a given year had some kind of illness in the following year. In later studies, various investigators demonstrated a correlation between the number and intensity of life events and the occurrence of minor physical illnesses soon after the life events. Other investigators (Rabkin, 1976) found similar associations between LCU's and sudden cardiac death, myocardial infarction, tuberculosis, leukemia, multiple sclerosis, diabetes, athletic injuries, and traffic accidents.

A number of people have studied the relationship between life events and depression. Paykel and his associates (1969) showed that depressed patients had three times as many life events before their depression as had the people in the control group in the same period of time. The depressed patients had many more undesirable life events than had the people in the control group. Most of the life events were everyday experiences rather than catastrophes. In what is perhaps the most methodologically sound study of life events, Brown and his associates (1973) showed that in the three weeks before their depression, 51% of the depressed patients, as opposed to 16% of the people in the control group, had at least one life event. Outside the three week period, the number of life events was the same for both groups. However, the depressed patients had *threatening* life events throughout the year, whereas the people in the control group rarely had threatening life events. Brown and his associates concluded that "over a third and perhaps much more of depressive disorders are the result of a formative environmental effect—in the sense that either onset would not have occurred anywhere near the time that it did without the event, or indeed might not have occurred at all." It has been shown (Brown, 1973) that, regardless of the treatment they received, patients who relapsed into a depression had significantly more life events in the three months before their relapse, especially in the month before the relapse, than had the people in the control group. An unusually high number of the life events were threatening ones.

Suicide attempters in one study (Paykel et al., 1975) reported four times as many events as were reported by depressed patients prior to the onset of depression. A substantial peaking of events occurred in the month before the suicide attempt. There were more events with threatening implications among suicide attempters than among depressives and more which were outside the respondent's control. The authors conclude that the findings indicate a strong and immediate relationship between suicide attempts and life events.

Brown and his associates (1973) found evidence that life events precipitate episodes of schizophrenia. Their study covered four three week periods. In the three week period immediately before an episode of acute schizophrenia, 46% of the patients had at least one independent (outside of the patient's control) life event, whereas in each of the three earlier three week periods only 12% of the patients had an independent life event. In the control group, 14% of the people had an independent life event in each of the four three week periods. Thus before the episode of schizophrenia there had been an increase in the number of life events that could not be explained by abnormal behavior on the patient's part. Brown and his associates suggested, however, that in schizophrenia, life events are less significant than they are in depression. In most patients with schizophrenia that they studied, the life event simply triggered an episode that was probably ready to occur.

Leff and his associates (1976) studied the occurrence of life events before relapses in schizophrenic patients who were being treated with drugs or with placebos. The people who had relapses while they were being treated with drugs were more likely to have had a life event than were the patients who had relapses while they were being treated with placebos and the patients who did not relapse. The authors concluded that drug treatment protects people with schizophrenia from the ordinary stress of social interaction and that some additional stress is needed to precipitate a relapse in schizophrenic patients who are being treated with drugs.

LIFE EVENTS AND PHYSICAL ILLNESS

Psychophysiological measurement and clinical observation have been used to study the relationship of life events, stress, and physical illness. The research is difficult because coping mechanisms may intercede and dilute an otherwise demonstrable physical response, a focus on physiological response often precludes the simultaneous analysis of psychological and social variables, and medical biases often result in an over-emphasis on negative response patterns and on disease.

Claude Bernard's concept of a constant internal physiological environment was the basis for studies of physiological and biochemical disequilibrium. Cannon de-

scribed an "emergency" catabolic reaction to stress that is mediated by the adrenal medulla and characterized by an increased production of adrenaline. Cannon's work led to further investigation (in the 1940's and 1950's) of the role of adrenaline and noradrenaline in emotional responses. In his "anger-in vs. anger-out" studies, Funkenstein (1955) demonstrated that the two substances are dissociated. An anger-in response, primarily an anxious response, could be correlated with an increase in a person's serum levels of adrenaline, whereas an anger-out response, primarily an aggressive response, could be correlated with an increase in a person's serum levels of noradrenaline. Since adrenaline is produced primarily by the adrenal medulla and noradrenaline is produced primarily by the sympathetic nervous system, the dissociation is not surprising. Studies of airline pilots and passengers— and of people subjected to gravitational stress—support Funkenstein's findings.

Levi (Gunderson and Rahe, 1974) refined the concept of dissociation of catecholamine responses. Levi measured the levels of adrenaline and noradrenaline in the urine of people shown films that were thought to elicit specific emotional responses from the people watching them (e.g., anxiety, aggression, sexual responses, laughter) and he demonstrated specific patterns of dissociation. For example, whereas an anxiety-producing film produced increases of both adrenaline and noradrenaline, an anger-producing film produced an increase in noradrenaline only, and a laughter-producing film produced decreases in both substances. More recently Selye, Mason, Brown and others (Mason, 1975) demonstrated important correlations between some emotional states and serum levels of some hormones and neurotransmitters.

The psychophysiological studies of physical response to stress are based on the hypothesis that prolonged activation of some substances causes disease. However, there is not proof that they do. Most of the mammalian studies that demonstrate a direct, causal relationship between stress, the release of hormones, and physical changes have not been replicated.

Studies based on clinical observation have attempted to show high correlations between stressful situations and specific organ systems. That tendency has its roots in the early work of Alexander (1950), who thought that the vulnerability of an organ to stress was determined genetically, and of Dunbar (1938), who thought that physical disorders were related to personality types.

Perhaps the most impressive study is that of Weiner and his associates (1957) which was inspired by the work of Mersky (1958). In a prospective study Weiner showed that people who had a predisposition to peptic ulcers (because they had high serum levels of pepsinogen) developed peptic ulcers when they were exposed to a stressful situation (a U.S. Army boot camp). People in the control group, who had low serum levels of pepsinogen, did not develop ulcers when exposed to the same situation. Using psychiatric assessments and tests of such things as a person's coping patterns, Weiner was also able to predict who of the people with high serum levels of pepsinogen would develop peptic ulcers.

Friedman and Rosenman (1959) showed that coronary artery disease and what they called the Type A personality were related. The Type A personality has been depicted by a forearm with a clenched fist and a watch strapped to the wrist, symbols that refer to such traits as conscientiousness, industriousness, a sense of urgency and competitiveness. The Type A person is also physically active and obsessive and compulsive. Friedman's and Rosenman's point is that people react to stress in a way that somehow (physiologically and biochemically?) affects their cardiovascular system. A number of other researchers have advanced similar ideas.

Engel and Schmale (1967) described an initial response to stress that makes the person so responding liable to develop a physiological and/or psychological dysfunction. They called the response the "giving up-given up" reaction. Engel and Schmale think that some people experience stress as loss and that those people feel helpless, inadequate, unable to cope, futile, confused about the future, and preoccupied with the misfortunes of the past. Such a state may be viewed as a grief reaction in the recoil-turmoil phase of crisis resolution. If the person grieves in a healthy way, he may recover at any point. If he does not grieve, he may decompensate physiologically, psychologically, or socially.

Engel (Arieti, 1974) described a somatopsychic-psychosomatic model. The term somatopsychic-psychosomatic conveys two ideas: the primary process in the genesis of a stress-related disorder is a physical one that not only is responsible for the physical disorder but also can contribute to the development of specific psychological features, and those psychological features determine what circumstances are stressful for the particular person and hence what psychodynamic conditions may activate the organic process.

Engel has described the clinical features that characterize the stress-related disorders. He lists a number of gastrointestinal disorders as examples of stress-related disorders: duodenal ulcer, ulcerative colitis, celiac-sprue syndrome, regional ileitis and colitis (Crohn's disease), irritable bowel syndrome, and achalasia. Engel thinks that Mirsky's work on duodenal ulcers provides a paradigm for the gastrointestinal disorders just listed. If a child has a genetically determined high serum level of pepsinogen, the relationship between the child and his mother is altered. As a result of the altered mother-child relationship, the child's oral-dependent needs are not satisfied and a conflict develops in the child. In a stressful situation in the person's later life (in Mirsky's work, stress in a U.S. Army boot camp) the person's conflict is reactivated. That fact, and the still high levels of pepsinogen, results in peptic ulcers.

The mechanism whereby stressful life events lead to physical illnesses has not been demonstrated in the laboratory or by clinical studies.

CRISIS THEORY

Crisis theory, which is basic to preventive psychiatry, has developed from the observations that life events play a significant role in the onset and course of a number of illnesses; and that life events provide the opportunity for the person to develop new ways of coping and thus can lead to personality growth, maturity and possibly even protection from some so-called psychosomatic illnesses.

Crisis intervention, a therapeutic technique, helps the person in crisis resolve the crisis and thus avert a lasting dysfunction.

Hirshowitz (1973) describes crisis as a state of temporary disequilibrium that is precipitated by inescapable life events. Crises are necessarily temporary because personality systems are self-sealing; that is, they tend to correct any crisis-induced imbalance in a few weeks after the crisis. Disequilibrium refers to a disruption of the person's steady state that requires the person to respond to an internal or external change. The disruption is manifested by cognitive uncertainty, psychophysiological symptoms, and emotional distress.

Caplan (1964) thinks that resolution of a crisis can lead to increased strength and personality growth. Using the concept of homeostasis, Caplan says that a person balances his emotional functioning with the adaptive techniques that he uses to solve everyday problems.

A crisis occurs when a problem is severe, when it is related to significant problems in the person, or when the person's adaptive skills are inadequate. When the person

in crisis realizes that his skills are inadequate, he may search for a new solution. If he is able to resolve the crisis, he has discovered that he has another potential. If he fails to resolve the crisis, that failure can lead to restriction of his personality, blocks in his development, or to an inability to function, and to illness.

Caplan described two patterns of reaction to threatening life events: dealing with the problem either by adjusting to the changed environment or by adjusting oneself, and evading the problem by pretending that the problem has been solved (e.g., the widow who acts as though her husband were alive). But whether the response one makes to the crisis is healthy or maladaptive, that response becomes part of one's coping repertoire, to be used in dealing with future problems. Thus Caplan considers a crisis as an opportunity for healthy growth and personality development or for lasting maladaptation, personality constriction, and illness.

The person in crisis can change significantly in a short period of time. During a crisis, one feels a greater need for help than he does when he is stable, and the signs of his distress usually move other people to help him. During a crisis a person is also more easily influenced by others. Although a person's responses to crises are determined partly by his experience, the psychological forces surrounding the crisis can shape its outcome.

Many authors have classified crises. Erikson (1963) in his theory of developmental crises described a life cycle that is made up of a series of stages. Each stage is characterized by a crisis in one's personal and social relationships, and resolution of those crises contributes to the development of one's sense of identity. Thus, according to Erikson, the child passes through successive crises: trust versus mistrust, autonomy versus shame and doubt, and initiative versus guilt. Those crises lead to the adolescent crisis of identity formation versus identity diffusion.

Each crisis may leave the person more capable or less capable of resolving the crisis of the next stage.

Accidental crises make up most of the items on life events scales. They are the threatening life events that, Caplan thinks, elicit adaptive responses or maladaptive responses.

Crisis theory may also help to explain the concept of critical role transitions. Teachers who become principals, salesmen who become sales managers, and lawyers who become business executives are examples of people undergoing critical role transitions. In describing the problem of the clinical psychiatrist who has taken on administrative duties, Levinson (1967) discusses how a person's old coping skills may fail him in a new job and how that failure may bring cognitive and emotional problems. The transition from one type of job to another necessitates change, just as disruptions of one's environment do. The person must give up ways of dealing with people and situations that may have worked before but are unsuitable to his new job. Difficulty in coping with role transitions may be manifested by "role stickiness;" that is, by a person's attempts to do his new job the way he did his old job. Like Erikson's developmental crises, critical role transitions provide challenges and opportunities for growth.

The transition state (originally described by Tyhurst in 1970) is another kind of crisis. The transition state describes the state of people who are literally in transit (e.g., after a disaster, during a migration) or figuratively in transit (e.g., in retirement). Parkes and others (1972) have expanded the concept of the transition state to describe the psychological changes common to all kinds of crises.

Crises are turning points. Crises may make the people involved in them better able or less able to deal with life's problems, and they can lead to health and maturity or to illness and blocks in development.

Hirshowitz (1973) synthesized the work of several authors who have written about crises. He divided crisis into four phases: (1) the impact phase, (2) the recoil-turmoil phase, (3) the adjustment phase, and (4) the reconstruction phase. That sequence applies to the four kinds of crises described in the preceding paragraphs. It is similar to Tyhurst's description of reactions to disaster.

The *impact phase* of a crisis may be described as a state of dazed shock that follows the distressing news. The impact phase is most severe when the change is unexpected and undesired ("I'm sorry, but your job has been phased out. We'll have to let you go"). The impact phase lasts from a few hours to a few days. The person affected feels numb. He exists very much in the present. He may have flight-fight responses; or he may show "frozen behavior." His thinking is disoriented or distracted. Dysmnesia, disorientation, perplexity, and impaired perception may occur. In old people, the reactions may mimic the symptoms of an acute brain syndrome.

As the distressing news sinks in, the person moves into the *recoil-turmoil phase*, which may continue for several weeks. He becomes preoccupied with the past, in a kind of mourning for a world that used to be but that has been permanently changed. His thinking becomes more organized, but his feelings are negative ones—anger, anxiety, depression, guilt, and shame. He may express those feelings by action or weeping, but more commonly he conceals them, and he appears overcontrolled and detached.

The *phases of adjustment and reconstruction* may last many months. The person begins to look to the future as he explores new relationships and tests new solutions. His painful feelings become muted, and they are tempered with hope.

In discussing reactions to illness, Kimball (1977) described a sequence similar to the one Hirshowitz described for crises.

The crisis phases of adjustment and reconstruction are labeled convalescence and rehabilitation when they are applied to illnesses. The convalescent phase begins with the stabilization of the patient's condition. It is also the phase in which the patient acknowledges that he has an illness and that the illness imposes limitations on him. The emotions that had been frozen or trapped during the recoil-turmoil phase can be released during the convalescent phase. Depression and anger are the most frequently occurring emotions during the convalescent phase. A grieving model seems applicable to the convalescent phase. If the patient avoids grief work, he may adopt a sick role that may become chronic. In the rehabilitation phase, the patient must master the tasks necessary for coping and adaptation. According to Kimball, the patient must:

(1) Maintain a sense of his worth.
(2) Keep his feelings of distress manageable.
(3) Maintain (or restore) his relationships with the people who are important to him.
(4) Enhance his prospects for recovery.
(5) Develop a socially acceptable lifestyle after recovery.

It is sometimes essential, and always desirable, that others who understand the physical, psychological, and social aspects of the patient's disease help him in the rehabilitation phase.

Every change involves a loss. When people lose something that is important to them, to recover from the loss they must undergo a period of grief or mourning. Thus Lindemann's description of bereavement may be considered a paradigm for many life events.

Kubler-Ross (1964) described the dynamics of loss in her studies of how people react to the news that they are fatally ill. As those people move toward giving up their attachment to life, they vacillate between denying and accepting the fact that they are going to die. Their predominant reactions are anger and depression; and bargaining behavior is characteristic ("If I live, I promise—").

In people who are not seriously ill but who must give up other kinds of attachment—to comfortable roles, to their neighborhoods, to old competencies—the same process unfolds. People who are in changing situations often feel angry. Frequently that anger, a part of the natural grieving process, causes long-term disruption as the person tries to settle into his new environment. According to Hirshowitz (1973) the anger is commonly displaced, and innocent bystanders such as the hospital staff are its targets. Or the person may repress his anger, and so become ill or exhausted or accident prone. Or the person may experience his anger as guilt and depression; or he may discharge his anger impulsively. Hirshowitz stresses that the person in crisis needs to express his negative emotions, to acknowledge the legitimacy of those emotions and the fact that he is temporarily dependent on others, and to direct his "aggressive energy" toward adapting. When he does not, he shows signs of unresolved grief.

COPING AND ADAPTATION

The concept of crisis implies that the person involved needs to make adjustment to a change. That adjustment involves adaptation and coping. The perception and definition of the tasks of people facing a crisis, as well as the selection of strategies for managing the tasks, are important parts of the resolution of the crisis. As mentioned, the person's patterns of adaptation may be primarily regressive and defensive (aimed at self-protection) or the person may attempt to master the changed environment and to achieve a new level of competence. Coping refers to the development of effective styles and strategies of mastery in crisis situations.

Studies of coping can be divided into

those that are concerned with intrapsychic mechanisms and those that are concerned with behavioral responses. The first group of studies centers on coping dispositions or traits. That is, they assess the person's tendency to use one or another coping mechanism—one that may or may not be relevant to the situation. The other group of studies centers on how one copes when he is in the midst of the crisis. Thus one who observes the person as he attempts to cope with a crisis may be able to identify his coping mechanisms.

Anna Freud's description of the ego mechanisms of defense (1966) was the basis for understanding the intrapsychic coping mechanisms. Anna Freud originally described ten ego mechanisms of defense: regression, repression, reaction formation, isolation, undoing, projection, introjection, turning against the self, reversal, and sublimation. The term ego mechanism of defense describes a habitual, unconscious mental process that one employs to resolve his conflicts between instinctual needs, internalized prohibitions, and external reality. The use of ego mechanisms of defense usually alters both internal and external reality, and it implies unconscious, integrated, dynamic psychological processes.

In a 30-year prospective study of 95 healthy American men, Vaillant (1976) demonstrated the relationship of one's choice of ego mechanism of defense to one's adjustment to adulthood. Vaillant's findings indicated that suppression (that is, the unconscious or semiconscious decision to postpone paying attention to a conscious impulse or conflict) and anticipation were the best defense. Projection and fantasy seemed to be the defenses most highly correlated with poor adjustment to adulthood.

Research on behavioral responses has involved the study of different kinds of coping mechanisms.

Chodoff and his associates (1967) studied coping behavior in parents of children who had a malignant disease. The defenses he noted most often in the parents were denial, isolation of affect, and excessive motor activity. He found a relationship between "anticipatory mourning" and strong denial. Hamburg and Adams (1967) reported that information seeking is an effective way to cope with major changes. They studied 17 major changes, including serious illnesses, school transitions, marriage, and pregnancy. They found that to cope with a crisis, people need to know the answers to the following questions:

(1) How can I relieve the distress?
(2) How can I maintain a sense of my own worth?
(3) How can I maintain my relationships with other people?
(4) How can I meet the task requirement?

Gal and Lazarus (1975) reviewed a series of studies that compared stress reactions in threatening life events. They studied how activity affects stressful situations, and they concluded that the person who takes action, instead of remaining passive, is much better able to cope with the stress. Perhaps that is so because activity gives the person a sense of mastery, or diverts his attention from his suffering, or discharges energy.

Several studies investigated denial as a coping mechanism in certain kinds of crises, such as life-threatening illnesses or surgery. According to Vaillant and others (1976) denial is a primitive, nonadaptive ego mechanism of defense, and it should not bring about adjustment. However, as Lazarus said (1973) a particular coping device may be helpful in some situations but not in others. For example, many parents of children who were dying from leukemia used denial "profitably" before the child's death, but they suffered more after the death than did parents who used other coping devices. Possibly, denial can be used more effectively by a person facing surgery because few of the fears connected with having an operation materialize.

Other authors have suggested that denial is important, perhaps critical, to the adjustment of seriously ill patients to their illness. Dudley and his associates (1969) showed that patients with severe pulmonary diseases used denial, repression, and isolation to protect their failing respiratory systems from environmental inputs. Failure to use those defenses led to physical and psychological deterioration. It may be that sometimes denial is necessary for survival. Studies of the coping behavior of people who have had a myocardial infarction support this hypothesis.

Hirshowitz (1973) summarized what is known about coping. He classified coping skills as general or specific. In regard to general coping skills, "low vulnerable individuals have the capacity, similar to ego strength, to orient themselves rapidly and plan decisive action in response to change." People who are highly vulnerable to change "become rapidly disoriented when confronted with change. They may experience paralysis of thought or will, unable to plan action or seek assistance." Hirshowitz described specific coping skills that, he thinks, derive from one's past experience with similar problems; but he thinks those skills are not applicable to dissimilar problems. Thus since people seldom have a series of identical crises, the opportunities for learning coping skills are limited.

SOCIAL SUPPORTS

The outcome of a crisis is affected by the nature of the stress, by the person's coping abilities, and perhaps most important by what Caplan (1974) described as "the quality of the emotional support and task-oriented assistance provided by the special network within which the individual grapples with the crisis event." Caplan's concept of a support system implies "an enduring pattern of continuous or inter-mittent ties that play a significant part in maintaining the psychological and physical integrity of the individual over time."

The epidemiologist Cassel (1974) reviewed a large body of human and animal research that concluded that some harmful environmental effects might be mitigated for those people who are part of small social networks. The reasoning is that the kinds of relationships with other people that are found in small groups act as a buffer against stressful life events.

According to Walker (1976) a person's support network includes his relatives, friends, neighbors, co-workers, and the professionals he pays to help him. The important characteristics of the support network are its size, the strength of the ties between its members, its density (how close the members are to one another), its homogeneity, and how its membership is dispersed (how easily they can contact one another). Those characteristics, Walker thinks, are particularly relevant to the proper functioning of the network.

Support systems may operate as buffers in two ways (Caplan 1974):

(1) By collecting and storing information and providing guidance for the person in crisis.
(2) By acting as a refuge to which a person in crisis may return for the rest from his encounters with the stressful environment.

Caplan (1979) has classified "natural support systems." The basic support system consists of a person's close friends and relatives. Ideally, those people provide continuing guidance, and they sustain their members in a crisis. In some crises, however, kith and kin supports may need to be augmented by the services of people in the community, who may be described as informal caregivers.

Informal caregivers may be either generalists or specialists. Generalists are considered by their neighbors to be wise about human nature. They tend to be gregarious and to have jobs that bring them into frequent contact with other people. (They are often druggists, hairdressers, bartenders, or policemen.) Their advice has been found good, and they have earned a reputation locally as being helpful.

Specialists are people who, having coped successfully with a threatening life event, are sought out by others who have had the same life event. In contrast to the generalists, the personality and helpfulness of the specialist may be less important than the fact that they have mastered a particular difficulty. In a study made of parents of premature babies who sought advice from other parents who had earlier had premature babies, a positive correlation was shown between making an effort to seek help in a crisis and a healthy adaptation to the crisis.

The outstanding characteristics of informal caregivers are that they are nonprofessionals and that their interactions with people are reciprocal. Helping others often reinforces their own feelings of competence.

The organizations that are counterparts of the informal caregivers are the volunteer service groups (generalists) and the various self-help organizations (specialists). The volunteer service groups generally help with a range of problems. The self-help groups assist with a specific type of problem, such as alcoholism or divorce. The purpose of the self-help group may be to help people break a dangerous habit, such as excessive drinking, or to provide a temporary community for people who have suffered a major loss, such as the death of a spouse. These groups offer immediate emotional support, and they have a body of concepts, values, and traditions that help people cope with specific problems.

Caplan (1974) thinks that religious denominations are usually the most widely available support systems in the community. He lists the following as "support-system" characteristics of religions:

(1) Most religions are organized in groups of neighbors (parishes, congregations or other types of communities).
(2) Most congregations hold meetings regularly, and they provide opportunities for their members to become friends.
(3) Most religions have a theology, value system, and body of traditions.
(4) Most religions enjoin their members to help one another, especially in times of need.
(5) Most religions have rituals for times of crisis, such as birth, marriage, illness, and death.

Several studies have been made of how social supports affect stressful life events. Nuckolls and her associates (1972) collected information about the life events scores and the social supports of 170 women (wives of U.S. Army personnel) before and during their pregnancies. The incidence of complications of pregnancy was high only in women who had high life events scores and poor social supports. Fifteen women who had many life events but good social supports had no complications in their pregnancies, presumably because of the buffer effect of their good social supports.

De Araujo and his associates (1973) showed that life events and social supports were related to the need for steroid therapy in a group of adults with asthma. The asthma patients who had high life events scores and good social supports did not need the high doses of steroids that the asthma patients with poor social supports did.

Gore's doctoral dissertation on unemployment (1973) demonstrated that social supports had a moderating effect on some physiological variables and some indicators of illness but not on others. Gore's most striking finding was that the men who had the poorest social supports had ten times more episodes of arthritis than had the men who had the best social supports.

Brown and his associates (1975) divided women with severe affective disorders into those who had a confidant and those who did not. A confidant was defined as a person with whom a woman had a "close, intimate and confiding relationship." The women who had threatening life events but no confidant were approximately ten times more likely to be depressed than were the other women. If a causal relationship can be assumed, the conclusion is that having a confiding relationship with another is somehow protective.

Lowenthal and Haven (1968) demonstrated that intimacy can help one adjust to threatening life events in old age, and Miller and his associates (1976) showed that people who had threatening life events but no confidant had more symptoms of illness than did people who had a confidant.

Speculating about a mechanism for the protective effects just described, Cobb (1976) defined social support as information that leads a person to believe that he is loved, that he is valued and/or that he belongs. That information might encourage a person to try to master a problem. It might also provide a climate in which identity changes can take place readily.

In a critique Walker made (1976) of Caplan's discussion of support systems, Walker maintained that social supports had different characteristics and functions and that three factors determine what the person in crisis needs:

(1) *The nature of the crisis.* For example, in a serious illness, a small, dense network of close ties may help the person; but when a person must undergo a major psychosocial transition, such a network may trap the person rather than help him make the change.

(2) *The stage of the crisis.* The kind of support system needed at one stage of a crisis may be quite different from that needed at a later stage.

(3) The *internal and external resources* of the person in crisis may determine his ability to use certain kinds of social supports.

There is evidence that social supports can protect people in crisis from a number of illnesses. Caplan (1974) thinks that mental health professionals should foster the development of support systems. We would go a step further to say that all health professionals—not only those in mental health—should be aware of the nature and quality of their patients' social supports.

REFERENCES

Alexander, F. (1938): *Emotions and Bodily Changes.* New York, Columbia University Press.

Arieti, S. (1974): *American Handbook of Psychiatry.* 2d ed. New York, Basic Books.

Brown, G.W., Harris, T.O., and Peto, J. (1973): Life events and psychiatric disorders. *Psychol. Med.* 3:159.

Brown, G. W., Bhrolcha, M.N., and Harris, T. (1975): Social class and psychiatric disturbance among women in an urban population. *Sociology.* 9:225.

Caplan, G. (1964): *Principles of Preventive Psychiatry.* New York, Basic Books.

Caplan, G. (1974): *Support Systems and Community Mental Health.* New York, Behavioral Pub.

Caplan, G. and Killilea, M. (1976): *Support Systems and Mutual Help.* New York, Grune and Stratton.

Chodoff, P. (1970): The German concentration camps as a psychological stress. *Arch. Gen. Psychiatry.* 22:78.

Chodoff, P. et al. (1964): Stress, defences and coping behavior: observations in parents of children with malignant disease. *Am. J. Psychiatry.* 120:743.

Cobb, S. (1976): Social support as a moderator of life stress. *Psychosom. Med.* 38:300.

Cohen, F. and Lazarus, R.S. (1973): Active coping processes, coping dispositions, and recovery from surgery. *Psychosom. Med.* 35:375.

Darbonne, A.R. (1967): Crisis: A review of theory, practice and research. *Psychotherapy: Theory, Res. Prac.* 4:49.

De Araujo, G., Van Arsdel, P.P., Holmes, T.H., et al. (1973): Life change, coping ability and chronic intrinsic asthma. *J. Psychosom. Res.* 17:359.

Dohrenwend, B. (1973): Events as stressors: A methodological inquiry. *J. Health and Soc. Behav.* 14:167.

Dudley, D.L., Verhey, J.W., Masuda, M., et al. (1969): Long-term adjustment, prognosis and death in irreversible diffuse obstructive pulmonary syndromes. *Psychosom. Med.* 31:310.

Dunbar, H.F. (1950): *Psychosomatic Medicine.* New York, W.W. Norton.

Edwards, J. (1976): Psychiatric aspects of civilian disasters. *Br. Med. J.* 1:944.

Engel, G. and Schmale, A. (1967): Psychoanalytic theory of somatic disorder. *J. Am. Psychoanal. Assoc.* 15:344.

Epstein, H. (1977): 12 heirs of the holocaust. *The New York Times Magazine,* June 19, p. 12.

Erikson, E., (1963): *Childhood and Society.* 2nd ed. New York, Norton.

Freud, A. (1966): *The Ego and the Mechanisms of Defense.* New York, International Universities Press.

Friedman, M. and Rosenman, R. (1959): Association of specific overt behavior pattern with blood and cardiovascular findings. *J.A.M.A.,* 169:1286.

Funkenstein, D. (1955): The physiology of fear and anger. *Sci. Amer.* 192:74.

Gal, R. and Lazarus, R. (1975): The role of activity in anticipating and confronting stressful situations. *J. Human Stress.* 1:4.

Gore, S. (1973): The influence of social support and related variables in ameliorating the consequences of job loss. Doctoral thesis. University of Pennsylvania.

Gunderson, E. and Rahe, R. (1974): *Life Stress and Illness.* Springfield, Ill., C. C Thomas.

Hamburg, D. and Adams, J. (1967): A perspective on coping behavior: seeking and utilizing information in major transitions. *Arch. Gen. Psychiatry.* 17:277.

Hirshowitz, R. (1973): Crisis theory: a formulation. *Psychiat. Ann.* 3:33.

Holmes, T. and Rahe, R. (1967): The social readjustment rating scale. *J. Psychosom. Res.* 11:213.

Kubler-Ross, E. (1969): *On Death and Dying.* New York, Macmillan.

Leff, J.P. (1976): Assessment of drugs in schizophrenia. *Br. J. Clin. Pharmacol.* 3:75.

Leif, A., ed. (1948): *The Commonsense Psychiatry of Dr. Adolph Meyer.* New York, McGraw-Hill.

Levinson D. and Klerman, G. (1967): The clinician–executive. *Psychiatry.* 30:3.

Lindemann, E. (1944): Symptomatology and management of acute grief. *Am. J. Psychiatry.* 101:141.

Lowenthal, M. and Haven, C. (1968): Interaction and adaptation: intimacy as a critical variable. *Am. Sociol. Rev.* 33:20.

Mason, J.W. (1975): A historical view of the stress field. *Journal of Human Stress.* 1.

Miller, P., Ingham, J.G., and Davidson, S. (1976): Life events, symptoms and social support. *J. Psychosom. Res.* 20:515.

Mirsky, I.A. (1958): Physiologic, psychologic and social determinants in the etiology of duodenal ulcer. *Am. J. Dig. Dis.* 3:285.

Nuckolls, K., Cassel, J., and Kaplan, B.H. (1972): Psychosocial assets, life crisis and the prognosis of pregnancy. *Am. J. Epidemiol.* 95:431.

Parkes, M. (1972): Components of the reaction to loss of a limb, spouse or home. *J. of Psychosom. Res.* 16:343.

Paykel, E. et al. (1969): Life events and depression: A controlled study. *Arch. Gen. Psychiatry.* 21:753.

Paykel, E., Prusoff, A., and Myers, J.K. (1975): Suicide attempts and recent life events: a controlled comparison. *Arch. Gen. Psychiatry.* 32:327.

Rabkin, J. and Struening, E. (1976): Life events, stress and illness. *Science.* 194:1013.

Titchener, J. and Kapp, F. (1976): Family and character change at Buffalo Creek. *Am. J. Psychiatry.* 133:295.

Tyhurst, J. (1970): *The Role of Transition States— Including Disasters—in Mental Illness.* Washington, D.C. Walter Reed Army Institute of Research.

Vaillant, G. (1976): Natural history of male psychological health. *Arch. Gen. Psychiatry.* 33:535.

Walker, K. et. al. (1977): Social support networks and the crisis of bereavement. *Soc. Sci. Med.* 11:35.

Weiner, H. et al. (1957): Etiology of duodenal ulcer. *Psychosom. Med.* 19:1.

FURTHER READINGS

Cobb, S. (1976): Social support as a moderator of life stress. *Psychosom. Med.* 38:300.

A review of studies demonstrating the protective effects of social supports.

Hirshowitz, R. (1973): Crisis theory: a formulation. *Psychiat. Ann.* 3:33.

An excellent review of crisis theory.

Kimball, C. (1977): Psychosomatic theories and their contributions to chronic illness. In: *Psychiatric Medicine.* Edited by G. Usdin. New York, Brunner/Mazel.

A description of illness stages as reactions to a life-threatening event.

Lindemann, E. (1944): Symptomatology and management of acute grief. *Am. J. Psychiatry.* 101:141.

The classical clinical description of reactions to a significant life event.

Rabkin, J. and Struening, E. (1976): Life events, stress and illness. *Science.* 194:1013.

A review of evidence linking life events and illness behavior.

Vaillant, G.E. (1977): *Adaptation to Life.* Boston, Little, Brown.

A fascinating and highly readable longitudinal study of coping behavior in North American men.

6

Biology, Behavior and Mental Functioning

Alexander Bonkalo and Gregory M. Brown

In earlier ages, philosophers searched for the seat of the soul in various parts of the brain. Then, in the early nineteenth century, awakening medical science redirected the quest for the seat of human personality traits. A group of physicians and laymen, the phrenologists, believed that certain personality traits, such as cautiousness, firmness, benevolence, were related to certain areas of the cerebral cortex and that their existence in a person could be identified through an examination of the bulges and depressions on the person's skull. That crude speculative approach to human behavior was soon replaced by objective research. In 1861 the French neurologist Broca made one of the first significant psycho-physiological discoveries. He discovered that the motor speech center was located in the frontal lobe of the dominant hemisphere of the brain. During the decades following Broca's discovery the cerebral organization of movement and perception were mapped out. In the early twentieth century, the areas of the cerebral cortex that are involved in elaborate semantic skills and their impairments (aphasia, agnosia and apraxia) were localized.

Progress in the understanding of heredity had a major impact on psychiatry. Twin studies, and the demonstration of clustering of syndromes in families suggested that certain forms of psychopathology had a genetic basis. Later on, the discovery of chromosomal abnormalities opened new perspectives, and contributed significantly to our awareness of the somatic causes of specific forms of pathological behavior, particularly in relation to etiological factors in mental subnormality.

Knowledge of the biological basis of behavior has advanced substantially during the last decades. This progress was facilitated by the discovery of the significance to behavior of certain subcortical structures and the role of neurotransmitters in synaptic transmission. It was discovered that certain subcortical structures (the limbic system and the reticular activating system) initiate and organize fundamental emotional, intellectual, and instinctual activities, and control certain cortical functions related to changes in consciousness and levels of attention. The research on the neurotransmitters has concentrated on identifying and otherwise investigating the *transmitter-substances* at the synaptic junctions in the central nervous system. This research found evidence that mental health depends primarily on the adequate conductive capacity of the synapses in the central nervous system.

THE LIMBIC SYSTEM

The limbic system is composed of a complex network of nuclei and fiber tracts located in both temporal lobes and in the midline area of the brain. Phylogenetically it is an old structure. It has several functions that involve basic mental activities that are carried out more or less independently of conscious control. The functions of the limbic system include the organization of emotional processes, fundamental instinctual drives, and certain memory transactions.

The limbic system is the "seat" of emotions. In the limbic system emotions are generated and subjectively experienced; and it is there that emotional responses establish connections with structures in the autonomic nervous system. Those connections form the channels through which emotions are expressed externally (e.g. by blushing, pallor, or sweating) and internally (e.g. by palpitation, adrenal and other endocrine changes, or by visceral responses).

The limbic system organizes the fundamental instinctual drives that are directed to the preservation of the self and the species. Thus, it regulates hunger and thirst and the activities involved in finding, consuming and utilizing food. Furthermore, the limbic system reinforces or restrains aggression and it initiates or inhibits fighting and fleeing behavior. Limbic function also regulates sexual behavior—its intensity and direction (i.e. heterosexual, homosexual or autoerotic), and it organizes activities that provide for the well-being of offsprings whose survival still depends on their parents.

Finally, the limbic system is involved in memory formation and recall. Memory, in general terms, preserves information in order to affect behavior. Limbic structures participate in the selection and encoding of new memories and in the recall and decoding of data from the permanent memory store, which is outside the limbic system.

THE RETICULAR ACTIVATING SYSTEM

The reticular activating system (RAS) is composed of a complex neural network in the brain stem that projects into the thalamus. The RAS acts as the sentinel at the crossroads where afferent tracts carry sensory stimuli upward and efferent tracts carry motor and autonomic stimuli downward. The RAS monitors and affects those tracts in both directions. The descending function of the RAS affects motor behavior and autonomic processes, which have only indirect implications for psychiatry. However, the ascending function of the RAS has a major impact on behavior in regard to the regulation of the states of sleep and wakefulness, the maintenance of alertness, the focusing and concentrating of attention, and the control of sensory stimulation.

The RAS initiates arousal and it organizes brain function in its transition from sleep to wakefulness. It maintains in the brain a state of graded alertness that is attuned to internal and external requirements. Sensory stimuli arrive at the cerebral cortex even when the brain is "asleep," but such stimuli fade away instantly and are not consciously perceived; in wakefulness, however, they become integrated with other stimuli instead of fading away unnoticed. Thus, in this context, the concept of consciousness has dual meaning. First, it means awareness. This is a subjective experience which everybody can understand but cannot fully describe. Second, it refers to the state in which stimuli and other mental contents are not isolated or prematurely extinguished but instead are related to one another to form a pattern and to be woven into thoughts and memories.* The RAS primes the cerebral cortex to maintain the state of consciousness. In fact, lack of consciousness, leading to a state of coma, may develop if the brain stem is damaged in a way that affects the functioning of the RAS.

Besides maintaining consciousness, the RAS controls the clarity, range, and scope of consciousness. In other words, the RAS, in a feedback relationship with intellectual forces, directs and sustains attention. The term attention in this context means a state in which a portion of the conscious mental processes is selected to stand out from the rest. Impairment of selectiveness in mental processing is a RAS dysfunction in a neurophysiological sense, and results in the inability to concentrate attention and in excessive distractibility.

The RAS can discriminate between important and unimportant sensory information. That function is unconscious and may continue during sleep. A common example is the mother who is wakened by a faint sound from her baby yet who sleeps undisturbed by much louder street noises. Habituation to certain noises may facilitate discrimination between stimuli. Thus, habituation may have a protective effect; for example, a person who is accustomed to the chiming of a grandfather clock sleeps through the night, whereas a visitor's sleep is disturbed by the chiming.

The harmonious functioning of the RAS depends on the availability of a consistent inflow of appropriately patterned sensory stimuli. Pathological disorders of consciousness may result if the inflow of the stimuli is deficient, ill-adjusted (e.g. excessively jarring or strident), or disorganized. The clinical examples of such disorders include confusional states, illusions and hallucinations brought about by toxic conditions, sensory deprivation, ex-

treme isolation, exhaustion, and the use of psychedelic drugs.

NEUROTRANSMITTERS AND BRAIN FUNCTION

There are seven known neurotransmitters: acetylcholine, norepinephrine, dopamine, serotonin, gamma-aminobutyric acid, glutamic acid, and glycine. There are also many other substances that are probably neurotransmitters.

The neurotransmitters are stored in vesicles in the presynaptic terminal of the neuron. The neurotransmitters are released on arrival of an action potential at the synaptic junction and they diffuse across the synaptic cleft. When the neurotransmitter arrives at the post-synaptic membrane, it acts on a specialized receptor. The receptors for the neurotransmitters have clear-cut specificity for the neurotransmitter and for agonists and antagonists. Each neuron appears to contain only one transmitter and that neurotransmitter is released from all its presynaptic terminals. However, usually there is more than one class of receptor for a given neurotransmitter and those receptors are found in different regions of the nervous system.

The drugs that are potent in neurotransmitter action affect neurotransmission at various levels. Thus, there are inhibitors of neurotransmitter synthesis, false transmitters, inhibitors of neurotransmitter inactivation, neurotransmitter-depleting agents, neurotransmitter-displacing agents, and drugs that act on the neurotransmitter receptors. The distribution of various neurotransmitters in the brain has been mapped. Serotonin neurons originate primarily in the raphe nuclei of the medulla pons and midbrain, and they ascend to diverse areas in the hypothalamus, limbic system, and cerebral cortex, and descend to the spinal cord. Norepinephrine neurons are found in two ascending pathways, both of which arise

*The Latin origin of the term "consciousness" (con + scio) implies "joint knowledge," "knowing things together."

from the pons and midbrain, and are distributed widely in the brain. Some noradrenergic neurons also terminate in the spinal cord. Dopamine neurons largely originate in the midbrain, and terminate primarily in the stratum and limbic system. The location of the other neurons sensitive to specific neurotransmitters is less well known.

DOPAMINE AND SCHIZOPHRENIA

One theory of schizophrenia holds that an excess of dopamine activity underlies this disorder. The major tranquilizers, which are effective antipsychotic drugs, are similar structurally to dopamine. These tranquilizers (or neuroleptics) can displace dopamine from the dopamine receptors in the brain, and they can block the action of dopamine at the dopamine receptors. Furthermore, the antipsychotic effects of the neuroleptics are directly proportional to their ability to displace or block dopamine. That is true even for those neuroleptics that block dopamine without affecting other neurotransmitters.

The nature of the dopamine abnormality in schizophrenia is not fully understood. Excessive amounts of dopamine may be released or there may be an increased sensitivity to dopamine. Or the basic defect may be in another organ or organ system in the body with the dopamine blockade by the neuroleptics modifying the schizophrenic symptoms by a secondary or compensatory effect. Moreover, the problem is further complicated by the fact that the neuroleptic drugs are ameliorative rather than curative, and the antipsychotic effects of neuroleptics may be more pronounced in other disorders, for example, mania.

MONOAMINES AND AFFECTIVE DISORDERS

A variety of theories about the causes of affective disorders are based on the fact that biologically active amines modulate the activity of the neurons in the central nervous system that may be involved in the regulation of mood and behavior. The somatic symptoms of depression, such as disturbances of sleep, appetite, gastrointestinal function, and sex drive, as well as the diurnal variation of the complaints and altered endocrine function support the theory that depression has a biological basis. The fact that drugs that alter the activity of the neurotransmitters have an antidepressant effect also supports the biological basis of depression. The catecholamine hypothesis of affective disorders proposes that some types of depression are associated with an absolute or a relative deficiency of catecholamines. Specifically, the supply of norepinephrine may be deficient at important adrenergic receptor sites in the brain. Elation, on the other hand, may be associated with an excess of catecholamines. However, because the catecholamine theory fails to explain all the known facts, other explanations of depression have been offered. Among them is the indoleamine hypothesis which proposes that in depression there is a deficiency of serotonin activity and in mania an excess.

ENKEPHALINS AND DRUG ADDICTION

A new chapter in the understanding of drug addiction began with the discovery in the brain of the opiate receptors and subsequent finding of the endogenous opiate peptides. Such receptors are also in the intestines. There are two forms of the opiate receptor: one type preferentially binds agonists and the other type preferentially binds antagonists. A variety of opiate peptides (endorphins and enkephalins) have been isolated from the brain that actively bind to the opiate receptors. These enkephalins and endorphins are similar to the opiate drugs in biological activity and in structure.

Opiate receptors are found in many areas of the brain, especially the areas that subserve pain and pleasure. Opiate peptides have also been found in the same regions. On the basis of those findings, it is reasonable to infer that these peptides may be neurotransmitters in pathways carrying pain and pleasure stimuli, and that the opiate receptors are the synaptic receptors for those neurotransmitters. Thus the following opiate peptide hypothesis of drug addiction has been proposed. In drug addiction, the administration of exogenous opiates activates the synaptic opiate receptors and alters their numbers. Simultaneously, the release of endogenous opiates decreases. Both those effects lead to drug tolerance. The withdrawal symptoms that occur when the administration of endogenous opiates is stopped are due both to the persistently reduced release of endogenous opiates and to the alteration of the synaptic opiate receptors. The withdrawal symptoms persist until normal quantities of endogenous opiate peptides are released and the sensitivity of the receptors returns to normal.

The discovery of the function of the limbic system, the RAS and the neurotransmitters, coupled with the increasing availability of sophisticated research techniques, has substantially changed the understanding of the biological basis of behavior and the theory and practice of psychiatry.

FURTHER READINGS

Ettigi, P. L. G. and Brown, G. M. (1977): Psychoneuroendocrinology of affective disorder: an overview. *Am. J. Psychiatry. 134*:493.
A review of the neuroendocrinology of depression.
Snyder, S. H. (1977): Opiate receptors and internal opiates. *Sci. Am. 236*:44.
A review of opiate receptors and endorphins.
Sourkes, T. K. (1977): Biochemistry of mental depression. *Can. Psychiatr. Assoc. J.,* 22:467.
A review of current chemical theories of depression.

CHAPTER 7

Being with the Patient
Stanley E. Greben

The physician and the patient come together, from their separate worlds, each with expectations of himself, and each with expectations of the other. When they meet a third entity is created: the physician-patient relationship. They meet for a specific purpose: so that the one, with his special capacities and training, will examine and understand the other, and, if indicated, institute some treatment. When the physician and the patient are together, there are three aspects to their relationship: *the real relationship* of two human beings, each with his own specific personal characteristics; *the therapeutic or working alliance* which develops between the two people, a cooperative attitude which enables them to work together; and, *the transference relationship*, in which their dealings with each other are affected by the residual unresolved personal conflicts which exist in each of them.

The Real Relationship. As described in earlier chapters, both the physician and the patient have personal qualities and backgrounds which influence the ways in which they carry out their roles. Each physician will have attitudes which lead to characteristic ways of dealing with all patients. But from patient to patient these will vary somewhat, depending on how the two personalities match or conflict.

The Therapeutic or Working Alliance. The physician and patient must develop a way of working together. They meet as strangers. As they continue to deal with each other, ideally trust and understanding grow between them, and their capacity to work together increases. That growth is essential to all physician-patient relationships. Even when the task is surgical, and the surgeon has a *much* more active role than the patient, the work proceeds best when a good therapeutic alliance has been established. In psychiatric medicine the therapeutic alliance is of even greater significance. And in that specific form of treatment which is called *psychotherapy* (see chapters 32 and 33) it is of pre-eminent importance.

The Transference Relationship. Every person has residual, unresolved conflicts which continue to affect his behavior as an adult. This applies both to physicians and to patients. One physician, for example, is made excessively angry by ungrateful patients. Another physician feels great distaste for obese patients. Another physician feels helpless in dealing with an aged, failing patient. One patient has an inordinate fear of an authoritarian physician. Another patient searches out and feels excessively needful of the maternal, or even infantilizing, physician. Another patient is enraged by the disorganized or unreliable physician. When these negative reactions go beyond certain bounds, they render the two people unable to work together. In usual physician-patient relationships the negative feelings are largely concealed. In the psychiatrist-patient relationship, especially during psychotherapy, they may be brought into the open by the physician, so that they can be understood and dealt with.

THE PHYSICIAN'S APPROACH TO THE PATIENT

The physician treats his patient as a good host treats a welcome guest. Let us consider the situation in which the patient comes to the physician's office.

The physician will, first of all, create an environment which is comfortable and receptive to the patient. This takes into account that often the patient is apprehensive, so that a physical atmosphere in which he feels that his general ease and right to confidentiality are considered, is essential.

The physician, ideally, deals with his patient in the following ways: he is respectful, concerned, interested, empathetic, objective but not distant, scientific but not de-humanized, helpful, friendly but not effusive, serious but not severe, courteous, and supportive. No physician, of course, achieves the ideal, but being aware of these factors offers the physician a goal toward which he can work.

All physicians gather information about patients in several ways; by taking the patient's history, by examining him physically, and by using special tests or procedures. With *all* patients the history taking is essential. However, with many medical and surgical patients, findings on physical examination or special tests may be of predominant importance. This may *also* be the case with psychiatric patients, but ordinarily it is not. Information gathering by interview including both history taking and assessment of the patient's mental status is extremely important for all psychiatric patients.

There are two types of interviews used in the treatment of psychiatric patients: *evaluative interviews* and *therapeutic interviews.*

Evaluative Interviews

This includes the consultation; it also includes the first or first few interviews when psychotherapy is being begun. The substance of the evaluation will be discussed in chapters 8 and 9, but some general comments will be made here.

Some physicians allot several interviews to the evaluation of the patient. Other physicians make every effort to come to some conclusion and plan of action after a single interview. In either instance, this evaluation includes eliciting the patient's complaint and the history of that complaint, taking the story of his life in overview, and making an assessment of the patient's mental status.

The first interview might be opened by a comment such as: "I understand that you have been having headaches," or "Dr. Brown tells me that you have been having attacks of anxiety." An expectant attitude of listening, with further questions as necessary, will then ordinarily lead to the presentation of the chief complaint and history of the present illness. When this information has been obtained in sufficient detail, the physician than questions the patient on the events and problems of his life in chronological order.

Therapeutic Interviews

Subsequent interviews, as part of psychotherapy, will have the purpose of shedding further light upon the patient's problems. They should help him come to some conclusions about what steps he might take to improve things. The interviewer may be more active or less active, more directing or more following, depending upon the nature of the psychotherapeutic method employed. Various methods will be discussed in chapters 32 and 33.

In the course of long-term psychotherapy, the relationship between the physician and the patient becomes more fully developed, and may itself come under close scrutiny as part of the therapeutic method. In psychoanalysis and the psychodynamic psychotherapies, the analysis of this relationship is one of the most important therapeutic tools.

THE SETTING

The atmosphere of the physician's office should help the patient feel at ease. The consulting room must be soundproof so that the patient need not fear being overheard. The physician and the patient might face each other in comfortable chairs. Some physicians do not sit behind a desk, preferring to use a more informal arrangement of chairs. Other physicians sit at a desk only during an initial interview to make note taking easier.

On this latter point there is a variety of practices. Most physicians take extensive notes during the first interviews, since a full record of each patient must be kept. When the patient comes repeatedly for psychotherapy, various approaches are used. Some physicians take notes during each interview, feeling that the patient soon learns to accept and even ignore the note taking. Many physicians feel that note taking interferes with the interview, and they make their notes when the interview is over.

Since the physician wishes his patients to see him as trustworthy and reliable, he considers it important that he, as well as the patient, keep appointments and keep them on time.

Equally, in order to have the patient feel free to talk about personal and even painful facts, he must feel that he has his physician's full attention. Thus the interview must not be interrupted, either by other persons directly, or by the telephone.

THERAPEUTIC ASPECTS OF THE RELATIONSHIP BETWEEN THE PHYSICIAN AND THE PATIENT

Throughout the contacts between physician and patient the basic aim is that the former should help the latter. Numerous attempts have been made to separate the psychological components of the therapeutic effect of the physician. Frank (1975) thinks that the physician's therapeutic effect is achieved by the physician's reawakening of hope in the patient. Marmor (1975) thinks that the therapeutic portion of their relationship can be reduced to the following ingredients which account for any improvement of the patient on psychological grounds:

(1) A good patient-therapist relationship, (2) release of tension, (3) cognitive learning, (4) operant reconditioning, (5) suggestion and persuasion, (6) identification with the therapist, (7) reality-testing, (8) emotional support.

The first of those ingredients listed above, namely a good patient-therapist relationship, has certain usual characteristics. These will depend in part upon the physician's qualities of character and personality, as well as his values, and, in part, upon the therapeutic stance which he assumes because of his professional training.

Greben (1977) thinks that the physician who is therapeutic has the following qualities:

(1) Empathy and concern for the patient, (2) a caring and protective attitude toward the patient, (3) a warm approach to the patient, (4) therapeutic forcefulness,

that is, the ability to reawaken hope in the patient who has given up, (5) the expectation that the patient will improve, (6) the absence of despair in the therapist, (7) reliability, that is, the therapist is "always there," (8) friendliness and respect toward the patient.

These qualities reflect the physician's innate personality and attitudes, which can be expected to be enhanced through appropriate training.

Further, there is a specific atmosphere which the physician should cultivate in his relationship with the patient. He is, on the one hand, concerned and involved, in the sense that he makes every effort to understand and help the patient. He is involved emotionally, in the sense that he does feel concern and regard for the patient as a person. But, on the other hand, he works in an objective, nonjudgmental, nonmoralizing way. This is essential, since, in order to perform his work successfully, the physician must have the patient's cooperation in making available all information, physical, emotional, and historical. The patient will not and cannot expose himself fully to a physician whom he sees as judgmental and derogating. But he will, in time, be able to be frank and open with a physician who is warm, objective, understanding, and nonjudgmental.

These are some of the characteristics, both in the relationship of the two people, and in the setting, which are significant when the physician meets every patient.

The situation in which the physician meets with the difficult patient is discussed in chapter 37.

REFERENCES

Frank, J. D. (1975): An overview of psychotherapy. In *Overview of the Psychotherapies*. Edited by G. Usdin. New York, Brunner/Mazel.

Greben, S. E. (1977): On being therapeutic. *Can. Psychiat. Assn. J.* 22:371.

Marmor, J. (1975): The nature of the psychotherapeutic process revisited. *Can., Psychiat. Assn. J.* 20:557.

FURTHER READINGS

Bruch, H. (1975): *Learning Psychotherapy: Rationale and Ground Rules.* Cambridge, Mass., Harvard U. Press.
  Chapter 1 entitled "When Strangers Meet," tells how the patient and therapist come together and begin to work.

Duguay, R. and Ellenberger, H. (1980): La relation médecin-malade. In *Manual de Psychiatrie.* Chicoutimi. Gaétan Morin et Associes, Ltée.
  A clear description of the doctor-patient relationship.

Friedman, L. (1975): Elements of the therapeutic situation: the psychology of a beginning encounter. In *American Handbook of Psychiatry.* 2nd ed. Edited by S. Arieti. New York, Basic Books.
  A description of the beginning encounter of patient and therapist, with a view of their roles and their relationship.

Greenson, R. R. and Wexler, M. (1969): The nontransference relationship in the psychoanalytic situation. *Int. J. of Psychoanalysis* 50:27.
  Whereas this article is written about the various elements of the patient-therapist relationship in psychoanalysis, much of what it says can help towards understanding the various portions of the relationship between any patient and his physician.

CHAPTER 8

The Examination: History

Sebastian K. Littmann and Gerald Shugar

It is on the quality of the psychiatric history, and on the thoroughness of the mental status examination that accurate diagnosis and good treatment in psychiatry depend. The basic tool used to obtain a psychiatric history and carry out a mental status examination is the psychiatric interview. Interviewing is a skill that must be learned.

Interviewing is a procedure designed to help the interviewer towards a full understanding of the interviewee's situation. It requires the use of language, mainly spoken, although at times written and on rare occasions sign language is involved. While numerous separate occasions may be required to obtain a comprehensive history, the single initial interview should enable the interviewer to arrive at a provisional diagnosis, formulation and treatment plan. This means that the interviewer has to recognize time limitations, and that even for this reason alone, he should undertake the interview in an organized and meaningful manner. The interview can be performed in an unstructured or in a structured manner. This is somewhat similar to a physical examination being carried out by the physician proceeding either from head to toe, or by system after system.

While the unstructured interview makes for greater spontaneity in the interview relationship, it is more difficult to use, particularly by those who carry out psychiatric interviewing but occasionally. The main place for unstructured interviewing is in ongoing psychotherapy.

In the initial interview, unstructured interviewing may be employed to let a person describe freely, without interruption, the development of his present problem. But for the major part of the interview, the structured approach is preferred. This means that the interviewer recognizes that the information required is grouped under a number of headings, and that these headings do not vary from interview to interview. The interview itself will most frequently be conducted by the interviewer's proceeding from one heading to another in order. Even when the sequence is not strictly maintained any information elicited is grouped under the appropriate heading.

PURPOSES OF THE INTERVIEW

The psychiatric interview has a threefold purpose.

Information Seeking. The interview is

an information seeking procedure on the part of an examiner who has a good understanding of what information is required by him to be of help to the patient. For answers to be to the point, meaningful questions need to be put in such a manner that the patient understands them. For example, not every patient will readily understand questions such as "Tell me about parental relationships and sibling rivalry in your nuclear family." A simpler version would be more appropriate such as "How did you get on with your parents and with your brothers and sisters?" Information seeking questions may be closed or open-ended. Open-ended questions by and large give the patient a greater opportunity to explain himself. For example, "Tell me about your father" is preferable to "Do you remember your father?" or "Is he still alive?" or "What was your relationship with him?" This type of question calls for single word, rather uninformative answers and makes for an interview that resembles an interrogation and prevents the patient from revealing his story and himself freely. It goes without saying that more focused questions are occasionally needed to seek supplementary information such as, for example, "You did not mention your father's job," or "it would be helpful to know how you got on with him."

The interview can be viewed as an intrusion into a person's life and even though the necessity of this is evident, it should proceed with tact and sensitivity. Tact, however, is not to be confused with seeking to avoid embarrassment at all costs. The interview is the verbal psychological equivalent of the physical examination. The physician has the same right and duty to intrude into areas which would be inappropriate in ordinary social interaction.

Observation. It is in the interview that the patient reveals himself and allows the interviewer to observe attitudes, feelings and appearance. The interview should allow a person to be himself. For this to happen, the interviewer is required to be warm, friendly and responsive. In other words, the interviewer should refrain from changing his own interviewing demeanor according to whether he likes or dislikes the patient. Indeed, it can be argued that politeness, consideration and friendliness are of particular importance when he is interviewing an unfriendly, and perhaps reluctant patient.

It is important that the interviewer use his own interviewing technique as a kind of yardstick by which to assess the personality and mental state of various types of patients.

Therapeutic. The third aim of the interview, even of the initial interview, is to establish a supportive relationship between interviewer and patient.

Most patients who are being interviewed for the first time are desirous of help and they expect some help to be forthcoming as soon as contact with the psychiatrist commences. That is to say, whereas both patient and psychiatrist recognize the importance of information gathering and observation, they also expect action, as it were in the form of emotional support, empathy, explanation, and advice. It is clear that without this understanding, the quality of the information gathered runs the risk of being either incomplete or distorted.

For example, the interviewer's refusal to answer an anxious patient's early question as to what is wrong with him on account of this being simply an information gathering initial interview, would likely make the remainder of the interview difficult and even impossible.

BASIC RULES OF PSYCHIATRIC INTERVIEWING

Interviewing can be made more effective if well-established rules are followed.

Make the Patient Feel at Ease. Making sure that the patient feels at ease includes greeting the patient by his name if possible and introducing oneself. "Good morning Miss Smith, I am Doctor Jones." It also means looking after his or her comfort. "Please come in, put your coat over there and have a seat in this chair." Whenever necessary, explain why certain questions are being asked or certain requests are being made. "To understand your present problem, it is helpful to me to know some of the important details of your early development."

Set Aside Enough Time. Perhaps nothing is more unpleasant to a patient than an interviewer who is obviously in a great hurry to come to the end of the procedure. Sufficient time should be set aside for the interview. The actual duration will vary with the skills and experience of the interviewer. It is better to set aside 60 minutes and have time left over than to set aside 30 minutes and run out of time. Ensuring that the interview can proceed without undue interruptions or other external demands and conveying to the patient the impression that this time is his time, are important points to observe.

Be Alert and Listen. The interviewer must be in good mental and physical condition, uninfluenced by adverse factors such as excessive fatigue, or serious personal or professional worries. Interviewing cannot proceed effectively in the absence of good listening. To be a good listener, one has to listen intently and well. This means concentrating on everything that is being said, how it is being said, and what is *not* being said. For example, a patient's long account of his family background may have gaps: He may not have mentioned his mother. He therefore needs to be reminded or prompted. Was the gap the result of an inadvertent oversight or does it herald problems in the patient's relationship with his mother? Similarly, repeated assertions or denials often denote problematic areas in the patient's life, for example, repeated, unsolicited attempts on the part of an impotent patient to reassure the interviewer that there is absolutely nothing wrong with his marital relationship.

Record the Information. Information collected from patients and observations made of their general demeanor should be regarded as valuables and as such, conveyed to safekeeping. In other words, data obtained must be recorded in writing during the interview so that at the end of the interview the interviewer is not left with incomplete portions of the history on account of his own faulty memory. Where appropriate, patients should be reassured as to the reasons for taking notes ("What you are telling me is important and it would be a pity if it were left entirely to the whims of my memory.") The confidentiality of the interview may require emphasis ("What we are talking about is between you and me and cannot be revealed to anyone else without your express written consent.") There are exceptions, such as when the interview is part of an assessment ordered by a judge. In this instance, it is proper to inform the patient *prior to* the interview that the details of the interview may be revealed to the legal authorities requesting it.

Remember That Each Patient Is Unique. The interviewer may be seeing numerous patients in the course of a working day and to him the whole procedure is therefore much more routine. However, each patient, and each history is unique. Each new patient sees the initial interview as a very special occasion and this deserves the respect of the interviewer.

Avoid Assumptions. The interviewer must avoid making assumptions or taking things for granted. Patients may use technical or semi-technical expressions such as "breakdown," "depression," "paranoid," or "feeling terrible." The very personal meaning of such expressions needs to be clarified by the interviewer.

Be Aware of Social Class and Ethnic Modifiers. The patient's social class and ethnic background need to be taken into consideration. Kinsey's researchers quickly discovered that college graduates could be asked about homosexual behavior early on in an inquiry, but that similar questions were best put later in the interview with blue collar workers. Similarly, school absenteeism in native Canadians living on isolated reserves may be the rule during the spring trapping season and should not necessarily be regarded as truancy.

Keep in Mind Language Difficulties. Decisions may have to be made about how well the patient speaks the language in which the interview is being conducted. As a rule, comments such as "he does not speak any English" should never be accepted until tested in the interview situation. Where a translator needs to be involved, non-family members are to be preferred since the presence of someone too close to the patient may at times inhibit the flow of the interview. In working with interpreters, it is better to address one's questions to the patient, both by word and by eye contact and not to the interpreter. At the same time, the verbal and non-verbal interaction between patient and interpreter deserves close scrutiny. Interpreters are not always willing to admit the difficulties they encounter in comprehending the patient and may produce perfunctory or approximate translations. Whenever interpreters are required, extra time allowances must also be made.

Special Communication Problems. Special attention is needed in difficult situations such as with the mute, the deaf and dumb, the deaf, the reluctant, hostile, or emotionally very upset patient. Again, these are difficult tasks; they call for special measures and sufficient time.

Terminating the Interview. An interview should never conclude without the interviewer thanking the patient and without the patient being given the opportunity to add or retract, or to ask questions about the interview. A suitable concluding statement might be "I think that is all Mrs. Jones. Thank you very much. Is there anything you wish to add, that would help me to understand your situation even better?"

"Do you have any questions?" When, as is not uncommon, the patient asks "What do you think is wrong with me?" the interviewer should be prepared to answer this question to the best of his ability. Replies such as "we can talk about it later" are not acceptable.

ORGANIZATION OF THE HISTORY

Information should be gathered in the following sequence or under the following headings:

1. Identifying data
2. Source of and reason for referral
3. Source of and reliability of information
4. Presenting complaint
5. History pertaining to the development of the presenting complaint
6. Previous history of illness (mental and physical)
7. Family history
8. Personal history
   a. early development
   b. childhood behavior
   c. schooling
   d. adolescence
   e. occupational
   f. psychosexual history
   g. marital history
   h. children
   i. use of alcohol, tobacco and other substances
   j. anti-social behavior
   k. present life situation
9. Personality

The subsequent part of the interview is then devoted to the more formal examination of the mental state as described in the next chapter. Finally the psychiatric history concludes with the diagnostic formulation, treatment plan and prognosis.

Identifying Data

This includes the family name, first name, sex, age, and address, and also elicits the basic information about marital status, religion, occupation, nationality, and previous contact with the agency or hospital. The interviewer should feel free at this point to seek additional information on these basic items, so as to familiarize himself more thoroughly with the patient's present situation. For example, the name of a street may take on more meaning if the interviewer knows in which part of town it is located. Being of one or the other religious denomination is of less interest than the meaning this has to the patient in terms of his everyday living. Similarly, it is more meaningful to an interviewer to know what exactly it is that a patient is doing than simply to content himself with knowing the name of the occupation.

Additional inquiries into these matters early on convey to the patient the interviewer's interest. This generally makes for a good start to the interview.

Source of and Reason for Referral

Here are the questions that the interviewer wants answered. Who is responsible for the patient's presence? What is the official reason? What is the real reason? Accompanying referral letters are of great interest, both on account of their content and form. The date on which the referral letter was originally written should be noted as considerable time may have elapsed, with significant changes in the circumstances of the patient as well as in the clinical state. If the patient refers himself, why did he come today rather than yesterday, or tomorrow, and why did he come here? Special attention should be paid to whether or not the patient is attending under some kind of duress, or pressure from, for example, his employer, or the police, or an angry spouse. Early acknowledgement of the circumstance prevents the interviewer from deliberately or accidentally creating the impression that he is acting on behalf of or in conjunction with

those forces responsible for the patient's presence.

Source of and Reliability of Information

It is easy to be misled by patients who are honest, but inaccurate, or by those who deliberately try to mislead. The interviewer has to estimate in his own mind how accurate, objective, and reliable the patient's account in fact is. On this estimate depends the need to seek additional corroborating information from outside sources. This is not to say that patients attempt to deceive, but it is to draw attention to the fact that, for example, an adolescent's account of an event would hardly ever agree with the account of the same event given by his parents. Similarly, a hypomanic patient always tends to minimize or rationalize some of his most outrageous behavior, whereas a severely depressed patient tends to overstate his misdemeanors because of the profound guilt he feels.

Where corroborating information is obtained, the interviewer must understand the relationship between the informant and the patient as well as the attitude of the informant towards the patient and the interviewer. It is important to remember that the patient who seeks help for a family crisis may not necessarily be the person most in need of help. It is best to take one's time to gather information, to observe, and to wait before making up one's mind about this.

Presenting Complaint

In the simplest form this is the reason the patient comes to the physician's attention. He may be able to state his complaint simply and succinctly. On the other hand he may require a great deal of help and assistance from the interviewer to help him tell his story. Questions which may help the patient to express his complaint are: "What brought you here today?" "How can I help you?" "What seems to be troubling you?" "What is on your mind today?" The patient should be allowed to state his complaint or complaints in his own words and these should be recorded. It is not important to force the patient to commit himself to a statement such as "depression" or "I have been feeling anxious." It is important to help the patient clarify the duration for which the complaints have been present. This is not always an easy matter and may require some discussion. A useful question is "When were you last perfectly well?" Another, "When did this illness begin?"

History Relevant to the Presenting Complaint

Virtually all presenting complaints have a specific time limited course which can be teased out and described and one should resist the temptation to see presenting complaints as lifelong incapacities or as being incapable of further definition. At the basis of the presenting complaint lie so-called stressors. The complaint can be seen as a response or modified response to those stressors. The information to be sought here can therefore be organized in terms of: stresses in the patient's present and recent life; and symptoms and signs (mental, emotional, behavioral, physical) each having its onset, each developing in a certain sequence that can be described, and following a course over a period of time (either continuous or intermittent). Any symptom that is discovered should be described in some detail, rather than simply being reported as present. Thus, stating that a patient has grown increasingly depressed over the past three months to the point where he now feels that life is not worth living, and that he is in constant torment, hopeless and sleepless, with his depression worse in the morning and unrelieved by distraction; and that he is pulled towards seeking relief in mercy killing and suicide, is much more meaningful than a simple statement to the effect that the patient has been increasingly depressed for the last little while.

The interviewer should make specific inquiry into symptomatology under a number of headings:

1. *Feeling*—How does the patient feel within himself? "Tell me how you feel today." Is there any experience of fear, anxiety, depression, irritability, suspicion, anger, or hopelessness? If present, what is their strength, their quality, their stability or lability, their periodicity if any?

2. *Thinking*—What type of thoughts does the patient report? What does the interviewer notice about the quality of the thinking process, the speed, the ease, the clarity, continuity, and relevance of thought? Does the patient complain about difficulties in his thinking? "Have you noticed any changes in your ability to think clearly?"

3. *Perception*—Does the patient experience any abnormality in any of the five senses, and in how his body feels to him and how he perceives the world? "Tell me about any unusual ways in which you see or hear things around you."

4. *Bodily functions*—Is there weakness, tiredness, insomnia, anorexia, weight loss, pain, or any other bodily disturbance? What help has the patient tried to obtain for these symptoms? Has he attempted to treat himself with alcohol or drugs, or both?

Mental and Physical History of Previous Illness

If the patient has had any previous illness, particularly mental illness, or treatment or hospitalization, much can be learned about his present situation from an account of the precipitation, presentation, duration, management, and response to treatment during previous periods of incapacity.

It is always possible that the current complaint has occurred before, but that the patient has never sought help for it. It is clear that many patients like to minimize previous episodes of illness, particularly mental illness, and to omit essential elements in the history. It may be necessary at this point to obtain permission to request information from the previous treatment settings. Phone calls are faster and more informative, and may help the interviewer to be of more immediate help to the patient at the end of the interview if for example he has information available about previously effective medication.

A full account of any past or present health problems also includes consideration of physical health. Specific inquiry should be made concerning accidents and head injuries as well as the patient's psychological adaptation to any form of ill health. It is also important to ask the patient about any medication recently or currently used by him.

Family History

The information sought focuses on the family into which the patient was born, and on the relationships in the earliest formative years. In cases of fostering, adoption, or step-parents, the records should include data concerning the biological and the social family. The current health of the nuclear family and the patient's involvement with this family are also of interest.

Parents. The information to be sought about the patient's father and mother should include mention of their present age or their age at the time of death as well as the cause of death. The parents' occupation, history of mental and physical illnesses and personalities should be included. Of particular importance is some definition of the patient's relationship to his parents in childhood and in adulthood, and his reaction to their death. A history of separation in childhood is important. The interviewer must be prepared to challenge gently the patient's description of his parents. Such descriptions are not infrequently highly idealized, and therefore deserve clarification. The simplest approach is to ask the patient to amplify answers such as "he was a good average father."

Siblings. These should be enumerated in chronological order of birth, present ages, marital state, occupation, and significant illnesses. Inquiry should be made into the occurrence of miscarriages or stillbirths in the nuclear family as these are often crisis points within the family unit. The patient's previous and current relationships with his siblings also deserve attention.

Extended Family. Other relatives should never be forgotten. Grandparents or aunts and uncles not infrequently have played more important roles in a person's life than the natural father or mother, and their death or illness can constitute a serious crisis in the person's life. In a more general sense, the patient should be asked about familial disease including alcoholism, or abnormal personalities, and mental disorders in the more extended family. If the patient says that he does not know whether or not any of his more distant relatives have had a mental illness, then this should be stated in the written history. Lack of information on the other hand is not equivalent to the absence of mental disorder in the family.

At the time that the patient and interviewer talk about the patient's family, an attempt should be made to understand the family atmosphere that prevailed in the patient's childhood, and early deaths, separations, illnesses or economic disasters deserve mention, with particular attention being paid to the patient's age at the time of the crisis.

Personal History

This is essentially a sketch of the patient's life sub-divided into the following sub-headings.

Early Development. Information is sought about the date and place of birth as well as the birth weight. Abnormalities during pregnancy and childbirth as well as early feeding difficulties or illnesses in infancy are asked about. Abnormalities of early milestones and, if possible the mother's attitude towards infant and child rearing, deserve mention here.

Childhood Behavior. This concerns itself with the specific inquiry into sleep difficulties, enuresis or encopresis, speech disorders, tics or mannerisms. Play activities and early fantasy life as well as the ability to make and get on with friends are inquired into. Any history of delinquency, truancy, antisocial behavior or hyperactivity should be mentioned under this heading. The same would go for overconformity, shyness and general unhappiness.

Schooling. This should include the age of beginning and finishing school, the types of school attended, the examinations passed or failed, including any mention of specific learning difficulties. It should also include a picture of how the patient fitted into school in a social sense, and how he got on with peers and teachers. An understanding of particular likes or dislikes for certain subjects gives insight into the patient's personality.

Adolescence. Under this heading the patient is asked to describe his attitude to growing up, to his peers, to his parents, and to authority in general. This is a period of frequent emotional turmoil. It may be the time when the patient first experiences drug, alcohol or tobacco abuse.

Occupational. Inquiry is made into details of training and the jobs held. Did the patient change jobs frequently? If so, for what reasons? Has he advanced in his chosen job? Ask about job satisfaction. Was there much unemployment? If so, how did the patient react to prolonged periods of being without work?

Psychosexual History. This includes an account of earliest sexual situations, often in early childhood. The age of onset of puberty should be defined as well as the

attitude thereto. The age at which masturbation started, the fantasies involved and associated anxieties should be elicited. The history of dating and heterosexual or homosexual relationships comes next, as well as an account of the early experiences involving such partners. The patient should also be allowed to talk about any dysfunctions such as impotence or anorgasmia, as well as any possible sexual deviations. An understanding of the current sexual practice is of importance, whether marital or other. Contraceptive measures, their satisfaction or associated problems should always be asked about.

Marital History. This should include the age, occupation, health, and personality of the spouse as well as mention of the duration of the marriage(s) and the circumstances leading up to the marriage or marriages. The quality of the marital relationship needs to be understood, and its strengths and weaknesses highlighted. Where applicable, dates of deaths of spouses, divorces, or separations should be ascertained.

Children. These should be listed chronologically with their names and ages, as well as their general state of health now, and in the past. It is important not to forget death, miscarriages, and stillbirths as well as therapeutic abortions. Attitudes towards children deserve attention as well as the couple's attitudes towards further child bearing. Are there any present difficulties associated with child rearing? Where the children are grown up, are they still at home? If not, what is the quality of the present relationship with absent children?

Use of Alcohol, Tobacco and other Substances. These should always be inquired into in some detail and the inquiry should never be a hasty one. The amount of tobacco consumed, the amounts of liquor and/or drugs used should always be discussed in some detail and attention should be paid to the duration of use or abuse. Any problems, whether psychological or physical, associated with the use of any of the above, or prescribed medication deserve particular attention.

Anti-social Behavior. This includes inquiry into the patient's history of conflict with the police or the courts, if any. "Have you been in any legal difficulties during your life?"

Present Life Situation. This description should supplement the identifying information collected at the beginning of the interview and include a full account of the patient's family's present socio-economic circumstances, including income, housing, circle of friends, financial obligations and debts, relationships with neighbors, parents, and inlaws.

Personality

Personality consists of those characteristics, attitudes and patterns of behavior which, together with his physical characteristics, make him the individual he is. Personality traits by and large are enduring and all pervasive, but personality may sometimes change as the result of serious illness. In addition, severe mental illness may at times obscure the premorbid personality. It is important, therefore, to obtain as clear a description of the previous personality as possible. An assessment of personality traits requires direct questioning of the patient himself, observation of his behavior during the interview, as well as additional information from those who have been close to him for a long period of time and who know him best.

Personality is best described in non-technical language and can be grouped under the following sub-headings.

Attitudes to Others. This includes the ability to trust, to make and to retain relationships and friendships. In addition, it includes the ability to be a leader or to be a follower, the capacity to participate and to assume responsibility, and to make decisions. It describes relationships in terms of warmth or coldness, and of dominance or submissiveness. It also mentions the ability to take on roles in the family, at work, and in emergencies.

Attitudes Toward Oneself. Basically, one is concerned here with finding out whether the patient likes himself or dislikes himself and whether in his relationship to himself, he is overly for or against himself. An assessment of his ambition and achievement levels also comes under this heading.

Moral and Religious Attitudes and Standards. Is the patient a rigid or permissive person? Is he over-conscientious or easy going? What are the forms of his religious beliefs, if any?

Affective Disposition. Are his moods stable, or is he changing moods quickly and often? Do people regard him as joyful or as a morose and depressive person? Can he feel pleasure? Is he an extrovert or introvert? Does he have a sense of humor?

Hobbies and Interests. The patient should be asked to describe these rather than to respond to the interviewer's checklist.

The Ability to Tolerate Stress. Inquire into the patient's reaction to certain developmental crises, such as puberty and marriage, as well as to other forms of stress such as examinations, illnesses, various losses and rejections.

Conclusions

The quality of the psychiatric history is very much influenced by the development of good interviewing skills. Like any other skill, theory must be complemented by practice. Every opportunity should be sought by students to interview different types of patients, in various settings, such as the office, the emergency room, the home, and even over the telephone. Having one's interviews observed directly or on videotape is a most helpful procedure for increasing one's skills. The same can be said of observing one's own tapes and observing the interviews or tapes of colleagues.

REFERENCES

Finesinger, J. E. (1948): Psychiatric interviewing. *Am. J. Psychiatry*. 105:187.

Mayer-Gross, W., Slater, E. and Roth, M. (1969): *Clinical Psychiatry*. 3rd ed. London, Cassell.

Walton, H. J. and Littmann, S. K. (1973): Interview methods. In *Companion to Psychiatric Studies*. Edited by A. Forrest. Edinburgh, Churchill Livingstone.

FURTHER READINGS

Balint, M. (1964): *The Doctor, His Patient and The Illness*. 2nd ed. New York, International Universities Press.

The author analyzes, based on his experience with medical practitioners, the intricacies of the developing relationship between interviewer and patient.

Ruesch, J. (1968): Communication and mental illness: a psychiatric approach. In *Communication*. Edited by J. Ruesch and G. Bateson. New York, Norton.

Ruesch attempts to describe the conceptual systems within which the psychiatric interviewer operates. The interviewer is seen as an expert in communication.

Sullivan, H. S. (1954): *The Psychiatric Interview*. New York, Norton.

This is one of the classic texts on the art of psychiatric interviewing and draws attention to the important variables in interviews.

9

The Examination: Mental State

R. Ian Hector and Sebastian K. Littmann

The examination of the mental state is an integral part of the psychiatric consultation, though its completeness will be determined by the purpose of the particular consultation. While the student is cautioned against adopting any format of examination in too rigid or dogmatic a fashion, the examination of the present mental state is critical in establishing the correct provisional and differential diagnosis. In the assessment of a patient in regard to mental competence under the Mental Health Act, careful attention to detail with rigorous testing of each area is mandatory. In other psychiatric consultations, such as in the case of emotional difficulties in response to troubled life situations, formal evaluation of the mental state may be much reduced or not done at all. In these situations a more empathic, sensitive attitude to the patient's needs and feelings should characterize the interview. However, no amount of common sense will substitute for broad clinical experience, and clinical impressions are inferior to a carefully considered differential diagnosis.

The focus is on both the verbal and nonverbal behavior displayed in the interview, as well as on subjective experiences. In certain cases the examination will also include a physical and neurological examination. Where a patient has been admitted to a hospital, additional information becomes available as he participates in the life of the ward.

A large part of the examination can be carried out unobtrusively as the interview proceeds. Just as the interviewer is advised to note on paper the basic details of the history, so he should write down, perhaps in the margin of the page, any salient observations concerning the mental state. One should avoid thinking of the psychiatric interview as consisting of two parts, viz. history taking and mental status examination. Most observations are made and questions asked during the history taking. Only a few additional questions may need to be asked specifically at the end to complete the mental status examination.

Where mental processes are examined by specific procedures (e.g. serial sevens, proverbs, memory tests) the interviewer is advised to explain the reason for such questioning. Many patients become offended or puzzled if examined in a routine way without any explanation. But do not apologize for conducting this part of the examination, e.g. as silly or routine. It is as serious to fail in the diagnosis of early dementia as it is to miss a cancer of the rectum.

The interviewer needs to determine the degree of congruence between what he observes and what the patient describes as his subjective experience. The same type of awareness applies to the congruence between what one can reasonably expect of a patient (on the basis of his background, education and experience in life) and his actual performance.

At the end of the interview, when the case history is written up or dictated, observations concerning the *history* are put down first and are followed by those on the *mental state. Diagnosis and treatment* decisions are concluded at the end of the examination.

The Mental Status examination is considered under a number of headings:

1. Appearance and behavior
2. Affect and mood
3. Speech and thought
   a) thought process
   b) thought content
4. Perception
5. The sensorium including intellectual functions.

APPEARANCE AND BEHAVIOR

These aspects are best described if the observer pretends to be a novelist and painter combined, the aim being to create a life-like picture of the patient with the free use of adjectives. It is a descriptive analysis of behavior and while such a description cannot be too long, it should be accurate.

Is the person able to communicate adequately in the language of the interview? How easily and how well is rapport established?

How does the person look, in a general sense? Observe the height, weight, hair, eye color, complexion, and general bearing. Does he look in good health? Does he look unwell? If so, what makes you think he is unwell?

Consider his dress and degree of self-care. What clothes does he wear? Are they appropriate, old or new, clean or dirty? Do they fit him, size-wise and otherwise? What about his care of himself: does he care for his hair, for his face, and his hands?

What is the level of activity? Is the person overactive or underactive, slow, hesitant, or repetitive? Does he respond quickly or in a delayed manner? Are there any abnormal movements, including tremor, tics, or mannerisms?

Observe the patient's attitude. How does he relate to you? Is he cooperative and friendly or antagonistic and hostile? Is he frightened, overly demanding, overbearing, or too friendly? Is he overly brief, general or abstract, rambling or vague? Is there a gross denial of problems? Is he withdrawn, preoccupied with himself, with his thoughts or his inner experiences?

AFFECT AND MOOD

While *affect* refers to the emotional state displayed by the patient in the course of an interview, *mood* describes the prevailing or dominant affect over a period of time. Assist the patient in describing his mood by developing a vocabulary of descriptive adjectives large enough to contain the complexity and variability of the feeling tone.

The patient's general appearance and demeanor will give some indication of his mood. Not only the type of affect displayed, but also its changeability should be observed. Note any physical reaction to emotions, such as a change of face, attitude or gesture, the injection of the conjunctivae as a prelude to crying, or the sudden blotching in the blush area when conflict issues associated with shame and guilt emerge. Subjective feelings are elicited by questions such as "How do you feel in yourself?" or "How are your spirits?" Does what the patient says reflect how he apears to you? For example, is a subjective report of sadness matched by a sad appearance? Patients who appear depressed, perplexed or frightened should always be questioned about any wish, intention or plan to injure themselves. An appropriate opening question would be "Do you find life worth living?" Another, "Have you ever been frightened that you might harm yourself?" If there is evidence of suicidal preoccupation, ask details of any plans already made and inquire about any previous suicidal behavior. Remember that seriously depressed people can sometimes have both suicidal and homicidal feelings. Ask after unreasonable irritability or sharpness of temper.

Remember to make specific inquiry into various somatic functions, such as sleep, appetite for food, libido, and menstruation, as these are frequently disturbed in affective disorders, as well as into any regular variation of the mood throughout the day.

SPEECH AND THOUGHT

Thought Process

In observing a person's thought process, the interviewer first concerns himself with the rate and form of speech rather than with the content. Is there pressure or retardation of speech? Does the person talk spontaneously or only in answer to questions? How long are the answers? Always record a verbatim sample of the stream of speech illustrating any abnormality.

Disturbances in the form of thinking present in a number of ways. If the disorder is mild, the interviewer may simply become aware of some difficulty of comprehension during the interview; difficulties which are not removed when clarifications are sought and obtained.

The patient's associations may be *loosened* and he may thus make *overinclusive* statements such as "I went to the exhibition with my wife. I was born in the month of June."

Tangential thinking keeps the speaker from focusing on his initial goal; the direction of his thinking is influenced by a peripheral happening. Thus, when asked to describe the death of a friend in a traffic accident, a patient kept on describing the flowers in the field at the side of the road and the make of a plane flying overhead.

The *circumstantial* thinker loses himself in minute, irrelevant details, makes frequent corrections and not uncommonly loses completely the thread of his thought.

There may be *thought blocking* "Did you know, doctor, that my mother told me to —," followed by a long pause, with the speaker unable to continue as if he had lost his thoughts.

Logical connections between ideas may be replaced by odd patterns of associative connections such as *clang associations, flight of ideas, rhyming and punning.* For example, "How have you been?" answered with "keen, my queen. Gertrude Stein was also seen in Maclean."

Motor aphasia may present with word finding difficulties. "Could I please have a —" (indicating he wants a light for his cigarette).

Perseveration may occur. "I have never been too fond of spaghetti. Somehow I just don't like spaghetti. I don't know why, but spaghetti just doesn't appeal to me. I just don't like it."

A young, single woman suffering an acute catatonic schizophrenia sat down at a typewriter on the mental hospital ward and spontaneously wrote the following paragraph. (The characteristic disturbances of thought process with loosening of associations between ideas, the unusual linkage by similarity of sound, and the peculiarity of symbolic meaning are obvious.)

"This is a typewriter. This is not 1959, or 1960, or 1961. I am honestly attempting to find truth, but am at sea (see) (C). This is the truth. I do not know "when" this is, but am sure that it is out of time, or I am out of x time, or that I am "in" some sort of fifth or sixth or seventh millennium or something where I shouldn't be. God knows, and I do not use that phrase xxx lightly, or 'the gods', or the powers that be, that I *was* genuinely confused when I came in here; I remember only fragmentary parts of 'visions' I had in the past; and of a great love I am sure I must have had for people and animals, and birds and things when young, or younger. But as a student I never studied the "right" way toward the 'Right' things. A few nights ago,—or Ages—as the case may be, all I felt I really wanted was to (not rush to my own destruction), but be utterly destroyed—somehow that if people or gods hacked me to pieces and ruined me, that would be my just desserts. This thought in itself is a despicable one; to wish such an xxxxxxxxxxxxx execution to be performed *by* anyone. I have lived in this House, for I know it is not merely the old Ontario Hospital, frightened, confused, incapable of xxxxxxxxxxxxxxx grasping what all the people were trying to make clear to me—not only the "people" I have never seen before, but the relatives, who were here with replicas of my old shoes, my father's shoes, old clothes, new clothes, xxxxxxxx coming and going and time whirling—this is beginning to lack all sense too—but I did not understand; I still do not understand. The only thing at this point that I *do* understand is this: xHaving not understood,—and I did sincerely try to understand; some mind or soul must know that—I felt I had utterly, utterly failed in an attempt to reach the understanding which evidently a child of two or less over here could reach—I was, because I am out of place I am sure—even unable to "let go" the "right" way. I am still unable to let go the right way. I do not know how. And at this point, I can not even feel shame for not knowing how to 'go' from here, or "come" to there, wherever "there" may be, because "I do not know". I say this not in anger, not in scorn, not in malice, envy or any other thing such as that, but simply as a statement of fact. I DO NOT KNOW."

Neologisms are a striking form of disordered thought. The patient uses a word that he has made up, and that cannot be found in any dictionary; it has significance to him alone. For example, a patient said he had a "stomaseal," meaning he could not talk. Another strange type of speech activity is referred to as *echolalia* in which a patient repeats the question put to him or part of the question, or *logoclonia* where he may simply repeat the last word. Extreme disorder of thought process results in *word salad*: there are no evident logical or coherent links and the patient talks gibberish.

Thought Content

The content of thought may be disturbed in a variety of ways. Preoccupations and worries are common and interfere with clear thinking. Anxiety may be experienced as a feeling of dread or anticipation related to a specific object, or as a rather vague feeling of disease or apprehension. In its most severe form it becomes a sense of impending doom and produces panic.

Derealization is experienced as the world outside oneself having a strange or distorted appearance, sometimes with special meaning for the patient. Depersonalization is the same phenomenon, now experienced as such change within one's self. The déjà vu phenomenon consists of the impression that an experience has repeated itself, often with an intense sense of familiarity.

Dreams may be remembered as pleasant or terrifying. They may be recurrent. Special significance may be attributed to them.

Phobias and obsessive phenomena, repetitive thoughts, feelings or impulses, while recognized as irrational by the patient, override an internal resistance but exert considerable influence on him, despite attempts to disregard them. They may occupy much of his waking hours.

Ideas of reference are experienced as happenings or remarks being specifically related to or aimed at a person when in fact they are not; e.g. persons seen on television appear to be addressing the patient with special meaning.

Ideas of influence or passivity feelings are experienced as one's thoughts or actions being controlled by outside agencies.

Thoughts may be experienced as repeated, withdrawn from or inserted into a stream of thinking, as broadcast to an external agency, or as heard as though spoken aloud inside the head.

Delusions are fixed false beliefs, not open to logical persuasion and lacking the consensual validation of the culture. Belief in *God* is not generally considered a delusion, but the belief that one *is God* would be viewed by many cultures to be a false belief and so a delusion. Primary delusions are experienced suddenly and they are usually preceded by a particular mood of bewilderment and perplexity. Or they may be secondary delusions as a result of elaboration of previous delusions or perceptual distortions. They may be experienced in relation to the environment, or to the body, or to the self. One should attempt to determine the content, the mode of onset and the degree of fixity of delusions. One should observe such characteristics as their absurdity, their internal consistency, their degree of systematization, their comprehensibility, and their susceptibility to change or certainty of conviction, as well as the presence of evasiveness and concealment, and the level of overall preoccupation. Delusions related to the environment include ideas of reference (attribution of special meaning to events as being related to the self), misinterpretations, and beliefs of being persecuted or singled out or being experimented upon. Bodily delusions take the form of false beliefs related to changes in the body such as the two halves being different, or that the stomach is rotting or the nose growing.

Delusions may be fleeting or they may be of long duration and quite systematized. It is important to be clear about the impact of a delusion on the person's daily life and on his plans.

Observe and record the affective accompaniment to these abnormal inner experiences, e.g. resigned, frightened, angry, depressed, ecstatic, apathetic.

ABNORMAL PERCEPTUAL EXPERIENCES

Perceptions may be distorted by *illusions* which are simply misinterpretations of sensory stimuli e.g. shadows being seen as animals, or by *hallucinations*, which are sensory perceptions independent of objective reality. These may be referred to the environment, to the body or to the self. All sensory modalities may be involved, though auditory and visual distortions predominate. To find out about such experiences, the interviewer should ask questions: "Have you ever had any unusual psychological experiences? Have you ever been wakened at night thinking that you have heard your name spoken, to find no one there? Have you ever had that experience in the daytime?" Somatic hallucinations are unusual and include such sensations as being sexually fondled, of electricity running through the body, or parts of the body having died, or sensations of smell which are most commonly of foul odors.

Perceptual disturbances may vary, not just in content, but also in intensity and reality. It is important to determine whether their occurrence is related to day or night, falling asleep or waking up. Similarly, actual perceptual deficiencies such as deafness or partial-sightedness need to be taken into consideration. It is wise to remember that such disturbances may occur in relation to alcohol or other substance abuse.

SENSORIUM

The sensorium should be briefly assessed in every patient, but expanded in detail in all older patients and in those with any suggestion of an organic cerebral disease. In testing, make sure that the patient understands the nature of the test being administered, e.g. in offering a proverb ensure that the patient understands the nature of proverbs, by example if necessary.

Orientation. A person's orientation for time (day, date, year) place and person (knowing one's own name) may be intact in all three areas or in one or the other, or it may be completely distorted. This may be readily apparent in the interview, but may also require specific questions. Note that disorientation for time of day is not common in organic states.

Attention and Concentration Span. The attention and concentration span is tested easily, but before doing so it is always appropriate to ask the patient about his ability to pay attention and to concentrate.

Serial Seven's is a simple test. The person is asked, starting with 100, to subtract 7 and to keep on subtracting 7. The amount of effort required and the speed and accuracy of the responses are noted. The average person can complete serial seven's in one minute with fewer than four errors. Where serial sevens prove too difficult, have the patient recite the months of the year or the days of the week backwards.

Memory. How good a person's memory is can often be easily assessed during the interview, but specific questions and tests may be needed, especially in cases of organic brain damage where specific testing is called for. Remote, recent, and immediate memory require assessment.

Remote memory is assessed by asking the patient to recall important dates in the distant past, such as birthdays or anniversaries. The patient may not remember at all, or may give correct, false or distorted answers. It is important, therefore, to check answers against reliable information. The recall of well-known historical events is an alternative procedure for testing remote memory, but presupposes a level of information or education not necessarily related to memory. Evidence of selective impairment of memory must be recorded in detail.

Recent memory can be assessed by asking the person to recall the events of the last hour or days, provided the interviewer has the opportunity to check the replies for their veracity.

A simple test consists of giving the person a name, address and phone number to remember. It is important that the person repeat the test data at once, so that the interviewer is certain that they have been heard and registered. The interview is then allowed to proceed. The patient is asked to recall the name, address and phone number, first after three, then after five minutes. Recall may be correct, absent or distorted, and the patient may be aware or unaware of any mistakes. Confabulation is said to exist when a person makes up answers to fill the gaps in his memory.

Immediate memory can be tested best by the *Digit Span.* Sets of digits, starting with three digits, are read to the patient one at a time. Each digit is pronounced clearly, at a regular rate. The patient is then asked to repeat the set aloud. When a mistake is made, another set of identical length is given. Where a set is repeated correctly, longer sets are given. The test is stopped after a second failure in a set of any length. When the test has been performed in a forward direction, it is repeated backwards, starting always with the shortest set.

An appropriate response level is seven digits forwards, and five backwards. It is useful to remember that the digit span, correctly performed, is a reasonable measure of overall intelligence.

Another test is the number of repetitions required for the accurate reproduction of one of the Babcock sentences, e.g. "The one thing a nation needs in order to be rich and great, is a large secure supply of wood." The pattern of response is also observed, e.g. perseveration of error in organic cerebral deficit, marked variability of response in high tension states.

Intelligence. Intelligence is best assessed on the basis of the history, the level of general knowledge as well as the school and work record and performance. Accurate measurement of intelligence involves the administration of intelligence tests. The student should be familiar with and able to administer such well standardized tests as the Mill Hill Vocabulary Scale and the Raven Progressive Matrices. Simpler tests that can be given during an interview focus on a person's level of information, vocabulary and ability to handle concepts, as follows:

Information. The following information is requested:

Name five provincial or state capitals, or the capitals of five countries.
Name the present Prime Minister of Canada and his predecessor or the present President of the United States and his predecessor.
Give an account of the most important recent public events as reported in the news media.

Vocabulary. This may need to be assessed where communication difficulties exist on account of either retardation, brain damage or insufficient language skills. Select five words from a standard vocabulary scale and become familiar with the range of responses in relation to socio-economic and educational backgrounds.

Concepts. The capacity to reason abstractly is often disturbed in mental conditions, especially in the organic cerebral deficits and in the schizophrenias. The student is cautioned to remember in testing for disturbance in the capacity to reason abstractly, that broader issues such as mental subnormality, a severely limited educational background as may be seen in certain socio-economic groups, and efforts to speak in a second or new language, can produce responses that may appear to reflect impairment of this function. Testing should not be performed in a rote fashion that fails to be sensitive to the personal and social background of the patient. The capacity to reason abstractly is tested in two ways:

1. *Proverbs*—the interviewer asks the patient to give the meaning of one of the following proverbs:

a. A stitch in time saves nine
b. A rolling stone gathers no moss
c. People living in glass houses should not throw stones
d. The apple falls under its tree.

Where the patient is not familiar with one of these, he should be asked to produce a proverb from his own background which can then be interpreted. The relevance of the answers is noted as well as the degree of concreteness or abstractness.

2. *Similarities and differences*—the patient is asked to state in what way the following are similar or different:
a. orange and apple
b. wall and fence
c. child and dwarf
d. reward and punishment.

Judgment, Competence and Insight. The patient's own view of his difficulties matters in more than one way. Lack of insight may be one of the major signs of a serious psychiatric disorder, as in some psychoses, or in severe personality disorders. Such impairment may already have been noticed by relatives, friends or colleagues. It may also be observed during the interview. Lack of insight may have a profound influence on the patient's attitude to any treatment planning.

Impaired judgment can be assessed further by asking the person about his plans for the future. Standard questions to test judgment include "What would you do if you were in a theatre and you detected a fire?"

Competence to manage one's affairs presupposes good judgment. One would expect the person to be accurately informed about his assets and possessions as well as about his duties and obligations. In addition, in the managing of his affairs the person should not be under the influence of harmful or deleterious delusions.

THE EXAMINATION OF ORGANIC CEREBRAL DISORDER

In all cases of suspected organic brain disorder a full physical and neurological examination is an essential prelude to more detailed study of the intellectual functions. Remember that for the patient with an organic brain disorder awareness of a defect may be partial or quite incomplete. You may assume that the patient will tire mentally and you must be careful not to exaggerate the defect by too hurried testing. Nonetheless, the examination must be precise, for an early organic cerebral deficit may be missed by allowing the patient to evade the question, e.g. "Do you know where you are?" "Yes of course." "Right." Be sure to obtain a satisfactory response to each question.

Begin by determining the *level of consciousness*, noting especially minor fluctuations during testing or reported by informants or nursing staff. Clouding may be evidenced by moments of minor disorientation, impairment of attention and concentration spans, and impaired performance on tests of recent memory. Gross change with drowsiness or somnolence is easily recognized, but minor fluctuations may be missed and require a sensitive touch in the examination. As in subsequent testing of speech functions, record the stimulus (command) and the response so that subsequent change in the mental state may be measured. Remember that the level of consciousness varies between full clear consciousness with accurate relation to reality, through mild clouding, characteristic of the swimming head of a bad cold, to delirium, stupor or coma.

Next, inquire into defects in language function, noting that to the extent that a person cannot use language in the interpersonal relationship he cannot use language within his own mentation and so is proportionately demented. Language function may be quickly assessed by testing and recording data regarding each of the following:

1. Spontaneous speech
2. Comprehension of the spoken word
3. Comprehension of the written word
4. Ability to name objects
5. Ability to read spontaneously
6. Ability to write spontaneously
7. Ability to write to dictation
8. Left–right confusion
9. Ability to draw pictures that involve the parietal lobes.

Then examine memory functions, as in the earlier sections but in greater detail with particular attention to recent memory and learning ability. Nonverbal memory should also be tested by having the patient reproduce simple figures after an interval of a few minutes. For patients over sixty, these are best tested by assessing:

1. Memory for recent personal events
2. Memory for past personal events
3. General information regarding current events
4. General orientation measured by his capacity to learn his way in a new place, e.g. the hospital ward.

During testing, pay particular attention to such performance difficulties as undue fatigue, inability to sustain or shift attention, perseveration of error or response pattern, concreteness of response, and especially note any lability of affect or indication of the catastrophic reaction. This is a sudden explosive emotional response with an abrupt cessation at all efforts to complete the task, seen when a patient with an organic cerebral disorder is pressed past the limits of his mental ability. Note any evasiveness concealing a defect, awareness of and reaction to the defect, gross denial or absolute lack of insight into the defect. Regular assessment of these characteristics will permit the required assessment of competence on admission to a psychiatric facility.

THE EXAMINATION OF STUPOR

This can be a very complicated issue in differential diagnosis and requires meticulous detail in clinical examination. A full physical and neurological examination is obligatory, remembering that inaccessibility and unresponsiveness do not equate with unconsciousness. Many patients have been deeply hurt by inopportune remarks made during their being examined.

When such a diversity of conditions as catatonic stupor in schizophrenia, depressive (or its opposite manic) stupor in the affective disorders, a psychoneurotic dissociative reaction, a severe motor dysphasia, and severe metabolic disorders with intoxications are included, one can appreciate that no system of examination can be prescribed that will satisfy every case.

The emphasis must be upon a broad orientation to the possibilities of the differential diagnosis with careful attention paid to the nuances of the doctor-patient relationship during the performance of the physical and neurological examinations.

ENDING THE INTERVIEW

At the end of the interview, thank the patient and ask him if there are any matters that he is concerned with which have not been mentioned so far. The patient should also be given an opportunity to ask any questions and the interviewer should be prepared to answer without undue evasiveness. It is rare that the interviewer does not have a reasonably clear idea of the diagnosis at the end of the interview, as well as of any further steps to be taken. These should be explained to the patient in language he can understand.

Diagnosis. The information gathered and the understanding gained are harnessed to group the patient's complaints according to the principles of the International Classification of Diseases (ICD-8) or to the Diagnostic and Statistical Manual (DSM II).

Provisional Diagnosis. This represents the interviewer's diagnostic impression as of the moment. It allows for modification or change as the result of additional information, for example, when the results of special investigations become known, or when the patient is able to give further information.

Differential Diagnosis. Under this heading should be listed all other diagnostic categories which have been considered in the patient's case. Mention should be made of the reasons which support or rule out their inclusion. For example, it is insufficient to state that a diagnosis of paranoid schizophrenia was considered, but ruled out. Reasons for doing so must also be stated such as for example, the absence of delusions and of auditory hallucinations.

Further Investigations. Additional information may be required to reach a final diagnosis. This may entail the use of laboratory or psychological tests or of additional interviews with family members, friends or colleagues. Any of the procedures recommended should be mentioned here.

Formulation. This consists of a comprehensive explanation of why *this* patient is experiencing *these* particular difficulties at *this* time. The formulation takes into account biological, social and psychodynamic factors and attempts to define whether they play a predisposing, precipitating, or perpetuating role.

Treatment Plans. The major treatment modalities are psychological, social, and somatic. Under this heading, the interviewer explains not only which treatments appear indicated in this case, but also why they, and not others are appropriate. He should also set objectives for each treatment recommended. Without this, evaluation of case management becomes haphazard.

Prognosis. Under this heading the interviewer attempts to forecast the outcome of treatment and the time it will take to achieve the projected results.

FURTHER READINGS

Jaspers, K. (1963): *General Psychopathology.* Chicago, University of Chicago Press.
This large textbook contains extensive descriptions of the phenomena of disturbed mental functioning. It should be used as a reference text for deeper understanding of particular phenomena such as delusional experience.

Mayer-Gross, W., Slater, E., and Roth, M. (1969):*Clinical Psychiatry.* 3d ed. London, Cassell.
This standard clinical text contains a most satisfactory description of the major psychoses and of organic mental states as well as a very full account of the procedure of the examination of the mental state and the physical and neurological examination of the mentally ill person.

10

The Examination:
Physical and Special Investigations
Paul M. Cameron

THE APPROACH OF PSYCHIATRY TO
THE PHYSICAL EXAMINATION:
A Psychosocial View of the
Functional Inquiry

To every psychiatrist, knowledge about the physical health of all his patients is crucial. Different psychiatrists may choose to obtain this information in different ways. Some may prefer to conduct a general physical and/or neurological examination themselves while others may prefer to refer patients to trusted colleagues more familiar with this aspect of the overall examination.

The psychiatrist may gain much useful information about patients by conducting a full functional inquiry himself as he reviews all systems of the body with a broad psychosocial perspective.

Patient's Attitude to Past Illnesses and Present Health. While conducting a thorough history of past illnesses, one looks for the basic emotional response of the patient to the threat of ill health. Ask about how the patient felt during the prodrome, the acute illness, and the convalescence. Lipowski (1975 a) writes of the personal meaning of illness to patients—illness can be experienced as a loss, a threat to intactness, or in a symbolic way.

Patient's Attitude Toward Medical Personnel During Past and Present Illnesses. This part of the examination gives valuable

information about how this patient relates to doctors, nurses and other care giving helpers. Look for a pattern of receiving help while in a dependent or regressed situation. One may see what David Mechanic (1968) has labelled 'deviant illness behavior', i.e. noncompliance with medical treatment, forgetting to take medication, gross denial of illness, hypomanic states, or apparent indifference to serious illness.

Patient's Attitude Toward Family and Work During Illness and the Attitude of the Family to the Patient. Look for secondary gain from illness, that is, to the use that some patients make of their illness, namely, deriving satisfaction of some neurotic need. So, for example, the patient may enjoy the extra affection and sparing of demands of family so much that his recovery is postponed. Also look for significant changes in the organization of the family or occupational status or other environmental influences which are the result of the illness. A person who is losing grasp of adequate functioning in a job may use illness as an opportunity to deny or avoid his failing abilities.

A change in dominance or division of

labor may occur in a family so that a masochistic person may only be relieved of unreasonable burdens when he is "ill."

A husband may help in parenting only when the wife is ill. Then the wife may learn that when relief from the demands of mothering is needed, illness is the only route to obtain this relief.

Psychosocial Life Events as Precipitants of Illness. This is an active area of research in psychiatry and many stress scales are available (Holmes and Rahe, 1967). Death of a spouse, loss of job, moving one's home, for example, are major stressful events and often result in psychophysiological illness soon after the event. Look for this kind of pattern in the patient's life or in his family.

Pain as a Common Symptom Which Demonstrates These Issues. Headache, (Friedman, 1975) and chest pain (Billings, 1977), or abdominal or low back pain are all very common symptoms frequently elicited on functional inquiry. A psychosocial as well as a psychophysiological view of pain is crucial for complete understanding of the symptom.

One often finds a family history of painful illness in the same body area as is affected in the patient. Identification with the family member's pain may be part of the mechanism of pain for the patient. Where the patient has a complex emotional reaction to his pain, it is useful to explore the circumstances surrounding the painful illness of the family members as well.

The issues of the meaning of the pain, symbolic concerns of the organ system involved and secondary gain should be explored.

PHYSICAL EXAMINATION: Common Clinical Findings in Psychiatric Patients

General Appearance. In patients who appear much older than their stated age, one may discover signs of arteriosclerosis or presenile dementia. Often their skin color and skin turgor is that of very elderly patients, although they may be only middle aged.

Head and Neck. There are rare congenital defects seen in certain organic forms of mental illness of childhood, for example, cataracts, or ear and skull defects. Copper deposits in the cornea will point to Wilson's disease. Psychiatric disorder is often seen in patients with thyroid dysfunction, particularly in hypothyroidism.

Neurological System. Lipowski (1975 b) has written extensively about the interaction between neurological and psychiatric disease. Broad categories of presentations are: psychological presentation of neurological disease, such as a change in affective state, a change in personality, or a conversion symptom; or psychiatric complications of neurological disease, such as an organic brain syndrome, a reactive syndrome, or deviant illness behavior.

Close collaboration with a neurologist is crucial where symptoms of neurological and psychiatric disease co-exist or are suspected. Some of the most difficult areas for management are temporal lobe seizures or severe migraine headaches.

Respiratory System. General lowered resistance to respiratory infection is a common finding in neurotic patients. Asthma (French & Alexander, 1941; Knapp, 1969) is a frightening illness, especially in children and often is associated with overprotective parenting. Paying attention to the use of medication in respiratory illness is imperative as excessive use can often provoke secondary symptoms of anxiety or depression.

Gastrointestinal System. Patients with a history of duodenal ulcer (Mirsky, 1958), ulcerative colitis (Engel, 1955), or irritable bowel syndrome, often have an excessive preoccupation with food and weight. Symptoms in the gastrointestinal system are not infrequently associated with disorder of body image, obesity, or anorexia.

Close cooperation with an internist is advisable in severe gastrointestinal dysfunction, especially in conditions associated with blood loss. These patients are often aware of a pattern of psychosocial stress in connection with symptoms.

Endocrine System and Metabolic Disorder. In all depressed patients the physician should consider a potential dysfunction in pituitary, parathyroid, thyroid, pancreatic, adrenal, or gonadal function, for disorders in these functions are often associated with significant depression. With dysfunction of some of these glands, not only a picture of depression may occur, but also one of confusion and anxiety. Furthermore, weight problems and body image disturbances are common in patients with endocrine disorder.

Dermatological System. Skin disease is often visible and may restrict the comfort of the sufferer with respect to being seen when the illness is not under control. Psychosocial stress often exacerbates skin diseases. Depression and phobic behavior are common. The skin is also commonly a focus of hypochondriacal preoccupation.

Musculoskeletal System. Disorders often involve pain, loss of function and, in addition, suffering due to the psychological meaning of these symptoms. In very active, athletic people, such problems may be more of a threat than in more intellectual patients. Also a threat of unemployment often becomes a key issue here.

Hematological System. Disorders of blood or marrow or hepatosplenic tissue are often associated with fatigue, depression, and anxiety. Life threatening illness is common in this system confronting the patient with the psychological issues of death and dying.

Cardiovascular System. In hypertensive patients, one must look for both the psychological reaction to the illness as well as external stress factors which may exacerbate their medical problems.

Lipowski (1975 c) revised the evidence for the contribution of psychological factors to the pathogenesis of coronary heart disease, myocardial infarction, and cardiac arrhythmia.

Cardiac side effects of psychotropic drugs are well documented, for instance, arrhythmia and hypotension, and must be considered in all patients receiving these medications.

INVESTIGATIONS IN PSYCHIATRIC PATIENTS

The assessment of psychiatric patients in a general hospital will often involve certain investigations:

Neurological Investigation

Most psychiatric patients should be assessed with regard to the need for skull x-rays, and EEGs. Any patient who has headache or possible signs of organic brain syndrome must have these tests. The interpretations of skull x-rays, and such other complementary procedures as pneumoencephalogram, or EMI scan should be done by a radiologist, neurosurgeon, or neurologist.

The EEG is a record of the electrical activity of the cerebrum. In analyzing the EEG one may consider three major components:

(1) The individual waves are evaluated as to frequency, form, amplitude; (2) series of waves, i.e. rhythmic qualities are analyzed; (3) the location of waves are studied, especially comparison of differences of one hemisphere to the other side.

The cerebral electrical activity of a normal awake adult consists of moderate voltage sinusoidal waves occurring 8½–13 cycles per second. These waves occur in rhythmic series that form spindle patterns.

Frequency. Activity slower than 8 c.p.s.

is abnormal. Generalized slow wave activity is suggestive of diffuse organic disease.

Focal slow activity is indicative of localized organic disease.

Activity faster than 13 c.p.s. is abnormal. Generalized fast activity is seen in some drug intoxications. Focal fast activity is usually indicative of organic disease which may be epileptogenic.

Voltage. Low voltage diffuse activity may be a manifestation of suppression of cerebral activity seen in *severe* cerebral disease. Low voltage of focal nature may be subdural hematoma. Very high voltage activity may precede seizure.

Spike Activity. Anterior temporal lobe spike activity is most commonly associated with psychomotor seizures. Other spike activity or spike wave activity usually indicates other forms of seizures.

Diagnostic Value in Organic Brain Disease. EEG patterns are not pathognomonic of specific disease with possibly the exception of petit mal epilepsy (3 c.p.s. spike and slow wave bilateral synchronous paroxysmal bursts).

Slow wave activity may be seen in tumor, vascular inflammatory disease, trauma, metabolic, toxic, and degenerative disease.

The EEG is of greatest value in diagnosing epilepsy.

EEG in Psychiatry. The EEG is currently of *relatively little aid* to the clinical psychiatrist. Specific EEG abnormalities do *not* correlate with specific illnesses. Research continues, however, and there may be useful approaches developed in the future.

Personality Disorder. Differences of opinion exist concerning the effectiveness of diagnosing personality disorders by the use of electroencephalography. European authors emphasize slow wave EEG abnormalities as evidence of immature development. Americans stress the association of 14 and 16 c.p.s. spike pattern (Gibbs & Gibbs) but this is disputed by many investigators.

Dennis Hill wrote a textbook on EEG in psychiatry. Abnormalities in EEG tend to be commoner as the population becomes more abnormal, particularly if the abnormality includes propensities for aggressive, explosive behavior.

In individuals selected for emotional stability EEG abnormality level is 5%:

In general population	15%
In neurotic population	26%
Aggressive psychopaths	65%
Murderers	73%
Murderers who were insane	86%

Anxiety causes a decrease in alpha rhythm (8 c.p.s.) and increase in low voltage fast activity. Obsessive neurotics have normal EEG as do people with psychosomatic disorder. Patients suffering from hysterical disorder have immature recordings.

Schizophrenia—EEG characteristics of schizophrenia are variable. Most have a normal EEG. However, 30–40% have an abnormal EEG. Sleep EEGs can be different in stages of the illness.

Some techniques will be mentioned for the use of electroencephalography in research only so those interested may pursue the references. The sedation threshold may differentiate endogenous from reactive depression.

Evoked potentials are being studied in all populations, retarded, neurotic, and psychotic. Depth electrode studies have been completed in schizophrenia and temporal lobe epilepsy.

In summary, the EEG is most useful in ruling out organic illness, epilepsy, and the troublesome borderline condition of temporal lobe epilepsy. It may have promise in the future through research.

Investigations of Patients Receiving Psychoactive Medication

Patients receiving psychotropic drugs should be examined for potential side effects.

Hematological. The blood picture (especially the white cell count) should be checked especially if symptoms of chronic infection or an acute infection which does not respond to treatment occur. Anemia should be considered in all patients who present with fatigue, depression and weight loss.

Renal. Renal disease can be the result of analgesic abuse for chronic pain problems. Lithium carbonate may produce renal dysfunction.

Ophthalmological. Patients receiving phenothiazines should be examined annually. Pigmentation of retina, and lens opacities have been reported. Mellaril is a particularly common drug to produce irreversible pigmentation of the retina in doses in excess of 400 mg per day.

Cardiovascular. Postural hypotension, hypertension and arrhythmia may occur with psychoactive drugs.

Metabolic. With lithium therapy in particular, special attention must be paid to electrolyte balance and the function of the thyroid.

INDICATIONS FOR FULL EXAMINATION OF PATIENTS WITH PSYCHOSOCIAL AND PSYCHOLOGICAL COMPLAINTS

Psychiatrists working in general hospitals routinely conduct a full functional inquiry, a full physical examination, and order investigations on all patients admitted to their units as well as on many outpatients. Sometimes psychiatrists who practise a subspecialty such as behavior therapy, psychoanalysis, or family therapy will assume that the patient has been assessed properly by the referring physician, prior to referral.

The author's rule of thumb is as follows: Do a full functional inquiry on *all* patients during the initial one or two visits. Then decide whether there is a need to examine and investigate one or more systems again (e.g. in headache, examine neurological, cardiovascular and endocrine systems). If

symptoms persist or change in quality over the next month, ensure that a full examination is done by a qualified family practitioner or specialist. This rule could be used or slightly modified by a non-psychiatric physician.

It is important to *always* consider that many diseases are known to present with psychological symptoms (especially depression and/or confusion) before the physiological symptoms become apparent.

Also when symptoms are puzzling, it is *not* safe to assume they are psychogenic; in fact, often when they are puzzling to psychiatrists too, masked or atypical presentations of organic disease are detected.

In short, the physician must consider the possibility that physiological illness may underlie all psychological complaints and also be aware of side effects of psychotropic drugs when treating psychiatric illness.

REFERENCES

Engel, G. L. (1955): Studies of ulcerative colitis: the nature of the psychologic processes. *Am. J. Med.* 19:231.

Freedman, A., Kaplan, H., Sadock, B. (1975): *Comprehensive Textbook of Psychiatry.* Baltimore, Williams and Wilkins.

French, T. M., and Alexander, F. (1941): *Psychogenic Factors in Bronchial Asthma.* Washington, D.C., National Research Council.

Friedman, A. P. (1975): Headaches. In *Comprehensive Textbook of Psychiatry.* Edited by A. Freedman, H. Kaplan, and B. Sadock. Baltimore, Williams and Wilkins.

Gibbs, E. L. and Gibbs, F. A. (1951): Electroencephalographic evidence of thalamic and hypothalamic epilepsy. *Neurology.* 1:136.

Holmes, T. H. and Rahe, R. H. (1967): The Social Readjustment Rating Scale. *J. Psychosom. Res.* 11:213.

Knapp, P. H. (1969): The asthmatic and his environment. *J. Nerv. And Ment. Dis.* 149:133.

Levene, D. K. (1977): *Chest Pain: An Integrated Diagnostic Approach.* Philadelphia, Lea & Febiger.

Lipowski, Z. J. (1975a): Physical illness: the patient and his environment. In *American Handbook of Psychiatry,* 2nd ed. Edited by S. Arieti. New York, Basic Books.

Lipowski, Z. J. (1975b): Psychiatric liaison with neurology and neurosurgery. In *Consultation-Liaison Psychiatry.* Edited by R. Pasnau. New York, Grune and Stratton.

Lipowski, Z. J. (1975c): Psychophysiological cardiovascular disorders. In *Comprehensive Textbook of Psychiatry*. Edited by A. Freedman, H. Kaplan, and B. Sadock. Baltimore, Williams and Wilkins.

Mechanic, D. (1968): *Medical Sociology*. New York, Free Press.

Mirsky, I. A. (1958): Physiologic, psychologic and social determinants in the etiology of duodenal ulcer. *Am. J. Dig. Dis.* 3:285.

Slater, E., Roth, M. (1969): *Clinical Psychiatry*. London, Bailliere, Tindall.

FURTHER READINGS

Arieti, S. (1975): *American Handbook of Psychiatry*, 2nd ed. New York, Basic Books.

This large volume is devoted to current data and theoretical concepts which describe complex interactions between physiological and psychological processes. The reader may select any disease process and read about the psychosocial aspects of this condition.

Melzack, R. (1973): *The Puzzle of Pain*. New York, Basic Books.

This short clearly written book describes pain from many points of view. It is the most commonly quoted single book about trying to understand pain mechanisms. The author is an excellent teacher and his writing is most useful in the field of psychophysiology.

Kaplan, H. I. (1975): Psychophysiological disorders. In *Textbook of Psychiatry*. Edited by A. Freedman, H. Kaplan, and B. Sadock. Baltimore, Williams and Wilkins.

This detailed account of psychosomatic medicine and the theories which explain the relationship between psychological and physiological mechanisms is complementary to the first reference. Although there are many similar classical references, the chapters, written by different authors, provide not only different points of emphasis, but new information.

11

The Examination: Psychological Testing

Gerald Shugar

When a physician first engages a psychiatric patient, he begins a process of defining complaints, concerns and problems which have brought the patient to him. He next undertakes an etiological survey, exploring the links between these presenting complaints, the patient's life situation, his personality and forces acting on it—biological, psychological, interpersonal or sociocultural. This investigation ultimately leads to a plan of management. The primary investigational tool is the physician's carefully taken history and his clinical skills. However, he will often wish to supplement or extend his own findings by ordering special investigations. One of the most useful is testing by a clinical psychologist.

A clinical psychologist is a licensed professional with a broadly based education in scientific methodology, sociology and human development, thinking, feeling, perception and behavior. Psychologists have special training and experience in selection, administration, scoring and interpretation of psychological tests. However, physicians in general and practising psychiatrists in particular should be familiar with the range of tests, their usefulness in individual cases and their validity and reliability.

Psychological tests are specialized assessment procedures based on a subject's responses to objective and standardized tasks. These may involve such tasks as answering personality questionnaires, completing unfinished sentences, interpreting ambiguous pictures or doing mathematical calculations. Some tests are designed to elicit very specific information about a limited area of functioning, e.g. reading level. Others attempt to sample more global phenomena, such as personality organization, unconscious conflicts, or interpersonal relationships.

Tests with specific aims usually require factual answers which permit numerical scoring and objective analysis. They include self-report inventories, aptitude tests and achievement tests. Tests which attempt to assess less objective issues—personality traits, structure and dynamics, attitudes, motivation or emotion—require specialized scoring and interpretation. These rely more heavily on the interpreter's art, skill, intuition, and clinical judgement.

Most tests, whatever their specific intention, provide clues about malingering. The manner in which the subject handles tasks in general may reveal considerable information about his personality to the skilled, practised observer.

Any physician who employs specialized tests will make best use of them only if he is informed about them. The following questions can usefully be asked about each psychological test. The answers can be found in standard textbooks. Exposure to the test can be gained by seeking permission from a psychologist to observe him administering them.

These are the questions to be answered:

1. What is the theoretical basis of this test?
2. Does it purport to measure a specific function, e.g. memory, or a general function, e.g. personality?
3. How was the test evolved, and by whom?
4. What materials are used, how is the test organized, and administered? What tasks must the subject perform, and how much time is taken?
5. How is the test scored?
6. How are the test data interpreted? How much of the interpretation is subjective and how much objective?
7. On what population was the test standardized and to what group does it apply?
8. What is the test's reliability, that is, does it achieve consistent results when repeated?
9. What is the test's validity, that is, does it actually measure what it purports to measure?
10. How relevant and useful are the results of this particular test?

Answering these questions about the various tests mentioned here will give the student a comfortable familiarity with the most frequently used and most useful psychological tests.

WHAT TYPES OF TESTS ARE USED?

Intelligence Tests

The most commonly used intelligence tests are the Wechsler Adult Intelligence Scale (W.A.I.S.) and Wechsler Intelligence Scale for children (W.I.S.C.). They measure basic intellectual capacity, and problem solving ability. They contain a number of discrete subtests which assess verbal and performance skills. They may contribute as well to detecting organicity or psychotic functioning.

This report substantiated a borderline I.Q. in a patient who presented with Atypical Schizophrenic symptomatology:

> "Intelligence testing using the WAIS indicated that Mr. M. is currently functioning in the borderline range, full scale I.Q. 74. Verbal abilities were in the dull normal range whereas performance scores were markedly lower in the defective range."

Tests for Organic Brain Dysfunction

Although results suggestive of organicity may be found on many psychological tests, there are, as well, specific tests for CNS inpairment. The Bender Visual Motor Gestalt Test assesses perceptual-motor coordination by requiring the subject to copy geometric designs. It can indicate brain damage. Special tests are available which, in expert hands, help to localize organicity, e.g. the Reitan battery, which consists of many subtests.

An 18 year old girl was referred for assessment of possible impairment due to brain damage following an automobile accident. She was doing poorly in school and was having difficulties with concentration and memory:

> "The results of the assessment clearly indicate intellectual and cognitive impairment attributable to brain damage. On the WAIS, Ruth performs to the dull-normal range of general intelligence (Verbal I.Q. 86, Performance I.Q. 93, Full Scale I.Q. 88). Her performance is quite variable, with impairment

in all areas of ability, including concentration and attention. The impairment is most severe, indeed almost catastrophic, in memory functioning. She is unaware of the most elementary aspects of general information.

Common sense judgement is impaired. She is simply unable to recall recent events, and has similar problems with remote memory. The assessment does indicate that visual-motor abilities are relatively intact. Perception seems unimpaired, and motor speed is adequate. However, when visual-motor functioning includes a memory component, significant difficulty is noted.

On the basis of present functioning and capacity Ruth cannot be expected to progress further in the normal high school situation. Her vocational choices will be limited to routine work, involving manual skills. Any training or work involving judgement, recall or learning of novel tasks will not be feasible unless there is considerable recovery from her present level. Ruth requires some counselling and feedback about her problems, and should be directed towards nonacademic pursuits.''

Projective Tests

In these tests the subject's underlying attitudes, feelings and needs emerge in response to ambiguous visual or verbal material. Conclusions can be drawn about personality structure, dynamics and conflicts. Among the most common tests are the Rorschach ink blots, sentence completion tests and the Thematic Apperception Test in which the subject sets stories to scenes pictured on cards. Their use is surrounded by controversy. In skilled hands they seem to yield useful clinical information, but recent research has cast some doubt on their objective value.

This is an excerpt from a report which correctly anticipated the development of a schizophrenic illness in a young man:

"The alternate, more malignant possibility is that Mr. M. is suffering from a schizophrenic disorder which is more than just the extreme form of unrelieved panic and confusion which he manifests. As evidence of this possibility, his first response on the *Rorschach* was sexual and inappropriate,

suggesting a schizophrenic disinhibition of impulses. His percepts were fluid, his thinking during the testing was confused and he suffered from sudden qualitative changes. There were several examples of idiosyncratic, symbolic thinking and numerous examples of loss of control sometimes resulting in bizarre content.''

Personality Inventories

These are self report questionnaires that detect particular categories of symptoms. The responses are scored to produce a personality profile. The Minnesota Multiphasic Personality Inventory (M.M.P.I.) is commonly used. It has a number of subscales and conclusions are drawn from the profile of responses revealed by the subject rather than from one single score.

This report, based on projective tests and personality inventories, helped differentiate a severe personality problem from a suspected psychotic illness.

"Results of personality testing are not indicative of a psychotic process. The most prominent features are rigidity, perseveration, constriction and concreteness. His inability to speculate on the Rorschach—to go beyond form in giving response determinants—highlight his rigid control, flatness and difficulty coping with ambiguity. Ambiguity arouses serious anxiety and he must constantly seek structure. Generally he has problems dealing appropriately with emotionally laden events, and the resultant anxiety typically is dealt with by denial, guardedness, and emotional withdrawal. As a result, spontaneity is lacking and capacity for relationships is limited. On the self report tests he does express concern about the implications of his illness and some continuing concerns about his limited academic and vocational success.''

Aptitude, Skills and Interest Tests

These are used in vocational assessment and counselling. The Strong Vocational Interest Blank assesses preferences for particular types of activities.

REFERRAL TO THE PSYCHOLOGIST

Clinicians refer patients for psychological testing to supplement and extend their clinical evaluations. In a few medical and psychiatric settings, all patients receive routine batteries which may include a brief intelligence test, e.g. a partial W.A.I.S., a personality inventory, e.g. M.M.P.I., and an unstructured or projective personality test, e.g. a Sentence Completion Test. Individual clinicians vary widely in the use they make of psychological testing, based on their training, theoretical orientation and the availability of competent psychologists. Some refer rarely for help with important and specific questions. Others refer virtually every case accepted into psychotherapy for an opinion regarding psychodynamics, conflict areas, ego functions and defensive operations.

When referring a patient to a psychologist, it is best to have one or more specific questions in mind. Ask these questions, but also tell the psychologist what problems or concerns have led you to ask them. Refer early in the assessment process, when answers to your questions are most likely to influence management decisions.

You can expect to receive information which will usefully supplement your clinical impression in the following areas:

1. What is this patient's intellectual capacity?
   Sample questions:
   "Is this patient retarded? Will he respond to a given rehabilitation program?" "Is his illness significantly impairing the use of his full potential?" "This child is falling behind his class. Does he have some learning deficit?"
2. Is there evidence of central nervous system pathology, acute or chronic?
   Sample questions:
   "He has undergone a progressive deterioration in function following a severe concussion one year ago. Are there signs of neurological deficit? Can it be localized?" "He has confusional symptoms for which I can find no obvious cause. Please let me know if you can find signs of C.N.S. damage."
3. "Can you describe areas of significant conflict in this patient's personality?"
4. "Can you assess this patient's personality and offer an opinion about his potential dangerousness in society?"
5. "Can you test this patient's aptitudes and interests and contribute to his career planning?"

In usual practice, the physician makes his questions as specific as possible, and the psychologist suggests the appropriate tests. His report is more likely to meet your needs if you make them explicit and if you provide him with baseline data about your patient. This should include name, age, sex, education, familial and occupational status, presenting problems and circumstances, your diagnosis and tentative treatment plans. Any treatment or condition which may interfere with testing, e.g. E.C.T., should be mentioned.

Search out one or two clinical psychologists with whom you can develop a working relationship. It is most helpful if they know where, how and with whom you work, and if their orientation complements yours. After you discuss your referral with the psychologist, you should prepare your patient so that misconceptions will not impede or undermine the test sessions. He should know that you are referring him in order to obtain information which will help you in treating him. He should not confuse psychological tests with classroom tests which he may pass or fail. He can expect to spend three to four hours and to be asked to do a number of different tests. Generally, the psychologist will not discuss the results with him, but will forward his report to you.

The psychologist will interview the patient and, based on your requirements, will select a number of appropriate tests which he will administer in a standardized fashion. He will score these tests, interpret them and draw conclusions from his interview and the integrated test results. He will send you a typed report containing the date of examination, the tests he used, and the patient's behavior and responses to the interview and the test situation. He will report the actual results of the tests used, and, finally, he will integrate these results to offer conclusions, recommendations and speculations in response to your questions. His conclusions may raise significant issues which you had not asked about. It may be difficult for you to know how strongly held the opinions expressed are, and it is often useful, where there is doubt, to discuss with the psychologist the basis of the conclusions he has drawn.

ADVANTAGES AND LIMITATIONS OF PSYCHOLOGICAL TESTS

Psychological tests should not be used as a substitute for careful clinical examination, but they can usefully supplement it. They may help with differential diagnosis, for example, where a patient's psychopathology appears to border on two syndromes. Occasionally more serious pathology will be revealed in a person who appears relatively well on the surface. Testing is clearly useful when one requires extensive information about a very specific area, e.g. memory impairment in an alcoholic patient. Psychological testing can also provide a rapid, broad survey of the patient's personality, his symptoms and psychopathology, suggesting specific areas for further detailed clinical study. Some clinicians use testing by a particularly talented psychologist as a second clinical opinion for difficult or problematic patients.

However, psychological tests are far from perfect tools. Broad conclusions drawn from a limited sample of behavior are subject to inaccuracy. At times it is difficult to differentiate factual from speculative statements. Tests of general personality functions are subject to both inspired and faulty interpretation. Any test which focuses on the individual subject will tend to underemphasize and underreport significant life circumstances. Lastly, psychological tests are poor predictors of suicide, homicide, or impulsive acts.

Clearly, the more familiar the physician is with the tests and their appropriate applications, the more useful they will be to him in his clinical practice.

FURTHER READINGS

Anastasi, A. (1968): *Psychological Testing*. 3d. ed. London, Macmillan.

Korchin, S. J. (1976): *Modern Clinical Psychology*. New York, Basic Books.

Goldenberg, H. (1975): *Contemporary Clinical Psychology*. Monterey, Cal., Brooks/Cole.

CHAPTER 12

The Examination: Formulation

Paul M. Cameron and Stephen A. Kline

A formulation is an hypothesis which integrates the relative importance of known biological, psychological and social factors that may contribute to the development of the patient's personality. An effective formulation must include a variety of perspectives. Phenomenology, the collection of historical data, and psychodynamic exploration are all essential to the formulation.

The diverse schools of psychiatry have polarized the approach to patients, often leading to the exclusion of relevant data. Several approaches to formulation have been suggested elsewhere, but these tend to bias the process of data selection into one of four major conceptual models: medical, psychological, behavioral, and social.

The approach to formulation that is suggested in this chapter consists of the following steps:

(1) a longitudinal data collection (history), (2) a descriptive cross-sectional evaluation (mental status examination), (3) an integrative evaluation including differential diagnosis, (4) a tentative prognosis.

These techniques have been described in detail in other chapters. We would like to focus on how the physician integrates the information he collects into an hypothesis which may help us understand and treat the patient. The following paragraphs comment briefly on the steps that make up a formulation.

Introduction. In one or two sentences, describe the patient, the illness or problem, and why this patient seeks assistance at this time.

Biological Considerations. These should be divided where possible into predisposing, precipitating or perpetuating factors. State explicitly if no biological factors have been elicited. [For a detailed description of these concepts see Kline and Cameron (1978).]

Psychosocial Considerations. Comment on the following aspects of the patient's condition:

1. Psychodynamic
   a. conflicts, defenses, and coping mechanisms.
   b. strengths and weaknesses.
   c. characteristic patterns of relationships with both men and women.
2. Social—important family and peer relations, as well as other significant social influences (community, cultural, religious).

3. Phenomenological—extract important findings from the mental status examination. Attempt to link these phenomena with the underlying biological, psychodynamic and social factors elicited in the history.

Construction of the Hypothesis. Seek internal connections between and within the biological and psychosocial areas. In simpler terms, past experiences may be linked to current difficulties, e.g. early losses can contribute to depression in an adult.

EXAMPLE OF AN INITIAL FORMULATION

The following pages give a sample initial formulation. Then the initial formulation is analyzed, and a sample reformulation is given. Since a formulation is an hypothesis. it should be evaluated and reformulated as necessary.

B is a 20 year old married Canadian female clerical worker who was referred by her obstetrician for unresolving depression in the post-partum period.

In June, three months before referral for therapy, she gave birth to a boy. In the ninth month of the pregnancy she began to feel depressed and during the post-partum period she was "upset", anorexic, insomniac, tremulous and feeling as if she were in a "bad dream." She felt guilty because she did not love her baby and did not even want to see him on the first day after the delivery.

Her mental status examination was characterized by subjective and objective depression, with passive suicidal ideation, and a phobia of trains. She had hypnagogic visual hallucinations for the first six months related to an uncle who committed suicide, but these ceased.

There is a history of suicide in the family. A cousin overdosed after repeated attempts connected with depression secondary to chronic disease.

The patient's milestones were normal, there were no childhood neurotic traits, her early object relations were satisfactory. Her socialization in latency and throughout adolescence was adequate and her adjustment to and performance in school was above average. She suffered one major loss at the age of 15 when she was in an accident in which a close girlfriend was killed by a train. This had had a tremendous impact on B, for she has a residual train phobia and thinks of the accident almost every day. This manifests as a fear of dying and a concomitant "live for today" attitude.

The end of the highschool period was the next stressful period. B and her mother were fighting a lot and she was trying to grapple with questions of identity. At this time, she seriously considered committing suicide and almost took an overdose, but resisted. In addition, she married for "all the wrong reasons"—to get out of the house, uncertainty regarding her future and because her family expected it.

Indeed, her marriage is one of her biggest problems at present. She does not love her husband and regards him as a burden who places unfulfillable expectations on her and yet who cannot keep up with her in terms of intellectual or physical activity.

A recurrent theme with the patient is "living up to other people's expectations." Her mother, with whom she maintains quite strong, yet ambivalent, ties, is the prime identified source of friction. As a critic of her desire to live "independently" and freely, mother is the focus of much hostility. In addition, family dynamics are confusing for B.

She knows that her father always wanted a son. Her two older sisters were and still are tomboys who went hunting, flying and fishing with father in order to gain his attention and affection. Even now, B can only talk to him about business, politics, science, or finance. Simultaneously, mother demands a decidedly feminine role for approval, and negatively reinforces any deviation from the housewife role.

Hence, the patient's conflict is around dependency needs and drives to autonomy. Her conscience instills guilt. The stress of social expectations and hostile impulses tax her ego, which is not helped by conflicting contradictory figures for identification. The result is anxiety, which the patient cannot effectively handle. She also represses and introjects her anger, which leads to signs and symptoms of depressive neurosis. And although she attempts to cover it by denial and rationalization, she has never really completed the adolescent task of emancipating herself from the family.

Set in this background, the precipitating factor seems to have been the birth of the baby. Delivery may have reactivated the conflict because the child represented the part of her which despises a feminine role. Or identification with the baby, secondary to unresolved dependency needs, may have led the patient to fear the same angry, greedy attitude from it, that she herself feels toward her mother. Hence, she must reject him, which in turn brings on guilt.

The patient's impaired functioning is manifesting as an identity crisis and marital discord. Her resources of intelligence, capacity for mastery and synthesis and ability to sublimate allow her to carry on in the sphere of work and play, but the last leads to a self-destructive pattern of avoidance and her repression and introjection leave her depressed.

Being young, psychologically-minded, capable of introspection, and well-motivated with a basically intact ego, B should be a good candidate for individual psychotherapy. The opportunity to ventilate and release her affect, as well as to explore her problems from a dynamic perspective should help her resolve her anxieties and result in a good prognosis.

If the vegetative accompaniments of her depression worsen or continue unabated, she may benefit from an adjunctive course of antidepressant medication at some point.

DISCUSSION AND REFORMULATION

Introduction. The introduction is clear and direct.

Comprehensiveness. The formulation is comprehensive in that it considers all areas of data. The abstraction, inferences, and integrative steps, however, are organized too loosely. The discussion of the sequence: external expectation, internal identifications, conflict, defenses, affective problems, could have been clearer. It could have been coupled with a description of B's losses and of the overall quality of her relationship with the therapist.

Biological Considerations. The discussion of milestones of her family history or affective disorder and suicide are good.

Psychosocial Considerations. PSYCHO-DYNAMIC. The formulation covers the most important areas. More continuity is needed in the developing of themes; for example, B's sensitivity to loss and her confusion about her identity. The defen-

sive operations which B uses to deny or avoid dependence in her object relations should be examined.

PHENOMENOLOGY. This area is well covered except for the relationship between B and the therapist.

Abstraction and Integration. This is quite a wide-scope formulation which shows skills in looking at historical information, interpersonal relations, family dynamics, and phenomenology. These observations are related to the intrapsychic concepts of defenses, conflicts, and identification. The formulation needs improvement in regard to showing the interrelationships between B's object losses, her dependency problems, and the quality of her relationships with others. The following sample reformulation shows how those defects can be corrected.

B is a 20 year old married Canadian female clerical worker who was referred by her obstetrician for sustained depression in the post-partum period.

Predisposing biological factors include a paternal first cousin who committed suicide after repeated episodic depressions. The particular precipitating event seems to have been the birth of her son, for prior to the pregnancy she was essentially asymptomatic, but since then she has been significantly impaired by depressed affect.

Dynamically, the patient's conflict is around dependency needs. Due to moves at the age of 13 and again at 16, she lost all her close friends, and at the age of 15 her best girlfriend was killed in a train accident. Thus sensitized, she has been trying to deny and avoid intimacy in relationships for fear of further disappointment. This she does by displacement, intellectualization and rationalization.

In addition, she suffers from identity confusion. She knows that her father always wanted a son, but instead he had four girls, of which the patient is the third. Her two older sisters have always been tomboys, and the only important men in her life have been either strong and distant (father), or weak and passive (husband). Her mother, on the other hand, has always expected her to be traditionally feminine. The patient's present relationship with her mother is characterized by strong, yet ambivalent ties.

The patient has adopted primarily masculine identifications, and has developed a driving quest for independence, which can really be seen as a defense against symbiotic ties, especially with mother. Her relationships as a whole tend to emphasize distance, attempts to isolate affect and preoccupation with mastery, competence and cognitive achievement. This mode of interaction applies to her relationship to the therapist as well.

There remain hostile impulses towards her parents, secondary to the pressure of their differing social expectations. B deals with these by repression and introjection of anger, which leads to anxiety and depression.

Her marriage is a contributing problem in the social sphere. Her husband whom she met and married before she could complete her emancipation from her family, burdens her with what she feels are unfulfillable expectations—primarily to be a devoted housewife. As a bright driving woman who is a competitive, ambitious, determined career person, she feels inhibited by his passivity and dependency on her. The situation is further complicated by the presence of her infant, who places further demands on her, and whom she therefore finds difficult to love.

Phenomenologically B demonstrated subjective and objective depression, with insomnia, anorexia, fatigue, decreased libido and menstrual irregularity. She had crying spells and occasional passive suicidal ideation. She also has a train phobia.

B's identity confusion may have led her to a premature choice of marital partner. All her present object relations are characterized by fear of dependence (fear of loss), and compensatory strivings for autonomy, which manifest as a rather obsessive emphasis on achievement and competence.

The birth of her baby has re-activated the conflict and upset the equilibrium because he represents her own unresolved dependencies, and places further demands on her in reality.

In the short term, the patient's basically intact ego should allow her to cope with the converging stresses. In the long term, her youth, capability for introspection, anxiety as a motivating force, and facility at verbalizing in therapy should reflect a favorable potential for change and readjustment. Her symptoms are not so severe that suicide is a threat, and her excellent vocational placement should also aid continuation of therapy.

The formulation is a complex task directed toward understanding a patient's psychological problems.

The crucial portion of the formulation is the *construction of the hypothesis.* The set with which the clinician approaches the interview is altered by the knowledge that he must formulate.

In addition, the process of formulation enables the clinician to select a treatment plan which is tailored to the individual patient.

FURTHER READINGS

Coleman, Jules, V. (1967): Social factors influencing the development and containment of psychiatric symptoms. In *Mental Illness and Social Processes.* Edited by T. J. Scheff. New York, Harper and Row.

Committee on Child Psychiatry (1966): Psychopathological disorders in childhood. In *Theoretical Consideration and a Proposed Classification. Group for Advancement of Psychiatry, Report No. 62,* 6:293.

Dewald, Paul A. (1967): Therapeutic evaluation and potential: the psychodynamic point of view. *Compr. Psychiatry* 8:284.

Feighner, John P., et al. (1972): Diagnostic criteria for use in psychiatric research. *Arch. Gen. Psychiatry* 26:57.

Gill, M., Newman, R., Redlich, R. (1954): *The Initial Interview in Psychiatric Practice.* New York, International Universities Press.

Kline, S., Cameron, P. M. (1978): Formulation. *Can. Psychiatric. Assn. J.* 23:39.

13

Common Psychiatric Disorders: Introduction

David M. Berger

Systems of classification attempt to group signs and symptoms into "units," or diagnostic categories, that demonstrate uniformity in their course, prognosis, and etiology. Their ultimate purpose is to arrive at discrete therapeutic interventions. In psychiatry, classification is based primarily on symptoms and secondarily on established causes. The latter refers especially to the organic brain disorders. A diagnosis is founded on the presence of a prominent symptom or symptoms, although it is understood that the disturbance in mental functioning pervades the individual's personality, interpersonal relationships, and social functioning. Often more than one diagnosis is necessary to present a more complete psychological picture of a patient (e.g., depressive reaction with an organic brain syndrome, involutional melancholia in an obsessive compulsive personality). A patient shares some characteristics with all human beings, some with members of his diagnostic class only, and still others—his unique characteristics—with no other patients. Diagnosis is a useful way to summarize the characteristics he shares with the members of a class at a given time (Rosen and Gregory, 1966).

Unfortunately in a given patient, the prominent symptoms may vary from time to time, so that a patient diagnosed as manic depressive on one occasion may on another be diagnosed as schizophrenic. As well, some patients simply do not fit neatly into categories such as phobic disorder or schizophrenia. Even when the clinical picture is stable and there is general agreement about the criteria of a given diagnosis clinicians may disagree on difficult cases due to differences in perception of actual pathology (Katz, Cole and Lowery, 1969).

In the light of these uncertainties and as more information and more sophisticated tools become available, classification systems are regularly being revised. Perplexing as this may be to the student of "syndrome psychiatry," he must realize that the classification of mental disorders is not as fixed, stable, or as universally agreed upon, as it may appear to be in a textbook. Some psychiatrists have even suggested that psychological symptoms do not lend themselves to categorization but are best viewed as fitting along a continuum, or as "reactions" (i.e., final common pathways reflecting a multiplicity of etiologies, the way in which "fever" is viewed in physical medicine).

In the longer standing classificatory systems, emotional disorders of *functional* origin (i.e., those which have no known physical causation) are grouped mainly within three broad categories: the neuroses, the psychoses, and the personality disorders. These terms merit discussion because they tell us something about the general characteristics of the syndromes grouped under their umbrella, and because they remain in general usage (anxiety disorder is often referred to as anxiety neurosis, manic depressive illness is often referred to as manic depressive psychosis).

The terms neurosis, psychoneurosis and neurotic reaction are used interchangeably. The syndromes within this subgroup include anxiety reaction, phobic disorder, obsessive compulsive disorder, conversion reaction, dissociative states, and the less severe depressive disturbances. The term neurosis refers to a functional emotional disorder characterized by experienced emotional pain (e.g., anxiety, disturbing fears and rituals) and is less severe than a psychosis.

The person suffering from a psychosis exhibits a disintegration of personality of considerably greater magnitude than the patient with a neurosis. For the psychotic, there is defective appreciation of reality, and confusion about the boundaries between the self and the outside world (e.g., the belief that one's inner thoughts have caused a certain news item to appear on the radio). The syndromes classified as psychoses include manic depressive illness, schizophrenia, involutional melancholia, and the paranoid states.

A patient diagnosed with the label, personality disorder, does not exhibit the disintegration of a psychotic. Compared with a neurotic, the person with a personality disorder does not present, relatively speaking, with an overt identifiable symptom, (e.g., subjective emotional pain) but rather with a constellation of maladaptive behavior patterns which are most apparent in interpersonal relations. The continuum of maladaptive behavior patterns ranges from distressing obsessional traits to compulsive criminal behavior and severe drug addiction. The distinction between a neurosis and a personality disorder however, is not a clear one. Indeed one may evolve from the other. An individual who has been compulsive all his life—neat, fussy, excessively orderly, and so forth—may one day develop a clinically identifiable and crippling compulsion (e.g., an elaborate handwashing ritual that interferes with daily functioning). This would be an example of an obsessive compulsive *neurosis* evolving from an obsessive compulsive *personality*.

In a personality disorder, the behavioral patterns are regarded by the individual as ego syntonic (i.e., as consonant and compatible with his sense of self). If the patient described above decides to seek help prior to the onset of the crippling compulsion, it would likely be on the basis of interpersonal difficulties. He might, for example, be distressed that others become easily irritated with him, or that he has difficulty establishing intimate relationships. In a neurosis, the symptoms, in this case, the excessive handwashing ritual, are regarded by the individual as ego alien (i.e., as incompatible with his sense of self). The latter individual might come to a physician complaining "I am not being myself." Because his appreciation of reality is not defective, the neurotic is aware that his mental functioning is disturbed.

Presently in the United States, an attempt is being made to revise the major groupings of psychiatric disorders and to define more accurately the characteristics of each syndrome. The changes include the abandonment of the broad categories neurosis and psychosis (this would bring the depressive disorders, whether of neurotic or psychotic severity, closer together under a subgroup), and the grouping together under the heading of anxiety disorders, those disorders in which anxiety is directly felt (e.g., anxiety disorder, phobic disorder) or secondarily experienced when the patient attempts to control his symptoms (e.g., obsessive compulsive reaction). Conversion reactions are felt to fit better within a separate subgroup associated with somatization, and dissociative states, conditions in which anxiety has been felt to play a role but is often not apparent, have been assigned a separate category. Whether this new nomenclature will bear fruit heuristically and therapeutically is presently uncertain; as with all nomenclatures, it is not meant to be a final and definitive nosological system but only a step along the path towards a better understanding of mental illness.

REFERENCES

Katz, M. M., Cole, J. O. and Lowery, H. A. (1969): Studies of the diagnostic process: the influence of symptom perception, past experience and ethnic background on diagnostic decisions. *Amer. J. of Psychiatry* 125:937.

Rosen, E., and Gregory, I. (1966): *Abnormal Psychology*. Philadelphia, W. B. Saunders.

FURTHER READINGS

American Psychiatric Association (1968): *Diagnostic and Statistical Manual of Mental Disorders*. 2d ed. Washington, D.C., American Psychiatric Association.

This provides a quick and easy-to-read overview of psychiatric classification and capsule descriptions of the major syndromes.

Spitzer, R. L., Sheeky, M., and Endicott, J. (1977): DSM III: Guiding Principles. In *Psychiatric Diagnosis*. Edited by V. M. Rakoff, H. C. Stancer and H. B. Kedward. New York, Brunner/Maxel.

Problems and issues pertaining to psychiatric classification are discussed by three psychiatrists mainly responsible for revising and changing the American classificatory system.

14

Anxiety and
Anxiety Related Disorders*

David M. Berger

The term anxiety is used to refer to (1) the anxiety that is part of everyday experience. Such anxiety is not severe or pervasive and it is not necessarily detrimental to one's ability to think and act. (2) The anxiety that is psychopathological. Such anxiety is usually severe and detrimental to one's ability to think and act. (3) A concept that is central to psychoanalysis. The three uses of the term anxiety are discussed in the following paragraphs.

ANXIETY AS AN EVERYDAY OCCURRENCE

The anxiety that is a part of everyday experience is usually mild. It is experienced by everyone, and it has both psychological and physiological components. In tolerable amounts it helps one to cope. The person who is anxious feels fear or an emotion closely related to fear, such as dread, panic, or alarm. The anxiety is unpleasant and "future oriented;" that is the person feels a threat of some kind, an impending danger.

*I am grateful to Dr. M. Rapp for his helpful comments on the learning theory point of view.

The physiological component of the anxiety includes some disturbances of physical function that are under voluntary control (for example, the person may feel an urge to run in panic, to scream, or to defecate) and some disturbances that are partially or completely under autonomic control (for example, the person may have a dry mouth, he may perspire, or he may experience tremors). These reactions vary from person to person. Thus one person may have tremors as the predominant physiological disturbance whereas another person may experience palpitations.

ANXIETY AS A PSYCHOPATHOLOGICAL CONDITION

Anxiety that is a psychopathological condition contains the features of the anxiety described above but is more severe and pervasive, and it is maladaptive. The person affected feels threatened, but either no observable threat exists or the danger is out of proportion to the distress that it evokes. Such anxiety may be a symptom accompanying any psychiatric syndrome. *Anxi-*

ety disorder refers to a syndrome in which the chief symptom is anxiety.

ANXIETY AS A PSYCHOANALYTIC CONCEPT

In psychoanalytic theory, the term anxiety refers to anxiety that may be unfelt, or unconscious. The person affected responds to the unconscious anxiety by warding if off, using one or more mental mechanisms to repress or control it. Unconscious anxiety may develop in the following way. An adult is faced with an event or a situation that threatens to arouse a wish he had repressed as a child because he felt the wish was unacceptable. Unconsciously he mobilizes defenses to ward off the arousal of this wish, because its arousal would cause him anxiety. The warding off may consist of a quantitative change in the person's usual character defenses (e.g., if he is compulsive, he may become more compulsive) and/or the appearance of a symptom (e.g., he may develop a phobia). This theory of the role of anxiety in the development of symptoms is supported by phenomena observed in the psychoanalytic setting; for example, a person suffering from a troubling symptom (such as a compulsion) but denying that he feels anxiety, may have an anxiety attack when the symptom is removed during treatment.

ANXIETY DISORDER

The person who has an anxiety disorder complains chiefly of an anxious overconcern and of recurring episodes of severe anxiety. The anxiety may begin suddenly or gradually. Often the patient also has somatic complaints. His anxiety is excessive, painful, unrealistic, and maladaptive. It is more pervasive and less restricted to specific situations or objects than is the anxiety of the person with a phobia. The anxiety is not related to a physical illness. The person may have symptoms other than anxiety but these are less prominent and less severe; the anxiety that accompanies a psychosis or an organic brain syndrome is not categorized as an anxiety disorder.

As a consequence or as a concomitant of anxiety, the person experiences a change in his sense of self, his view of the world, and his relations with others. He may feel unable to make decisions and to cope with his day to day life. He may have feelings of shame, guilt, or inadequacy. Often he is worried about his physical health. For example, the person with "cardiac neurosis" (Da Costa's syndrome) has chest pains and he suspects that he has heart disease.

The hyperventilation that occurs in some persons with anxiety can lead to respiratory alkalosis and other symptoms may appear, such as lightheadedness, numbness of the extremities and muscle twitching.

The person with an anxiety disorder may have a low tolerance for frustration and a tendency to view the world as threatening. He may find intimacy stressful and often this feeling is associated with sexual conflicts.

Incidence of Anxiety Disorders

Anxiety disorders are common. They occur in 10 to 15% of the people who consult cardiologists and in 27% of the people who consult general practitioners. Six to 27% of psychiatric outpatients have anxiety disorders. Studies suggest that among the people who are being treated by general practitioners, about 65% of those with anxiety disorders are women, whereas among the people who are being treated by psychiatrists about as many men as women have anxiety disorders.

Anxiety disorders occur mainly in young adults; the usual age of onset is from 16 to 40 years of age. Anxiety that first appears when the person is older is often associated with a depression (Marks and Lader, 1973).

Causes of Anxiety Disorders

The etiology of anxiety disorders is both *multi-determined* (that is, biologic, psychological or social factors may be causal agents) and *multi-dimensional* (that is, the factors may predispose the person to the anxiety disorder, may precipitate or perpetuate the disorder, or may influence the person's symptom choice; that is, his unconscious choice of an anxiety disorder rather than a phobia). Thus a biological factor, heredity, may predispose a person to a high level of anxiety. If that person then experienced emotional trauma, a psychological factor, the trauma might precipitate an anxiety attack. If the same person is then given a pension, a social factor, because he has an emotional disability, being given the pension might perpetuate his condition.

In regard to the etiology of anxiety disorders, it is not known whether the various neuroses should be studied together or separately. Is there, for example, a hereditary disposition towards all neuroses? If this is so, it would make the problem of symptom choice (that is, why one patient suffers an anxiety disorder and another a phobia), a secondary, albeit important issue.

Biological Determinants of Anxiety Disorders. In one study of monozygotic twins, the correlation coefficient for the degree of neuroticism was shown to be 0.85; in dizygotic twins it was shown to be 0.22 (Eysenck and Prell, 1951). This study did not separate the various neuroses. The data suggest that heredity is involved in neurosis, but how it is involved is not clear.

Studies of the somatic factors in anxiety disorders have shown that sympathetic and parasympathetic activity is increased in some people with anxiety disorders. A distinction has been made between high anxiety and low anxiety subjects in a general population. People who are anxious have been shown to respond pathognomonically with a drop in their systolic blood pressure to an injection of mecholyl. In some people, an infusion of lactate brought on an anxiety attack. This finding has led to the postulation that people who are anxious have an excessive production of lactate after they exercise, although this hypothesis has been disputed (Ackerman and Sachar, 1974). The effect of adrenergic blocking agents on the autonomic symptoms of anxiety is presently being studied.

Psychoanalytic Theory. In psychoanalytic theory, the progression of events that lead to a neurosis is described as follows. In his early childhood, the neurotic or anxious adult had repressed a conflict related to both the lack of satisfaction of a "forbidden" wish and the expectation, real or imagined, that his parents would punish him for harboring that wish. The person repressed the wish because he may have had a fear of abandonment (separation anxiety) or of physical punishment (castration anxiety) or because he had feelings of guilt or shame (superego anxiety). During that person's adult life, an anxiety attack is precipitated when an event or a new situation occurs that threatens to arouse the forbidden wish in a real or symbolic way.

> A single woman in her early 20's consulted a psychiatrist because of anxiety, hyperventilation attacks, and chest pains. The year before, her mother had died of a heart attack. Before her mother's death, the patient had lived away from home. After her mother's death, she moved back home, ostensibly to care for her father. In therapy, it was discovered that her anxiety was related to a wish she had had as a child to have her father to herself. She had repressed the wish because she had feared her mother's disapproval. Her mother's death and the patient's move back home created a situation that aroused both the wish and its prohibition. This led to anxiety. The prohibition or "mother's wrath" appeared symbolically in the chest pains. The patient feared that she too would die of a heart attack.

It is thought that neurotic symptoms have several functions. They attempt to manage and diminish anxiety. In the case of the woman just described, the chest pain did not manage the anxiety entirely successfully. The anxiety associated with this new symptom was considerable. Neurotic symptoms may also be symbolic; indirectly and metaphorically they may reveal something about a repressed conflict. The psychoanalytic model suggests that there is a dynamic equilibrium in the unconscious. When a new situation such as the mother's death and the move back home to the father disrupts an old equilibrium (the repression of the infantile conflict), a new equilibrium (new defenses and new symptoms, such as the chest pain) is established. The new symptom, the chest pain, contains elements of both the infantile wish and its prohibition. The wish is evident in the fact that the chest pains allowed the woman to remain with her father. The prohibition of the wish is evident in the patient's concern about having heart disease and dying.

Neurotic symptoms may also provide secondary gain (i.e., advantage accruing from the neurosis that is secondary to the original illness); the chest pains allowed the patient to be dependent on her father.

Learning Theory. Conditioned reflex theorists regard anxiety as an unconditioned inherent response of the organism to a painful or a dangerous external stimulus. Through conditioning, such a response can be attached to a stimulus that originally was neutral, such as being in the parents' home. An apparently innocent stimulus can become a source of intense anxiety because of its learned association with distressing or painful feelings. However learning theorists rely not only on stimulus-response but also on a variety of "sociolearning" concepts, "cognitive learning" or "social modelling" models to explain how maladaptive learning may occur. According to these models, the person imitates important figures in his environment, and he aspires to social norms of behavior in the wider environment. From such learning, he may derive ideas about

proper behavior and about roles. According to this model, the woman's self concept in the case described above is an essential factor. She returned home to care for her father, perhaps because she perceived herself as inadequate and not able to function on her own. She looked on her return home as a defeat, and the breakdown of her idea of herself as a strong independent person gave rise to anxiety.

Learning theory provides a model for understanding how neurotic symptoms are formed, and it provides a rationale for treating certain disorders (e.g., phobias). Learning theory is less helpful in explaining the origin of neurotic anxiety; but then learning theory is less concerned with causes than with a direct "behavioral attack" on symptoms.

Social Factors. Social upheaval may precipitate the development of anxiety disorders. In times of economic distress, the number of psychiatric patients treated in clinics increases. Anxiety may be "communicable"; so-called epidemics of anxiety in girls' boarding schools have been reported. The nature as well as the incidence of neurotic symptoms varies considerably from culture to culture and era to era. It has been suggested that symptom choice depends to some degree on how culturally acceptable a particular symptom is. In Western culture, anxiety disorders are most prevalent in people in the middle socio-economic groups (Hollingshead and Redlich, 1958).

Treatment of Anxiety Disorders

Anxiolytic medication and relaxation techniques may be used to diminish anxiety. If a focus for the anxiety can be discerned, progressive desensitization techniques can be used.

The goal of psychoanalytic psychotherapy is to bring unconscious conflicts to the patient's awareness. These conflicts cannot simply be pointed out to the patient. Intellectual awareness without at least an element of the affective component does not cure the patient. Since the patient continually wards off the affective component of his illness, the therapist must continually point out the defenses that the patient uses to accomplish the warding off. Once the patient gains insight into his disorder, the effect of the conflict on his current symptoms and behavior is diminished.

PHOBIAS

Phobia refers to the persistent expectation of panic some people have when they meet a situation or object considered by most people to be safe or harmless. The phobic person knows that his fear is unrealistic, but he still tries to avoid the situation or object. If he does encounter it, he has an attack of severe anxiety.

The phobic person will often restrict his activities. When he is in the company of someone he trusts, his phobia may diminish or disappear; hence the phobic person often becomes dependent and helpless. Phobias usually begin suddenly and they may become generalized. For example, a phobia may begin as an irrational fear of ascending a staircase and then expand to include a fear of elevators.

The term phobia refers to either a symptom or a syndrome. As a symptom, a phobia can be a concomitant of other psychologic disorders, such as schizophrenia or organic brain syndrome. In the syndrome labelled phobic disorder or phobic neurosis, the major symptom is a phobia. If other symptoms are present, they are neurotic, not psychotic. Phobias sometimes occur in conjunction with obsessions and feelings of depersonalization.

A phobia can usually be distinguished from an obsessive-compulsive idea. In a phobia, the fantasied danger is seen as coming from an external source *towards* the phobic person. Thus he may perceive animals, open spaces, or heights, for example, as threatening. He can diminish his anxiety by avoiding the situation he fears. In an obsessive-compulsive idea, the direction of the fantasied injury is reversed—namely, the obsessive is usually concerned that *he* will harm *others.* He has trouble escaping the persistent and forceful intrusion of the idea into his consciousness. He often feels the need to make reparation to undo the fantasied harm.

There are however a number of symptoms which seem to fall between obsessive ideas and phobias. A phobia of knives can be associated with fear of actively doing harm. A fear of dirt suggests that the person fears being harmed by an external agent, yet this fear may have the persistence and forcefulness of an obsession, which in turn may generate compensatory symptoms such as repetitive rituals aimed at diminishing the obsessive fear (e.g., compulsive behavior, such as the repetitive washing of hands).

The major difference between a phobia and an obsessive-compulsive idea is that in a phobia the person must avoid something in order to ward off his anxiety, whereas in an obsession, the person must do and/or think something to ward off his anxiety.

In a paradoxic response to phobic terror, a person may exhibit a persistent need to engage in activities that are dangerous; for example, sky diving, and stock car racing. Such behavior is termed counterphobic. The counterphobic person denies that he has any fears, and he exhibits a persistent need to engage in dangerous activities.

Incidence of Phobias

The incidence of mild phobia is 76.9 per thousand people and severe phobia, 2.2 per thousand people. The incidence of common fears is high in childhood; it is lower in young adult life, except for fears about death, injury, illness, separation, and crowds. Mild phobias occur more often in men than in women (Agras and Oliveau, 1969).

Causes of Phobias

The etiology of functional disorders is both multidetermined and multidimensional. In regard to phobias the following causative factors are particularly relevant.

Trauma. A frightening experience may become a nidus for an excessive conditioned phobic reaction—suggesting a behavioral model—anxiety is attached by conditioning to a stimulus that originally was neutral. It is not known, however, whether a trauma is a necessary determinant of a phobia. Sometimes a phobia appears immediately after a frightening experience. At other times there is a symptom-free interval of weeks, months, even years, between the frightening experience and the onset of the phobia. But often the phobia cannot be traced to a frightening experience at all. Even when it is known that a trauma has preceded a phobia it is not clear whether the trauma predisposed the person to the phobic disorder, precipitated the development of the phobia, or secondarily affected symptom choice in a person who would have suffered a neurosis anyhow.

Psychoanalytic Theory. According to psychoanalytic theory, a person forms a symptom in response to a new situation in which he feels a threat that an unconscious forbidden infantile wish will be aroused. The person adopts the phobic symptoms in an attempt to establish a new dynamic equilibrium of his unconscious forces. As a "compromise formation," the phobic symptom contains in disguised form symbolic representations of both the repressed wish and its prohibition. It helps to re-repress the conflict by displacing anxiety on to an external situation, which the person can then avoid. The person may become more dependent (secondary gain). It is not understood why a person resorts to one group of symptoms, (e.g., a phobia) to ward off anxiety rather than to another group of symptoms (e.g., an obsessive-compulsive idea).

Though it was not her chief complaint, a young woman in therapy was discovered to experience anxiety at the sight of a kite. Her free associations in therapy led her to recall that ten years before she had had a brief, stormy relationship with a man who was an avid kite flyer. The man was associated in the patient's unconscious with a younger brother, whom she had had to take care of when she was a child. She had envied and hated her brother because, she thought, her parents had preferred him to her. In the patient's dreams about kites, they appeared elongated, suggesting a phallus. It became apparent during therapy that the woman's feelings towards her brother had been generalized to include all men and that the phallus had become the major symbolic representation of these feelings. As a child, she had repressed her hostility towards her brother because she feared her parents' censure. When as an adult she became involved with men the conflict was aroused once more. She had displaced the attendant anxiety and translated it symbolically into a fear of kites.

Treatment of Phobias

Psychoanalytic psychotherapy attempts to remove a phobia by bringing the unconscious conflict to the patient's awareness. As mentioned psychoanalytic psychotherapy is a cooperative venture, one in which the patient and the therapist sift through dreams, free associations, affects, behavior patterns, and timelinks between events and the exacerbation of symptoms to arrive at an understanding of the phobia.

Behavior theorists point out that once a phobia develops, it is perpetuated by the phobic person's avoidance of the object he fears. In the woman just described, avoiding kites brought on a pleasurable sensation, relief from anxiety. The phobic person comes to perceive avoidance itself as rewarding, and the avoidance positively reinforces the phobia and maintains the symptom. Behavior therapy is directed at the "maintaining" cause—the avoidance. A variety of techniques that make avoidance impossible (e.g., desensitization and flooding) have been effective in treating relatively healthy people who have one or two disabling phobias. Generally, the more specific the phobia, the healthier the person appears to be otherwise, and the less the person has to gain from being ill (i.e., secondary gain) the more successful is the behavioral approach.

Anxiolytic medication may improve the phobic symptom by diminishing the underlying anxiety.

OBSESSIVE-COMPULSIVE DISORDERS

Obsessions and compulsions usually occur together, although when they do, one may be more prominent than the other.

An obsession is an idea or a thought that obtrudes itself persistently into one's consciousness. A compulsion is an impulse to action, and a compulsive act is the action that derives from the impulse. The obsessive idea and the compulsive impulse and action are ego alien. The person who has an obsession or compulsion realizes that it is absurd and he finds it unacceptable. Yet he cannot control it. When he tries to resist it, he cannot, and it persists.

A mild or transient obsession or compulsion, a common phenomenon, should be differentiated from a symptom that interferes with a person's functioning. The term obsessive-compulsive can refer to a symptom that occurs as part of another disorder (e.g., schizophrenia or organic brain syndrome) or to a syndrome (obsessive-compulsive disorder). In the syndrome, the most prominent symptom is an obsession or a compulsion or both. Other neurotic symptoms may be present, but they are less prominent.

In general, the person with an obsessive-compulsive disorder has a persistent fear that he may harm himself or others and he feels that he must ward off this possibility by performing reparative actions. The unacceptable idea contains an element of omnipotence. For example, a

person might express the idea that if he does not wash himself every hour, he might spread disease throughout the country. Touching and washing rituals are common compulsive acts. Doubting, ambivalence, and excessive ruminations are special forms of obsessive-compulsive symptoms. The person is often paralyzed because he cannot make decisions. This inability stems from his need to balance each impulse with a counter measure. The need to balance exists because the person perceives his impulses as harmful.

> A young girl developed a persistent fear that her mother might die while the girl was away at school. To ward off this obsessive thought, the girl developed a countermeasure—on her way to school each day she touched trees compulsively. The girl's obsessive thought had changed. If she touched trees on her way to school, her mother would not die while she was at school.

Personality Traits

The person with an obsessive-compulsive disorder often has a premorbid personality variously labelled "obsessional character," "anal personality," or "anancastic personality." Such a person is controlled and controlling, rigid, inflexible and cautious. He tends towards dryness and pedantry. He emphasizes logic at the expense of feeling. He may have secret "islands" of disorderliness. Such people tend to be cool and distant in their relationships with others. Acquaintances might describe them as being slow and sticky. Freud described obsessional characters as being perfectionistic, obstinate and parsimonious.

Obsessional character traits may be assets. They are pathological only when they interfere with the person's ability to function. Obsessional character traits are far more common than are obsessive-compulsive symptoms. Many people who have obsessional characters do not develop obsessive-compulsive symptoms.

Obsessive-compulsive symptoms do not always evolve from obsessional character traits.

Incidence

Obsessive-compulsive disorders occur in 1 to 2% of psychiatric outpatients. In about 65% of patients with obsessive-compulsive disorders, the disorder first appears before the age of 25, slightly earlier than the age of onset for other neuroses. In contrast to other neuroses, obsessive-compulsive disorders are found more often in people of the upper socio-economic groups and in people of superior intelligence. About 50% of the people who have obsessive-compulsive disorders do not marry.

Causes

Psychoanalytic Theory. Development of neurotic symptoms in general was discussed in the sections on anxiety disorders and phobias. Although symptom choice is not completely understood, it is somewhat better understood in the case of obsessive-compulsive disorders. In general, symptom choice is thought to be affected by the nature of the infantile wish, the childhood developmental period that the conflict is associated with, and the defenses the person uses to ward off the conflict.

Obsessive-compulsive symptoms are thought to stem from wishes and conflicts that belong to the period of toilet training (about the ages of 2 to 3 years). At that period, the conflict between a child and his parents often centers around control and aggression. This view of the derivation of obsessive-compulsive symptoms is consistent with the finding that these symptoms often focus on cleanliness and murderous impulses. Because of the relational difficulties the obsessive-compulsive person had with his parents during the period in which toilet training was a significant

event, he either became fixated at the anal phase of development (that is, his unconscious conflicts centered on wishes and prohibitions pertaining to the period of his toilet training) or he regressed to the period in which toilet training was a significant issue and abandoned the genital competitive impulses of the next phase of development.

An example of regression is provided by the obsessive-compulsive person with a handwashing ritual who could not tolerate wishes and fantasies about masturbation. To him, masturbation was associated with fears he had as a child about messiness and about damaging himself or others. He substituted for masturbation a handwashing ritual that symbolically retained both the wish to masturbate, in that the ritual was repetitive and urgent, and the prohibition against masturbation, in that the ritual led to cleanliness.

Such a person is in contrast to the phobic and the person with conversion symptoms, who use different defenses and whose repressed conflicts derive to a greater extent from the oral stage of development, not from the anal stage.

The major defense mechanisms of the obsessive-compulsive person—isolation, undoing, and reaction formation—are discussed in the following paragraphs.

ISOLATION. The defense mechanism known as isolation protects the obsessive-compulsive person from anxiety. Ordinarily a thought has both content and affect. When isolation occurs, the content is retained in consciousness but the affect is repressed. Thus the person is able to speak blandly about, for example, an impulse to commit murder. An obsession is, in fact, an idea that contains in a distorted form a repressed forbidden impulse that has been separated from its affect. The absence of affect permits the patient to disown the idea. Hence the obsessive idea is ego alien.

UNDOING. If the affect threatens to break through the isolation and connect with the idea (that is, if the "whole" repressed impulse threatens to become conscious) further defense mechanisms are required. In one of these mechanisms, undoing, the person performs a repetitive action that unconsciously undoes or repairs the imagined harm. Although the action is reparative, like other neurotic symptoms, it still contains an element of the forbidden wish.

REACTION FORMATION. Refers to manifest patterns of behavior and consciously experienced attitudes that are the opposite of the underlying impulses; for example, the obsessive-compulsive person may feel and show excessive concern about the person against whom he unconsciously harbors murderous wishes.

A 38-year-old dentist consulted a psychiatrist for treatment of a troubling compulsion. Every time the dentist turned on his drill, he felt impelled to tap it three times against a metal surface. The impulse and the act had begun three months after the death of the dentist's father. Before his father's death, the dentist had had fleeting ideas that his drill would slip and injure his patients. The ideas were bland and not too troubling, and since the dentist could hide them from others they did not affect his work or other relationships. At that point, by isolation, the dentist was able to ward off his repressed impulses towards sadism that stemmed from his childhood. The dentist had always been a slow meticulous worker, characteristics that demonstrate reaction formation. His excessive concern helped ward off his sadistic impulses. The tendency to be meticulous can be viewed as containing both sides of the conflict, the sadistic wish and its prohibition. The prohibition was contained in the dentist's overconcern; the sadistic wish, less apparent, was contained in his subjecting his patients to the discomfort of the dentist's chair longer than necessary.

It was discovered in therapy that the death of his father had aroused competitive feelings the dentist had felt towards his father in the genital period of his development (that is, the patient was about 4 or 5 years old). The death also aroused the guilt that had been associated with those competitive feelings. The competitive feelings were infused with issues of control and aggression that stemmed from the earlier anal phase of the dentist's development. The threat that these forbidden impulses and prohibitions might come to consciousness necessitated a shift in the dynamic equilibrium of his unconscious. The dentist's ideas about harming his patients became more forceful, his anxiety increased (his isolation defense was failing) and he became more and more meticulous to the point that he was almost incapacitated (he used reaction formation more and more to offset the increased urgency of the impulses). Finally he had to institute a secondary defense mechanism, undoing. Thus he tapped his drill three times on a metal surface. This new symptom was a compromise formation in that it symbolized both the aggressive act and its prohibition. Psychotherapy for the dentist concentrated on looking at how conflicts of control and aggression from the anal period had affected the genital competitive phase of development.

Other Causative Factors. Although electroencephalographic examination has revealed some neurophysiologic abnormalities in obsessive-compulsive people, the role of neurophysiologic factors is not fully understood. Also, it has been suggested that heredity is less important in obsessive-compulsive disorders than in anxiety disorders.

Learning theorists regard an obsession as a conditioned stimulus to anxiety. Because it becomes associated with an unconditioned anxiety provoking stimulus, the obsessive thought, originally neutral, arouses anxiety. They explain the development of a compulsion as follows. The compulsive person has discovered that a certain action diminishes the anxiety that is associated with an obsessive idea. The relief from anxiety that the action brings reinforces the action and leads to its repetition. Eventually the action becomes a fixed, learned response to anxiety of any kind.

Although there is a statistical correlation between the prevalence of obsessive-compulsive disorders and the prevalence of certain social factors (a high socioeconomic status, a superior intelligence, and a tendency to remain unmarried) social factors are not felt to be primary causative factors in the development of an obsessive-compulsive disorder.

Treatment of Obsessive-Compulsive Disorders

Treatment of obsessive compulsive disorders by psychotherapy has unique problems. The patient tends to intellectualize, doubt, and argue. Such behavior is an attempt to ward off the underlying anxiety and feelings, and to defend against gaining insight into the unconscious origins of conflict. Severe cases of obsessive-compulsive disorder have been treated with anxiolytic and antipsychotic medication, electroconvulsive therapy, and, when all else has failed, lobotomy.

REFERENCES

Ackerman, S. H. and Sachar, E. J. (1974): The lactate theory of anxiety: a review and re-evaluation. *Psychosom. Med.* 36:69.

Agras, S., Sylvester, D., and Oliveau, D. (1969): The epidemiology of common fears and phobias. *Compr. Psychiatry.* 10:151.

Brenner, C. (1973): *An Elementary Textbook of Psychoanalysis.* 2d ed. New York, International Universities Press.

Eysenck, H. A. and Prell, D. B. (1951): The inheritance of neuroticism. *J. Ment Sci.* 97:441.

Hollingshead, A. B. and Redlich, F. C. (1958): *Social Class and Mental Illness.* New York, J. Wiley.

Marks, I. and Lader, M. (1973): Anxiety states (anxiety neurosis): a review. *J. Nerv. Ment. Dis.* 156:3.

FURTHER READINGS

Freedman, A. M., Kaplan, H. I., and Sadock, B. J. eds., (1975): *Comprehensive Textbook of Psychiatry.* 2d ed. Baltimore, Williams and Wilkins.

A chapter in volume one provides an in-depth, albeit psychoanalytically slanted review of anxiety disorders.

Lewis, A. (1970): The ambiguous word anxiety. *Int. J. Psychiatry.* 9:62.

A scholarly review of the meanings of the term anxiety, historically and linguistically.

Marks, I. and Lader, M. (1973): Anxiety states (anxiety neurosis): a review. *J. Nerv. Ment. Dis.* 156:3.

A good overview from the British diagnostic point of view with an emphasis on epidemiology and genetic factors.

15
Dissociative Disorders and Depersonalization
David M. Berger

In the past, dissociative states and conversion reactions were sometimes listed together as hysteria or hysterical neurosis. At present, the inclination is to classify them as separate entities. In the proposed U.S. classification system DSM III, dissociative states will also be removed from the larger category "anxiety disorders" on the grounds that a person in a dissociative state experiences little conscious anxiety. However, many psychiatrists still feel that anxiety as an unconscious mechanism plays a role in the genesis of dissociative states.

Dissociative disorders are psychogenic conditions in which "alterations may occur in the patient's state of consciousness or in his identity, to produce such symptoms as amnesia, somnambulism, fugue, and multiple personalities." The dissociative disorders start and end abruptly, and are made up of a cluster of related mental events that the person cannot consciously recall but that can, under certain circumstances, return to the person's conscious awareness.

Dissociative states apparently occur spontaneously or after an emotional trauma. They may follow a head injury that is so slight that it seems insignificant physiologically, or a head injury that is so severe that it is difficult to separate the physiologic from the psychogenic components. It has been reported that dissociative states have followed electroconvulsive therapy, hypnosis, and even, in an early report, crystal ball gazing.

Though good statistical studies are lacking, most observers feel that dissociative disorders are rare.

KINDS OF DISSOCIATIVE DISORDERS

Dissociative disorders have been categorized according to the ways they manifest themselves. The clinical manifestations, however, do not always fit neatly into a single category. The following paragraphs discuss some of the common dissociative disorders.

Amnesia. Amnesia is the most common and least complex dissociative disorder, and all dissociative states contain, as a minimum, the features of amnesia. The person with amnesia is suddenly aware of a total loss of memory. The loss of memory

131

may be for a circumscribed period, as in localized amnesia, or for the person's whole life, as in generalized amnesia. The person with amnesia usually gives no indication to observers that anything is wrong. He appears alert. He is not, for example, in a trance, although at the onset of the amnesia, he might have a brief period of disorganization.

In rare instances, the person may be amnesic for only a specific event (such as the death of his child), or for a specific aspect of his mental functioning (e.g., amnesia after having read a book, or "automatic writing" in which the written content later seems foreign to the author).

Somnambulism. The patient who is somnambulistic exhibits an altered state of consciousness. He seems to be in a trance or a "zombie"-like state. He may seem upset, he may speak excitedly, or he may engage in repetitive behavior that seems to have meaning but that is hard to interpret. During the episode of somnambulism the person may be able to recall a past traumatic event vividly that he could not remember during his waking state. This fact suggests that the person in a somnambulistic episode is re-experiencing an earlier trauma that he normally represses. When the somnambulistic episode is over, the person does not remember it.

Fugue. The person in a fugue state exhibits purposeful wandering (e.g., to another part of town or even to another country)— as if he is looking for something. He does not seem to others to be in a trance or in any other unusual state. During the fugue, the person forgets his past, but he remembers it when he emerges from it. When he recovers, he is often in strange surroundings. He does not remember the fugue.

Multiple personalities. The person with multiple personalities is dominated by any one of two or more distinct personalities. Each personality is highly complex, fully integrated, and in itself, not odd or abnormal. The person's behavior, thoughts, and feelings are determined by the dominant personality. The person's transition from one personality to another is sudden. The person is usually amnesic for the nondominant personality or personalities. A nondominant personality may appear spontaneously, or during hypnosis or hypnotherapy, or after an emotional or physical trauma. The film *The Three Faces of Eve* and the television drama *Sybil* are based on case reports of women who exhibited multiple personalities.

CAUSES OF DISSOCIATIVE DISORDERS

Earlier explanations of these disorders were based on the similarity of dissociative states to the hypnotic trance. The induction of posthypnotic suggestion provides a model that parallels some of the features of dissociative disorders. For example, during an hypnotic trance, the subject may be told that the next day he will go to a store or hear a concert. On awakening, the person has forgotten the hypnotic suggestion, but the next day, he does as he was told, or he experiences a vivid sensory hallucination, as if he were in a somnambulistic or a fugue state. Unfortunately, the way hypnosis works is itself poorly understood.

Psychoanalysis has proposed as an explanation of dissociative disorders the mechanism of repression; namely, the removal of painful mental contents from the person's conscious awareness (Fenichel, 1945). The current explanations of dissociative disorders are based on psychoanalytic concepts. The repression of mental contents that is associated with amnesia and other manifestations of dissociative states is seen as a mechanism that protects the person from emotional pain that comes either from disturbing external circumstances or from the person's disturbing inner impulses and feelings. The amnesia of soldiers exposed to the trauma of battle is an example of the total repression of memories of a distressing event. It appears that in somnambulism, a previously repressed trauma has become conscious during the dissociative state but at the cost of the person's having to forget his usual self.

It has been noted that fugue is sometimes related to a person's search for a lost parent. This observation suggests that the fugue is a breaking through of a wish that the person represses when he is awake (Stengel, 1941).

In the person who has multiple personalities, an impulse that he usually represses or behavior that he normally controls often emerges as a feature of the new personality. The example that is often cited is that of the prim schoolteacher who during a dissociative state acts in an erotic manner.

THE PSYCHOANALYTIC THEORY OF SYMPTOM CHOICE

Freud recognized that a splitting off from consciousness of painful feelings and the associated ideas was the basic process in the various dissociative states. It was Freud's view that in obsessions and phobias the affect became separated from the painful idea and was displaced to a neutral (painless) idea, or to a neutral external situation, and that in conversion, the affect was converted into physical symptoms. The clinical symptoms of dissociation, he felt, represented the effect the splitting had on the personality as a whole. It is still not understood why a person resorts to one set of mechanisms rather than another.

TREATMENT OF DISSOCIATIVE DISORDERS

Psychoanalytic psychotherapy, aimed at diminishing the conflict underlying the dissociative disorder, attempts to achieve a better integration of the personality. Special techniques, such as narcosynthesis and hypnosis have been used to relieve symptoms of dissociative disorders rapidly.

DIFFERENTIAL DIAGNOSIS

Organic brain syndrome. It is often difficult to distinguish a dissociative state from an organic brain syndrome, especially when the person has had a severe head injury. Signs of organic brain dysfunction and abnormal physiological findings, such as those found by electroencephalographic examination, point to the presence of an organic brain syndrome.

Epileptic fugue. The twilight states associated with the ictal and post-ictal periods of an epileptic seizure and with petit mal can be mistaken for a dissociative state. In epilepsy, there appears to be a diffuse impairment of those mechanisms that are central to discriminative consciousness. When no focal signs of epilepsy are present, the diagnosis must be based on the electroencephalographic findings.

Schizophrenia. Although the labels schizophrenia and dissociative disorder both imply a splitting of the mind, and although the two disorders are sometimes hard to distinguish from each other, certain features set them apart. In the dissociative disorders, the splitting results in two or more *integrated* states or personalities. Each state has an internal consistency. In schizophrenia, the split is "molecular" rather than " molar;" there is disintegration of the personality rather than separation into two or more integrated and consonant states. For example, the thoughts the schizophrenic patient expresses may not be consonant with the feelings he expresses (e.g., he may laugh as he describes a tragic event) or he may express contradictory feelings only moments apart. Finally, the physician can communicate with and feel a sense of relatedness to a patient suffering from a dissociative disorder, whereas he often cannot communicate or empathize with a patient suffering from schizophrenia.

Childhood somnambulism. Although episodes of hysterical somnambulism may arise during sleep or waking, they are distinct from and unrelated to somnambulism in children. Somnambulism in children differs from hysterical somnambulism in that it is not necessarily pathological; it occurs during, and is associated with, stage 4 sleep; and it is poorly integrated and nonpurposeful.

DEPERSONALIZATION AND DEREALIZATION

Depersonalization and derealization usually occur together. In depersonalization, the person feels as if his body or a part of his body, or his personal self is strange or unreal. In derealization, the person feels as if the external world is unreal or strange. Variations in the clinical picture include déjà vu and the curious phenomenon of "doubling." In doubling, the person feels that his self is outside his body. Feelings of depersonalization and derealization usually begin suddenly. They are associated with anxiety and dizziness, and they may cause the person to think that he is going insane. Mild forms of depersonalization are common. DSM II recognizes a category labelled "depersonalization neurosis" but severe forms of these disorders are often associated with a psychosis. Depersonalization and derealization differ from dissociative states in their clinical manifestations, particularly in the fact that as the feelings of depersonalization and derealization occur, the patient is aware of them and feels pain and concern about them.

REFERENCES

Fenichel, O. (1945): Conversion. In *The Psychoanalytic Theory of Neurosis*. New York, Norton.
Stengel, E. (1941): On the aetiology of the fugue states. *J. Ment. Sci.* 87:572.

FURTHER READINGS

Kirschner, L. A. (1973): Dissociative reactions: an historical review and clinical study. *Acta Psychiatr. Scand.* 49:698.
Sargant, W., and Slater, E. (1941): Amnesic syndromes in war. *Proc. R. Soc. Med.* 34:757.
Stengel, E. (1941): On the aetiology of the fugue states. *J. Ment. Sci.* 87:572.
Taken together, the above three papers not only elaborate on our understanding of dissociative states but also illustrate three diverse approaches to the puzzling elements of these phenomena: the first from the sociocultural roles point of view, the second from a diagnostic point of view, and the third from that of a perceptive psychologically minded clinician.

CHAPTER 16

Somatization, Conversion and Hypochondriasis
David M. Berger

SOMATIZATION

Somatization, a broad term, refers to a person's *tendency* to experience, conceptualize, and/or communicate psychological states or psychological conflicts as physical sensations, functional changes, or somatic metaphors (Lipowski, 1968). To the extent that a physical or bodily complaint—whether it is a physical pain, a change in motor or sensory function, or an exacerbation of an actual medical illness—is felt to be a result of, or associated with psychological factors, it is a type of somatization. Somatization refers not to a syndrome, a symptom or a specific mechanism, but encompasses all those mechanisms by which psychological stress is translated into physical illness or bodily complaints.

The following are types of somatization phenomena:

1. Physiological changes accompanying emotions (e.g., the palpitations and sweating of anxiety and the anorexia and insomnia of depression).

2. Conversion symptoms or somatic changes that are symbolic representations of ideas.

3. Manifestations of illness that are described by the psychosomatic-somatopsychic model. Although biological factors must be present in a physical illness, psychological factors can affect the course and prognosis of an illness. The psychosomatic-somatopsychic model considers the effects psychological events have on the pituitary-adrenal axis and the autonomic nervous system. Physical changes lead to psychological changes; psychological changes affect the pituitary adrenal axis, leading to further physical changes, and so on.

4. Hypochondriasis, or an excessive preoccupation with normal or abnormal physical sensations and functions. Hypochondriasis includes nosophobia, a morbid dread of illness.

5. Somatic delusions, or fixed beliefs about one's body. Somatic delusions occur in schizophrenia, paranoia, psychotic depression, dementia, and

delirium. The delusions are usually bizarre (for example, the belief that one's organs are melting, that insects are crawling under one's skin, or that one's genitals are missing).

6. Malingering, or a conscious simulation of illness, especially in settings in which there is an obvious gain to being ill. The physician treating the malingerer should realize that in most instances of malingering, complex issues in the patient's unconscious may have contributed to his simulating illness.

7. Chronic self harm, which includes a rare group of syndromes variously labelled Münchausen's syndrome, hospital addiction syndrome, and chronic factitious disease. The person affected goes from hospital to hospital, presenting dramatic symptoms that intrigue the physician. He willingly submits to painful diagnostic and therapeutic procedures. Even when there is evidence of self-inflicted injury the person denies having injured himself or having taken toxic agents. The person has a pathological need to lie, and although he seems to be aware that he is lying, he cannot stop.

8. Communication of emotional distress in somatic metaphors, which includes situations in which the mechanism is not clear. This kind of somatization may overlap with one of the types described in items 1 to 7. This category includes the "alexithymic" person who it is said does not express his feelings through words, gestures, and facial expressions, but through physical symptoms.

Often there is no clear division between the various types of somatization, nor are they mutually exclusive. In many instances the mechanism is not clear. Each case of somatization must be studied indi-vidually. For example, psychosomatic-somatopsychic factors are more prominent in some illnesses, such as asthma, and less prominent in others, such as renal tumors. Moreover, in some patients with asthma, for example, psychological factors acting on the pituitary-adrenal axis, in the psychosomatic-somatopsychic model, affect the course of the asthma. In other patients with asthma, that seems not to be the case. In yet other patients with asthma, the respiratory symptoms have taken on the symbolic representation of the patient's unconscious impulses; their asthma is a conversion mechanism.

CONVERSION DISORDERS

Conversion disorders and dissociative disorders were at one time considered a form of hysteria. The loosely used term hysteria referred to a poorly defined syndrome of certain personality traits, such as flamboyance, emotional lability and sexual provocativeness; and to certain disorders (conversion reactions, dissociative states) felt to occur more often in individuals with hysterical personality traits. Hysteria was felt to be more common in women than in men. Although not associated with distinctive organic changes, hysteria was described as the great imitator of organic illness. The newer diagnostic systems tend to separate conversion disorders and dissociative states from hysteria and to classify those personality traits once associated with hysteria under the label "hysterical personality" (Berger, 1971).

A conversion symptom can occur as a concomitant of any psychiatric illness. The term conversion disorder refers to a syndrome which is described as a neurotic condition in which the patient complains chiefly of a conversion symptom or symptoms. It is defined as a syndrome in which "instead of being expressed consciously . . . . the conflict causing anxiety is 'converted' into functional symptoms in organs or parts of the body, usually those that are mainly under voluntary control. The symptoms serve to lessen conscious (felt) anxiety and ordinarily are symbolic of the underlying mental conflict . . . they are to be differentiated from psychophysiological autonomic and visceral disorders.''

This definition proposes a specific mechanism by which an emotional upset may lead to physical symptoms. As discussed, psychological problems may lead to physical symptoms in a variety of ways. The term conversion as used to describe a symptom implies that a mental conflict has been repressed and is expressed symbolically as a physical symptom. The following features suggest that the symptom has evolved by way of a conversion mechanism.

1. The symptom symbolically expresses a feeling conflict or forbidden wish. The body can express thoughts and feelings without words (for example, through dreams, pantomime, the game of charades). Verbal metaphors that use physical terms can also be used to express feelings (e.g., "I have a lump in my throat," and "thinking of that makes me sick to my stomach").

2. The symptom communicates to another person, real or imaginary, the person's distress and the nature of the hidden conflict.

3. The symptom has a model. The model for a conversion symptom is a physical sensation that the person experienced in the past or that he has observed in others (e.g., in his parents or in people he read about). To be a model, the sensation must be observable. Thus abdominal cramps may contribute to a mental representation that the person can use as a conversion metaphor, but an increase in the secretion of gastric acid, an unobservable phenomenon, cannot.

4. The symptom is multiply deter-

mined; that is, usually more than one event or mental representation causes the person to choose a symptom. For example, a patient who suffered from attacks of breathlessness had sat at the deathbed of her mother-in-law. The labored breathing of the dying woman was the immediate model for the patient's breathlessness. But in the past, the patient had had other significant experiences related to breathing: hearing the heavy breathing of her father when he was angry at her mother; hearing her parents breathing during sexual intercourse; holding her breath so that she would be better able to hear the sounds of intercourse, an experience that made the patient fear that she would not be able to breathe again; feeling suffocated when her father had held her during the administration of an anaesthetic for surgery; and inhaling the fragrance of her mother's bosom, a pleasant experience that had been coupled with the fear that she would be suffocated (Engel, 1970).

5. The symptom is precipitated by psychological stress. According to the psychoanalytic model, psychological stress may bring unconscious conflicts of forbidden wishes into one's consciousness. A new psychodynamic equilibrium is thus established that, in turn, leads to a conversion symptom. Because unconscious mechanisms, including repression, are at work, the patient does not connect his symptom with the psychological stress, nor does he regard his symptom as psychological in origin.

6. The symptom is reported ambivalently by the patient. He describes and displays the suffering and disability vividly; but also he may subtly display pleasure with and attachment to the symptom—La Belle Indifference. The term *"belle indifference"* refers to the patient's attitude towards his conversion symptom, not to his general mood.

7. The symptom is inconsistent with physical processes. The symptom is fashioned by the psychological needs of

the patient and not by anatomical factors. There are often inconsistencies in the anatomy and physiology of the symptom. The physical effects that should accompany the symptom are not present and the laboratory findings are negative. The clinical course of the illness is inconsistent with the course of the physical illness that it resembles.

8. The presence of hysterical traits and a history of conversion symptoms or multiple phobias suggest that the present complaint may be a conversion disorder.

9. The patient derives secondary gain from the symptom. In psychoanalytic theory, the primary gain refers to how well a person's conversion symptom symbolically expresses a repressed wish and keeps the underlying conflict from coming to the person's consciousness. The term secondary gain refers to the advantages the person gains from the illness itself. Any illness provides some gains for the ill person, but the person with conversion symptoms tries to gain as many privileges as possible from his illness; for example, as much attention, sympathy, or avoidance of responsibility as he can get.

The above features provide presumptive evidence that a particular symptom is caused mainly by a conversion mechanism. The symptom is proved to be a conversion disorder when the unconscious symbolic meaning of the symptom is discovered, for example, by psychotherapy or hypnosis, and the discovery has a significant effect on the symptom.

Features of a different nature suggest that a mechanism other than conversion plays a prominent role in a physical complaint deriving from a psychological conflict. In psychosomatic disorders, the somatization process is felt to be mediated by way of the pituitary-adrenal axis. The symptoms are felt not to require a mental representation; they do not have primary symbolic meaning, and do not primarily serve a specific psychological function. It follows that unlike conversion symptoms which are limited largely to organs connected to the voluntary motor and sensory nervous systems, including the special senses, psychosomatic disorders tend to be limited to organs innervated by the autonomic nervous system. Systems or organs can of course be innervated by both the voluntary and the autonomic nervous system, suggesting that the line of demarcation is not clear.

Clinical Manifestations of Conversion Disorders

The following are some of the clinical manifestations of conversion disorders:

Abnormal movements such as gross rhythmic tremors of the hands and limbs. The tremors are usually more pronounced when other people pay attention to them, and they are usually more organized and stereotyped than the tremors caused by neurological disorders, such as chorea. The person with psychogenic pseudo-epilepsy may have convulsive tremors throughout his body, but the characteristics of pseudo-epilepsy differ clinically from those of neurogenic epilepsy. In psychogenic pseudo-epilepsy the body thrashes about wildly without the rhythmic clonic movements of the extremities that occur in neurogenic epilepsy. Attention from other people seems to exacerbate the thrashing. The patient rarely hurts himself, voids or bites his tongue. He seems unresponsive, but he does react to stimuli although negatively; he often resists the examiner's attempts to open his eyes or to move his limbs. During the pseudo-epileptic period the patient's state of consciousness may be altered, but the alteration is more like a dissociative state than like the changes that result from gross disturbances in brain function.

Astasia-abasia is a disturbance of gait. The person affected seems to stagger, has pseudo-ataxic movements of the trunk and holds on to walls or furniture to steady himself. He rarely falls and if he does fall he is able to avoid injury.

Paralysis and paresis. Monoplegia,

hemiplegia, or paraplegia of the extremities are common forms of paralysis. Paralysis is usually characterized by flaccidity or sustained contracture of antagonistic muscles. The paralysis conforms to popular ideas of how a part of the body should be affected rather than to the anatomy of the nervous system. The paralysis is more severe in the proximal part of a limb whereas in neurogenic disorders the opposite is the case. Examination of the paralyzed part shows no genuine impairment of function. If the examiner tries to move the part, he feels resistance from the patient's antagonistic muscles. The patient's reflexes including his plantar responses are normal and he does not react abnormally to electromyographic stimulation.

Hysteric aphonia is a localized paralysis of the muscles that affect the vocal cords. The person affected can whisper without difficulty but he cannot vocalize sounds. Examination shows that the muscles are normal.

Sensory disturbances usually occur in the extremities and may accompany motor disturbances. All modalities are involved and, as in the motor dysfunctions, the distribution of the disturbance is determined by the person's idea of how the part should be affected and not by the anatomy of the nervous system. One may find stocking and glove anesthesia or hyperesthesia, anesthesia of a limb that stops at an anatomically visible articulation, or hemianesthesia which stops at the midline of the body.

The patient may manifest unilateral or bilateral deafness and loss of vision. A not uncommon syndrome is gunbarrel or tunnel vision, a concentric diminution of the person's visual field that leaves only his central vision intact.

Testing usually shows that sensation is not absent and that peripheral stimuli are being received, transmitted and registered centrally. What appears to be an unawareness of sensation is in fact an active denial of sensation by the patient. Some patients asked to close their eyes during the physical examination volunteer that they do not feel anything exactly at the moment that the disturbed area is touched.

Pain is a common sensory disturbance. Since the pain is frequently vague and hard to diagnose, it sometimes leads to unnecessary surgery.

Conversion symptoms that simulate physical illness. Conversion symptoms may express feelings in somatic metaphors, for example a heartache that represents emotional pain or a paralyzed arm that represents an inhibition of the wish to masturbate or strike someone. Conversion symptoms may also replicate a physical illness that the patient previously experienced or that he observed in others. Often a patient takes on the symptoms of a terminal illness that caused the death of someone he loved. The patient who is suspected of having a conversion symptom should be examined exhaustively since conversion symptoms can mimic almost any physical illness.

Conversion mechanisms intensifying genuine illness. Sometimes when a patient is genuinely ill, his physician may think that his suffering is greater than his illness warrants. In such a case, a conversion mechanism may have intensified the symptoms of a genuine illness. Genuine symptoms can take on symbolic meanings and the patient can extract secondary as well as primary gain from them.

Complications. Conversion symptoms can cause genuine organic illness. For example, a longstanding paralysis can cause muscle atrophy and contracture; hyperventilation can cause respiratory alkalosis, and nausea can cause weight loss and inanition.

Epidemiology

It is often said that conversion symptoms occur less frequently than they did 80 to 100 years ago, but it is difficult to substantiate that observation. Gross and dramatic symptoms such as paralysis and pseudo-epilepsy probably occur less often but sub-tler symptoms such as vague pain still occur frequently. A Swedish study showed that 5% of the Swedish population had conversion symptoms. Engel suggested that 20–25% of patients admitted to a gen-eral hospital had experienced conversion symptoms at one time or another. Three times more women than men have conver-sion symptoms. The more uneducated and unsophisticated the patient is, the more likely it is that his conversion symptoms will be dramatic and bizarre (Engel, 1970).

Causes

The psychoanalytic model is particu-larly applicable to conversion. The con-cept of conversion has in fact been derived from the findings of hypnosis and psycho-analytic therapy, and it has helped to fash-ion the psychoanalytic model. An event or situation is thought to awaken childhood impulses. Because these impulses caused conflict in childhood, they had been re-pressed. To re-repress the impulse a new equilibrium is established and a conver-sion symptom appears in which the con-flict is expressed symbolically, yet kept from the person's awareness.

An illustration of this mechanism is a case of a young man who found one day that he could not move the fingers of his right hand. The paralysis developed after he had had an argument with his employer. During the argument the young man had clenched his fist and almost struck his employer. It was discovered in therapy that the incident had triggered memories in the patient of repressed rage towards his father, who had been a violent man. Discovering the patient's childhood conflict relieved the paralysis and thus provided evidence that the paralysis was a conversion disorder.

It is not known whether psychological factors are sufficient to cause a conversion disorder. Early psychiatrists such as Janet suggested in addition an hereditary pre-disposition. Pathogenesis and symptom choice in the neurotic disorders has al-ready been discussed. Conversion symp-toms occur more often in people who when tested achieve high ratings on extraversion and neuroticism scales. It is not known whether these scales measure an heredi-tary or a biologic tendency (Templer and Lester, 1974).

It is thought that social factors affect a person's choice of symptoms, although to a lesser extent than does early experience. Certain symptoms seem to be more accept-able in one culture or setting than in another. In Western culture, for example, vague pain is considered less pathological than is paralysis of a limb. It is likely that the more unacceptable a patient's symptoms are within his social setting, in-cluding that of his childhood, the more disturbed the patient is.

Treatment

In addition to psychoanalytic psycho-therapy that uncovers the underlying con-flicts, certain specialized techniques employing suggestion and catharsis, such as hypnosis and the sodium amytal inter-view have been used to manage conversion symptoms. These two techniques are most useful shortly after a symptom appears, if its appearance was sudden, and if the event that precipitated it was clearly trau-matic.

Differential Diagnosis of Conversion Disorders

Conversion symptoms must be differ-entiated from hypochondriacal states, somatic delusions, and malingering. In hypochondriacal states the patient is alarmed rather than indifferent about his physical symptoms. The hypochondriac does not hope to discover an organic cause for his symptoms as does the person with a conversion disorder, nor is he resigned to his suffering.

Somatic delusions are more bizarre than are conversion symptoms and they often occur during psychotic and toxic states.

The malingerer is usually hostile, suspicious, and secretive, and shows apparent concern about his symptom. The patient with a conversion symptom is more dependent and appealing than the malingerer and he shows less concern about the symptom than one would expect. The symptoms of the malingerer are calculated and so his condition often resembles genuine illness more closely than does the condition of the person with a conversion symptom.

The similarities and differences between conversion symptoms and those medical illnesses in which pituitary-adrenal factors are most prominent are discussed in the section on psychosomatic illnesses.

HYPOCHONDRIASIS

Hypochondriasis has a venerable history, but in recent years it has been demoted from the status of syndrome and the term now is used to describe a cluster of symptoms.

The word hypochondriasis comes from the Greek with the literal meaning of "below the cartilage." Hypochondriasis has been described as the male counterpart of hysteria. In Greek the word hysteria means womb. Hypochondriasis is defined as an excessive preoccupation and concern with one's body or state of mental or physical health—and with the communication of these concerns to others (Kenyon, 1976). The hypochondriac may go to great lengths to avoid disease. He directs his attention towards himself; his caring and concern for others are diminished.

Hypochondriasis lies between normal concerns about one's health and ineradicable somatic delusions. Its borders are not clear and so it presents a problem in measurement and epidemiology. Its incidence increases with a person's age. Hypochon-driasis differs from conversion symptoms in that the hypochondriac is agitated and concerned about his symptoms rather than indifferent to them.

As mentioned earlier, the term hypochondriasis does not refer to a syndrome. It describes a state that may occur with almost any psychiatric syndrome. The psychiatric conditions in which symptoms of hypochondriasis are not uncommon include depressive disorders, especially severe, psychotic depressions, paranoid psychosis, organic brain syndrome, personality disorders, especially those associated with paranoid trends, severe obsessional neurosis, certain phobic anxiety states, and neurasthenia. Neurasthenia is an old term that is applied to a cluster of symptoms; in addition to hypochondriacal concerns, the symptoms include weakness, the tendency to fatigue easily, and a lack of tolerance for minor stress (Berger, 1973).

Hypochondriacal symptoms usually indicate a poor prognosis. The mechanism is not well understood; it is probable that the term refers to a heterogeneous group of symptoms. However, in severe cases, the nature of the hypochondriacal symptoms suggests a unique psychological formulation: the symptoms appear to express in body language the patient's concern that his sense of self is falling apart. This may be a reaction to an organic brain syndrome, to illness and old age, or to the onset of depression, or psychosis. The metaphoric expression is such as to suggest that the difficulties encountered by the patient tend to fall more within the psychotic rather than the neurotic range of disorders. As has been discussed earlier, it is in psychotic disorders that the integrity of the sense of self is threatened, and that the boundaries between one's self and one's environment become blurred. Hypochondriacal concerns may metaphorically represent the patient's attempt to ward off a psychotic disorder.

The treatment of hypochondriasis is

aimed at the primary condition that the hypochondriacal symptoms accompany.

REFERENCES

Berger, D. (1971): Hysteria: in search of the animus. *Compr. Psychiatry.* 12:277.

Berger, D. (1973): The return of neurasthenia. *Compr. Psychiatry.* 14:557.

Engel, G. L. (1970): Conversion symptoms. In *Signs and Symptoms.* 5th ed. Edited by C. M. Mac-Bryde and R. S. Blacklow. Philadelphia, J. B. Lippincott.

Kenyon, F. E. (1976): Hypochondriacal states. *Br. J. Psychiatry.* 129:1.

Templer, D. I. and Lester, D. (1974): Conversion disorders: a review of research findings. *Compr. Psychiatry.* 15:285.

FURTHER READINGS

Berger, D. M. (1971): Hysteria: in search of the animus. *Compr. Psychiatry.* 12:277.
An historical overview of hysteria.

Engel, G. L. (1970): Conversion Symptoms. In *Signs and Symptoms.* 5th ed. Edited by G. M. Mac-Bryde and R. S. Blacklow. Philadelphia. J. B. Lippincott.
An excellent in-depth discussion of conversion.

Lowy, F. H. (1975): Management of the persistent somatizer. *Int. J. Psychiatry Med.* 6:227.
A general overview of the problem of somatization with practical advice for physicians.

CHAPTER 17

Psychosomatic Mechanisms

Harvey Moldofsky

Psychosomatic medicine has its roots in the age old philosophical controversy on the relationship between mind and body; that is, whether operations of the psyche (mind) and soma (body) operate in dualistic or monistic systems. Contemporary thinking affirms that the proper understanding of man involves a holistic approach where man in health and disease functions as a psychosomatic unit (WHO Expert Committee on Psychosomatic Disorders—1964). Psychosomatic medicine is now considered to be a science of the relationship between psychological, biological and social variables as they pertain to human health and disease; *an approach* to the practice of medicine which advocates the inclusion of psychosocial factors in the study, prevention, diagnosis and management of all diseases; *clinical* activities at the interface of medicine and the behavioral sciences subsumed under the term "consultation—liaision psychiatry" (Lipowski, 1976).

PSYCHOSOMATIC CONCEPTS IN THE INITIATION OF DISEASE

Psychological Specificity. During the second quarter of this century, the early workers in the psychosomatic field were, for the most part, influenced by psychoanalytic theory and therapy. Freud's concepts of conversion and symbolism which led to the understanding of the formulation of hysterical symptoms were applied by psychoanalysts to the study of organic disease. In those diseases of unknown etiology, but in which anecdotal evidence suggested significant emotional influences, psychoanalytic theory suggested that specific psychological problems initiated the disease. Specific personality structures (Dunbar, 1943) or specific emotional conflicts, e.g. dependency-independency (Alexander and French, 1963) were thought to affect the onset of seven diseases: bronchial asthma, peptic ulcer, ulcerative colitis, thyrotoxicosis, neurodermatitis, rheumatoid arthritis and essential hypertension. The treatment of such psychosomatic disorders by psychoanalysis did not produce results which supported the exclusive use of psychotherapeutic measures. These early workers are now considered to have been rather naive and uncritically biased. Their psychogenetic orientation has been replaced by a theory of multiple etiology. In some instances, personality type may be one important factor among a variety of key factors in the genesis of disease. For example, such personality traits as intense competitiveness, achievement striving, time urgency and aggressiveness, termed by Rosenman and Friedman as Type A behavior pattern, have been implicated as a risk factor in the etiology of coronary artery disease (Rosenman et al. 1975).

Psychological Nonspecificity. For centuries physicians have commented on passions of the mind or varied emotional disturbances that seemed to herald the onset of illness. This ancient concept has had renewed interest in the light of psychologic/medical investigations. For example, major bereavement, particularly the death of a spouse or child, is followed by a deterioration in health in 25% of men and women under age 65 (Parkes, 1970). Situational distress, namely a psychological set of "giving up–given up" (Schmale and Engel, 1967) where there is failure of previously effective coping mechanisms and a sense of helplessness and hopelessness is claimed to be a common setting for facilitating the emergence of a variety of diseases, e.g. cervical cancer (Schmale and Iker, 1966), rheumatoid arthritis (Meyerowotiz et al., 1968) and leukemia. However, these psychological concepts fail to explain how situational distresses become translated into disease.

Stress and Disease. Selye's formulation on the theory of stress as a mediator of disease onset has had an important influence on psychosomatic medicine. Stress as a precipitating factor in chronic disease is now a widely held concept. Selye (1976) considers "stress to be the nonspecific response of the body to any demands. A stressor is an agent that produces stress at any time. The general adaptation syndrome (G.A.S.) represents the chronological development of the response to stressors when their action is prolonged. It consists of three phases: the alarm reaction, the stage of resistance, and the stage of exhaustion." Selye proposes that stress mediates in a nonspecific way between a variety of possible noxious agents (e.g. marital disagreement, frustration by a boss, combat fatigue, burns) and psychiatric or medical illness. The variability in response of individuals to comparable stressors is dependent upon endogenous conditioning (e.g. genetic predisposition, age, sex) or exogenous conditioning (e.g. drugs, environmental, or social factors). Therefore, the observation that a broad range of physiological changes occurs in stressed animals and humans does not support the earlier contention that a specific physiological change can be correlated with a specific emotional state (Weiner, 1977). Individuals identified as psychiatrically disturbed in a general practice population seem to be subject to all forms of physical morbidity (Eastwood and Trevelyan, 1972) and possibly both medical and psychiatric disorders occur in some people at the same time.

Psychobiologic Mechanisms. While there is much evidence to support a relationship between operations of the limbic-hypothalamic-pituitary systems and emotions, there is no understanding of how sensory pathways provide sensation with psychological meaning or convert to emotional experience. Moreover, no experimental method has been devised to demonstrate how an emotional experience is transferred into physiological responses. Much of the evidence for psychobiologic mechanisms depends upon covariant studies where relationships are drawn between psychological and physiological behavior. The association of emotions and physiological functioning has been known since Beaumont's (1833) observations through a fistulous opening that stressful events affected the functioning of Alexis St. Martin's stomach. Later Cannon (1932) observed how emotional distress was related to changes in physiological function under the control of the autonomic nervous system. Cannon viewed these psychophysiological responses to be adaptive and responsive to "flight" or "fight" situations. Other investigators have followed in Cannon's and Selye's footsteps and with sophisticated techniques have demonstrated the influence of psychological adaptation on physiological changes in both animals and man. For example, Brady (1958) demonstrated that if one of two monkeys, both trained to avoid shock stimuli, were placed in a shock avoidance situation for both of them, the "executive" monkey—that is the monkey which had to make the movements to avoid the shock—developed gastric and duodenal ulcers. Wolff and his colleagues in the 1940s and 1950s studied a variety of autonomic physiological responses to emotional distress. They conceptualized that a stressful life situation generated a protective reaction pattern that was either "defensive" or "offensive." The protective pattern was characterized by disturbed affect, e.g. anxiety and anger or sadness and fear, and was associated with altered organ activity, e.g. increased blood flow, lysozyme activity and mobility of the colon. In a maladaptive life situation the predisposed vulnerable organ may undergo structural change, e.g. colonic dysfunction might eventually progress to ulceration and hemorrhage. In a unique study where a genetic marker for disease predisposition was used to forecast disease onset in a controlled stressful situation, Weiner et al. (1957) showed that those U.S. army draftees with a relatively high level of serum pepsinogen and specific "oral" emotional conflicts developed peptic ulceration in the course of army basic training. Recent psychophysiological and psychoendocrine studies highlight the heterogeneity of psychosomatic disease (Weiner, 1976). That is, different mechanisms may produce the same physiological disturbance or disease. For example, varied combinations of allergic mechanisms, infection, and psychological factors trigger asthmatic attacks. Or, the same mechanisms may have variable effects, e.g.

some patients with chronic duodenal ulcer are hypersecretors of pepsin and hydrochloric acid, while others are normal secretors of these substances

Psychosocial Mechanisms. Evidence for the interplay of psychological and social factors on disease comes from broad based social-epidemiologic studies where connections are drawn between stressful life events and disease onset or frequency. The social event rather than the type of disease is of prime concern. Holmes, Rahe, and colleagues (1967) have demonstrated that the greater the social stress requiring change in the life situation, the greater the risk for becoming ill. On their Social Readjustment Rating Scale, those life events characterized by the necessity for a relatively intense and/or prolonged readjustment (e.g. death of a spouse) were more likely to be followed within a set time by the occurrence of medical or psychiatric illness. Furthermore, situations of social status incongruence have been suggested as a mediating factor to the frequency of illness. Hinkle et al. (1974) found a high incidence in illness and work absenteeism in New York City telephone employees whose social-economic background was inappropriate to the level of work responsibility. Finally, social isolation as a result of poverty, lack of family neighborhood affiliations, or ethnic minority status has been claimed to be harmful to health. But, the studies are inconclusive for they do not answer whether those individuals in such situations are self-selected or whether premorbid conditions predispose to both the social pathology and to the subsequent somatic and psychological pathology (Rabkin and Struening 1976).

PSYCHOSOMATIC PATTERNING IN THE COURSE OF DISEASE

Studies on the psychobiologic pattern of the disease may differentiate those who manage well from those who manage poorly during the course of their disease.

Such studies require longitudinal evaluation of psychological, biological and social variables and do not concern themselves with the uncertainties of disease onset mechanisms. Moldofsky and Chester (1970) found that those patients with rheumatoid arthritis whose severity of peripheral joint tenderness coincided with their emotional state (anxiety or hostility) demonstrated a favorable course of illness over the next two years. On the other hand, those rheumatoids, whose increased joint tenderness coincided with a sense of confidence and optimism, and decreased pain coincided with an increase in hopelessness and despair, had an unfavorable course of illness. Such patients (paradoxical responders) were exposed to more hazardous forms of treatment, complications of their disease and, in some cases, death. Furthermore, the "paradoxical" pattern group were contrasted to the "synchronous" pattern group by their perceived lack of adequate family-social supports. Education might alter an unfavorable illness-behavior pattern. Green (1974) showed a decrease in utilization of hospital emergency services by chronic asthmatics who were exposed to an education program directed to improve self care.

PSYCHOSOCIAL EFFECTS OF DISEASE

The clinical presentation of illness might be more dependent upon the meaning of the illness to the sick person, rather than on the biological process of interest to the physician. Illness behavior depends upon the manner in which people differentially perceive, evaluate and respond to their symptoms (Mechanic, 1966). The varied individual responses are products of social and cultural conditioning, coping repertoire to alleviate the symptoms, and the usefulness derived from behaving in a sick manner. Some patients might exaggerate their complaints in order to achieve financial gain or escape from an untenable domestic or work situation. Unconscious motivation might equally color symptom presentations through previously frustrated needs for attention, affection or sympathy.

In summary, psychosomatic medicine can be viewed as an extension of medical theory and practice that takes into account the role of psychological and social processes in the functions of the body in health and disease. This multifactorial orientation permits the evaluation of the interrelationship of biological, psychological and social processes in the comprehension and management of disease.

REFERENCES

Alexander, F. and French, T. M. (1948): *Studies in Psychosomatic Medicine.* New York, Ronald Press.

Brady, J. V. (1958): Ulcers in executive monkeys. *Sci. Am.* 199:95.

Dunbar, H. F. (1943): *Psychosomatic Diagnosis.* New York, Hoeber.

Eastwood, M. R. and Trevelyan, M. H. (1972): Relationship between physical and psychiatric disorder. *Psychol. Med.* 2:363.

Green, L. W. (1974): The effect of exposure to culture change, social change and changes in interpersonal relationships on health. In *Stressful Life Events.* Edited by B. N. Dohrenwend and B. P. Dohrenwend. New York, Wiley.

Holmes, T. and Rahe, R. (1967): The social readjustment rating scale. *J. Psychosom. Res.* 11:213.

Lipowski, Z. J. (1976): Psychosomatic medicine: an overview. In *Modern Trends in Psychosomatic Medicine.* Vol. 3. Edited by O. W. Hill. London, Butterworths.

Mechanic, D. (1966): Response factors in illness: the study of illness behavior. *Social Psychiatry.* 1:11.

Moldofsky, H. and Chester, W. J. (1970): Pain and mood patterns in patients with rheumatoid arthritis. *Psychosom. Med.* 32:309.

Parkes, C. M. (1970): The psychosomatic effects of bereavement. In *Modern Trends in Psychosomatic Medicine.* Vol. 2. Edited by O. W. Hill. London, Butterworths.

Rabkin, J. G. and Struening, E. L. (1976): Social change, stress and illness. In *Psychoanalysis and Contemporary Science.* Vol 5. Edited by T. Shapiro. New York, International Universities Press.

Rosenman, R. H., Brand, R. J., Jenkins, C. D., et al. (1975): Coronary heart disease in the western collaborative group study: final follow-up experience in 8½ years. *J.A.M.A. 233:872.*

Schmale, A. and Engel, G. (1967): The giving-up—given-up complex illustrated on film. *Arch. Gen. Psychiatry.* 17:135.

Schmale, A. and Iker, H. P. (1966): The affect of hopelessness and the development of cancer. *Psychosom. Med. 28*:714.

Selye, H. (1976): Forty years of stress research. *Can. Med. Assoc. J. 115*:53.

Weiner, H., Thaler, M., and Reiser, M., et al. (1957): Etiology of duodenal ulcer: relation of specific psychological characteristics to rate of gastric secretion (serum pepsinogen). *Psychosom. Med. 19*:1.

Weiner, H. (1976): The heterogeneity of psychosomatic disease. *Psychosom. Med. 37*:371.

Weiner, H. (1977): *Psychobiology and Human Disease.* New York, Elsevier.

18

Psychosomatic Disorders

Graeme J. Taylor

Psychosomatic medicine emerged during the 1920's as a reaction to the increasing mechanization of medical practice. From the start, psychosomatic medicine looked at the patient as a whole person and considered the role of emotional factors in all diseases.

The meaning of the term psychosomatic has changed during the past forty years and it has been difficult to maintain a satisfactory and consistent system for classifying so-called psychosomatic disorders. Despite Alexander's view (1950) that every disease is psychosomatic, early workers in psychosomatic medicine soon restricted their attention to seven diseases that are now called the classical psychosomatic disorders or "Alexander's Holy Seven": bronchial asthma, peptic ulcer, ulcerative colitis, thyrotoxicosis, neurodermatitis, rheumatoid arthritis, and essential hypertension. In North America these seven diseases are usually classified among the psychophysiologic disorders, and they are misleadingly defined as "physical disorders of presumably psychogenic origin" (American Psychiatric Association, 1968). During the mid-1950's, psychosomatic workers turned their attention from the patient's internal conflicts to his external en-

vironment. The term psychosomatic again broadened to encompass a wide variety of medical illnesses ranging from cancer to the common cold.

While "psychosomatic disorder" remains a nosological concept, the core concept, psychosomatic, now represents an approach to the understanding of the etiology of disease and to the clinical practice of medicine. Contemporary psychosomatic medicine, which uses a biopsychosocial model of disease, is a viable alternative to the prevailing concept of illness, which uses a biomedical model of disease that has molecular biology as its basic scientific discipline (Engel, 1977).

The psychosomatic viewpoint is not reflected in current classifications of illness. It has been proposed that a diagnosis modifier that indicates the degree (probable, prominent, or unknown) to which psychological factors play a role could be attached to the *International Classification of Diseases* (Lipp et al., 1977).

Several diseases are discussed in this chapter. Their selection is not intended to support the idea that some physical illnesses are psychosomatic and others are not. Most of the illnesses discussed here are outside the primary province of psychiatry, but they are illnesses in which the effects of psychological and social factors have been intensively studied.

BRONCHIAL ASTHMA

Bronchial asthma (dyspnea and wheezing due to bronchial obstruction) appears to be a heterogeneous illness in which the influence of psychological and social factors varies in different subgroups of asthma. It is now widely accepted that the asthma sufferer has a somatic substrate for bronchial hyper-reactivity which is presumed to be inherited. The lability of the bronchial system that causes it to overreact to both constricting and dilating stimuli is relative, and all patients do not have the same degree of lability. In some patients the defect in their bronchial system seems to be a deficiency in beta-adrenergic receptor activity which creates an imbalance with alpha-adrenergic receptor activity and parasympathetic activity.

In a person who is biologically predisposed to bronchial asthma, bronchospasm may be precipitated by various factors including inhalation of allergens, bronchial infections, prolonged exercise, situational stress and excitement, anger, or fear (Pinkerton, 1973). Although many factors may be involved in an asthmatic attack, one factor may be the most important one and the other secondary. The importance of each factor may change, and it may vary according to the sex of the patient as well as to the patient's age when the illness began (Weiner, 1977).

Through reinforcement and generalization, asthma can become a conditioned response. After the patient's first attack of asthma, precipitated by allergens, for example, subsequent attacks may occur in a similar situation even when the allergens are absent (Groen, 1976). The patient's attitude towards his illness in general and his emotional responses to the attacks of asthma may increase his distress and activate physiological mechanisms that exacerbate the attacks. In children an oper-

ant conditioning influence is established when parental responses, such as increased attention and affection, reward the asthmatic behavior. Hospitalization may improve a child's asthma because the hospital staff is less anxious than the parents when the child has an attack.

Although no single personality type is prone to asthma, it has been said that conflicts that stem from an exaggerated need to depend very often are associated with asthma. Without predictive studies it is not conclusive that these conflicts always precede the onset of asthma. French and Alexander (1941) identified the longing of the person with asthma to be protected and engulfed by his mother. This longing differs from the dependency conflict in the patient with a peptic ulcer, who has the unconscious wish to be fed by his mother. In Alexander's view, fear of separation from one's mother can initiate attacks of asthma which may represent a repressed cry for the lost mother. In other patients, the wish to be engulfed causes a fear of fusion so that closeness to their mothers seems more dangerous to them than does separation. If such a patient is separated from his mother his symptoms may disappear rapidly.

Although the mechanism by which psychosocial factors cause attacks of asthma is not well understood, two psychophysiological pathways have been proposed (Stein and Luparello, 1970): stimulation of the vagus nerve causes bronchiolar obstruction so that emotions may directly affect bronchiolar physiology through the central nervous system (independent of allergic mechanisms), and emotions may also modify the immunologic or allergic mechanisms involved in some cases of asthma. The two pathways may be involved simultaneously to cause asthmatic attacks.

HEART DISEASE

The heart may be directly affected by psychosocial stress. Congestive heart failure, angina pectoris, myocardial infarctions, cardiac arrhythmias, and sudden death have all been studied from the viewpoint of psychosomatic medicine. Hemodynamic changes are an integral part of all emotional reactions, but stress may also alter the balance of water and electrolytes, blood fats, and clotting mechanisms and so secondarily affect the heart. Persons whose hearts are already damaged are particularly vulnerable to sudden emotional arousal, and the frequent occurrence of nocturnal angina or of myocardial infarction during REM sleep has been attributed to the autonomic disorganization that accompanies dreaming.

Chambers and Reiser (1953) found that sudden, overwhelming emotional experiences often preceded congestive heart failure in patients who had depleted cardiac reserves. Other investigators found that the excretion of sodium and water decreases during periods of discouragement and hopelessness suggesting that depression can precipitate cardiac decompensation. Studies have shown that victims of sudden death were often depressed for a long time, and then were subjected to sudden emotional arousal by psychosocial events which were impossible for them to ignore. Such events included sudden losses, personal threats, and even happy experiences or times of triumph (Dimsdale, 1977). Although emotional stress may cause arrhythmias in otherwise healthy people, myocardial ischemia increases the chance that an arrhythmia may occur. Biofeedback has been used successfully to train people to control their atrial and ventricular arrhythmias. A specific behavior pattern, called the Type A personality by Friedman and Rosenman (1960), has been associated with fatal and nonfatal coronary artery disease (independent of the usual predictive coronary risk factors). The Type A personality is competitive, ambitious, overly aggressive and has a chronic sense of the urgency of time. Groen (1976) proposed that inability to discharge the feelings of frustration brought on by the failure to advance in one's career or to obtain affection from one's family can also precipitate myocardial infarction. Possible psychobiological mechanisms include elevated serum levels of triglycerides and cholesterol and the increased diurnal secretion of norepinephrine that is associated with the Type A personality. Stress may also increase the platelet stickiness that contributes to arterial occlusion. Patients in the coronary care unit of a hospital are often depressed and anxious but they are seldom psychotic. Occasionally they develop delirium but the delirium has been attributed partly to sensory monotony and sleep deprivation. The psychological defense of denial may protect the patient and reduce mortality during the acute phase that follows a myocardial infarction.

ANOREXIA NERVOSA

Anorexia nervosa, a condition of self-inflicted starvation, is not a specific nosologic entity. Primary or true anorexia nervosa must be differentiated from secondary, atypical, anorexia nervosa, although the physical condition produced by both types is similar. Secondary anorexia nervosa may occur together with any of a wide range of psychiatric disorders and the person usually suffers a real loss of appetite. She lacks the restlessness and desperate struggle for an independent identity that is seen in the person with primary anorexia nervosa (Bruch, 1977).

Primary anorexia nervosa usually develops during adolescence and is more common than it was previously thought to be. The disorder occurs ten times more frequently in women than in men (Hill, 1976). The basic psychopathology in primary anorexia nervosa is a body image disturbance that is accompanied by the need to maintain a pathologically low body weight (Crisp, 1977a, 1977b). Fearing that she will become fat, the person relentlessly pursues thinness. She maintains a low subpubertal body weight through abstinence, abulimia[*] and vomiting or (and) purging. The person's fear of fatness has been attributed to serious maturational conflicts of adolescence. The conflicts affect both the person and her family. Conflicts about separation and individuation and about sexuality are often present, but they are not specific to anorexia nervosa. Anorexia nervosa may be a brief illness and remit spontaneously, or it may be recurrent or chronic. The mortality for five years is 5%. Death usually results from suicide or inanition. Termination of the birth control pill sometimes precedes primary anorexia nervosa. Some people with anorexia have Turner's syndrome. There seems to be a functional anterior hypothalamic defect in anorexia nervosa, but it is not known whether the defect precedes, coincides with, or is caused by the illness.

The clinical features of anorexia nervosa include emaciation, cessation of menstruation, reduction of the basal metabolic rate, bradycardia, hypotension, peripheral vasoconstriction, hypothermia and hyperactivity. The axillary and pubic hair are retained but after some time downy lanugo hair may appear on the arms and legs. Patients who purge themselves excessively may develop abdominal pain and peripheral edema. The differential diagnoses include panhypopituitarism, granulomatous diseases of the small intestine, and tumors of the frontal lobes, diencephalon, and fourth ventricle. People with anorexia nervosa rarely want to change and they seldom seek help themselves. Because they are secretive about their diet (for example, they may hoard food instead of eating it) the condition is difficult to diagnose and treat. Information must be sought from parents and other outside informants as well as from the patient. Restitution of normal body weight alone does not constitute successful treatment. The psychosocial conflicts in the patient and her family should be identified and resolved through therapy.

DUODENAL ULCER

That stress affects gastric function has been known since 1833, when Beaumont observed the gastric fistula of the Canadian voyageur, Alexis St. Martin; now it is believed that emotions may affect the formation of duodenal ulcers more than they affect the formation of gastric ulcers. A genetic factor predisposes people to duodenal ulcers. People who are so predisposed are more likely to belong to the blood group O, and nonsecretors of ABH antigens have a significantly higher incidence of duodenal ulcer than do secretors. Duodenal ulcers occur more often in men than in women, and they are usually (but not always) associated with an increased secretion of hydrochloric acid and pepsin. Many adults who have intense, unresolved conflicts of dependency have a predisposition to duodenal ulcers. Alexander (1950) proposed that the person who develops a peptic ulcer has a deep-seated wish to be loved, cared for, and fed like an infant and that the person defends himself against such urges and conceals them with the traits of pseudo-independence. Mirsky (1958) proposed that infants with increased sucking needs have an increased production of pepsinogen and are more prone than others to oral frustration in their early mother-child relationship, even when the mothering is adequate. The child whose oral needs are frustrated may develop the character structure described by Alexander, and he may be predisposed to duodenal ulcers. A frustrating life event or interpersonal situation could reactivate the repressed oral conflict of such a person. Weiner and his associates (1957) could predict accurately that certain U.S. army recruits would develop ulcers under the stress of basic training. Weiner and his associates took into consideration the recruits' character structure and their motivations as well as their levels of plasma pepsinogen. Their study supports the idea that many people have both psychological and physiological predispositions to

[*] abulimia - morbidly decreased appetite.

duodenal ulcers. The ulcers may appear when the person is subjected to psychosocial stresses which threaten the gratification of his dependency needs.

Alexander's idea that the activation of dependency needs causes the secretion of gastric acid to increase has not been proved. It is now known that there are several neural and hormonal mechanisms by which emotions can alter the gastric and duodenal functions. There are different kinds of duodenal ulcers, and they may have different predisposing and initiating mechanisms (Weiner, 1977). The physician should consider the dependency needs and the immediate life situation of the ulcer patient so that he can provide comprehensive medical care.

DIABETES MELLITUS

Emotional factors may affect the onset, course and control of diabetes. Stress, especially disruptions in one's relationships with others, may reveal previously unrecognized diabetes, or it may change prediabetes to diabetes. There appear to be subgroups of diabetics, some of whom are more prone than others to react to stressful life events by decompensation of their metabolic equilibrium. For example, people with "super-labile" juvenile diabetes rapidly develop ketoacidosis in response to specific stress. The metabolic decompensation is mediated by endogenous catecholamines, and it may be averted by beta-adrenergic blockers. The investigation and resolution of the conflicts within the patient's family that create the stress are essential to the comprehensive treatment of patients with "super-labile" diabetes (Baker and Barcai, 1970). Some people with diabetes adjust poorly to their chronic illness, and some may use their illness to deal with unpleasant life situations by abandoning the diabetic regimen. Diagnostic confusion may arise in regard to neurotic patients with diabetes who have episodes of pseudohypoglycemia

that are caused by hysterical identification with the symptoms of true hypoglycemia. Evaluations of the patient's sugar levels, rather than of his responses to the oral or intravenous administration of glucose, are necessary to clarify the diagnosis.

ULCERATIVE COLITIS

This is an inflammatory disease that affects primarily the mucosa of the rectum and colon. It has alternating periods of exacerbation and remission. It may occasionally involve the ileum and it is not always easily distinguished from Crohn's disease with which it shares many common immunopathological and psychological features. Genetic, endocrine, allergic, infective, enzymatic, auto-immune, and psychogenic factors should all be considered as possible causes. It is not easy to separate the emotions that precede ulcerative colitis from the psychological reactions that follow it. Studies of groups that may be predisposed to ulcerative colitis have yet to be done. Two main categories of psychosocial events that precede the onset of ulcerative colitis have been identified. The categories are separation by death or other life events from a person on whom the patient had depended, and frustration of a person's urge to accomplish something coupled with his fear that he will fail to accomplish it. Engel (1955) and others have attributed a person's psychological predisposition to ulcerative colitis to his unresolved symbiotic relationship with his mother. The maternal relationship determines the quality of all future relationships. The patient cannot adapt to disruptions in his highly dependent relationships, and he responds to disruptions with despair and a feeling of powerlessness. These emotions are associated with the "giving-up" reaction which may trigger the predisposing biological mechanisms and so exacerbate the illness. Engel (1956) also noted the frequent occurrence of headaches as an alternative symptom during the periods of remission from ulcerative colitis. During remission, the patients studied were also more active, aggressive and capable of solving problems. Persons who have colitis often have obsessive-compulsive traits, including perfectionism, neatness, orderliness, conscientiousness, stubbornness, and a great sensitivity to real or imagined slights. They may develop a psychotic depressive or schizophrenic illness and occasionally ulcerative colitis alternates with psychosis. The prognosis is worse for people who have severe psychiatric disorders (O'Connor, 1970). Patients who receive psychotherapy in addition to medical and surgical treatment do better than patients who do not receive psychotherapy. The type of psychotherapy must be suited to the patient's symbiotic needs (Karush et al., 1977). The extreme vulnerability of the patient to disruptions in his relationship with his physician must also be considered.

CANCER

Cancer has a strong emotional impact on the patients, their families, and the health professionals, who often are no more sophisticated philosophically or emotionally than the lay person in regard to death and dying. Psychosocial factors may affect the onset and course of cancer. Loss, separation, depression and despair may precede the physical manifestations of cancer (LeShan, 1959). Some studies have observed that people who have cancer are often inhibited, bland, unable to express hostility, and make extensive use of repressive and denying ego defenses (Bahnson and Bahnson, 1969). Studies of the effect of psychological factors on the progression of cancer suggest that people who externalize their hostility and develop a fighting attitude fare better than people who do not externalize their hostility (Stavraky, 1968). The former group of people may represent the antithesis of the

"giving-up" reaction. Observations of patients with diseases of the reticuloendothelial system led to an early formulation of the "giving-up" reaction as a psychobiological state that seems to facilitate the onset of many diseases (Schmale, 1972). Adults and children with leukemia and lymphoma reported that they had many object losses. These losses were followed by the depressive feelings of helplessness and hopelessness that immediately preceded the apparent onset of their illness (Greene and Miller, 1958). Schmale and Iker (1966) evaluated the potential for hopelessness and/or the recent feelings of hopelessness in women with abnormal cervical cytology. They were able to predict with a high degree of accuracy those women who would show carcinomatous changes when a cone biopsy was done. There are methodological problems in trying to determine the exact onset of cancer; the feeling of hopelessness could be a concomitant of cancer rather than a precursor. Studies with improved methodology have not always supported the idea that cancer patients have suffered significant losses that preceded the development of the malignancy (Schonfield, 1975). Further investigation of psychosocial settings of the patients is required for the study of the rare but well-documented cases of spontaneous regression of cancer.

The immune system, and possibly a surveillance mechanism, is a crucially important biological element in the development of cancer. Researchers who worked from the viewpoint of psychosomatic medicine demonstrated that stress and emotional distress may affect the immune processes. The hypothalamus may mediate through its control of the activity of the neuroendocrine and the autonomic system (Stein et al., 1976). Behavioral conditioning may cause immunosuppression (Ader and Cohen, 1975).

Psychological symptoms such as depression, anxiety and premonitions of doom may be the earliest signs of cancer of the pancreas or stomach or of other abdominal malignancies. The mechanisms for these symptoms is completely unknown.

TREATMENT OF PSYCHOSOMATIC DISORDERS

Psychosomatic therapy is based on the biopsychosocial model of disease. The psychosomatically oriented physician combines physical treatment with the appropriate psychological and social treatment. He selects from a variety of psychiatric treatments, including psychotropic drugs, behavior modification, and individual, family, and group psychotherapy. Psychoanalysis or other kinds of interpretative psychotherapy is no longer the preferred treatment for the classical psychosomatic illnesses, but it may be necessary for the treatment of concurrent neurotic or character problems. Coincidentally the physical disorder may improve, but many people who have psychosomatic disorders have little contact with their inner psychological lives (McDougall, 1974). They are often less able to fantasize and to verbalize their feelings, a cognitive style that is referred to as alexithymia (Nemiah et al., 1976). Studies suggest that alexithymic persons may develop iatrogenic illnesses unless the physician recognizes their tendency to communicate emotional distress through physical symptoms. Certain patients may benefit from modified psychoanalytic treatment, but for most patients who have psychosomatic disorders the most useful psychotherapeutic approach is one that increases their awareness of the relationship between stress and the onset or exacerbation of their illness and improves their ability to cope with stress (Wolff, 1968). To help the patient realize that his mind and body are not separate it is better for supportive psychotherapy to be provided by the patient's primary physician rather than by a psychiatrist. The primary physician should consult with a psychiatrist if necessary. Group psychotherapy that educates patients about their illnesses is valuable for people with physical diseases.

REFERENCES

Ader, R. and Cohen, N. (1975): Behaviorally Conditioned Immunosuppression. *Psychosom. Med.* 37:333.

Alexander, F. (1950): *Psychosomatic Medicine.* New York, W. W. Norton.

American Psychiatric Association (1968): *Diagnostic and Statistical Manual of Mental Disorders.* 2d ed. Washington, D.C.

Bahnson, M. B. and Bahnson, C. B. (1969): Ego defenses in cancer patients. *Ann. N.Y. Acad. Sci.* 164:546.

Baker, L. and Barcai, A. (1970): Psychosomatic aspects of diabetes mellitus. In *Modern Trends in Psychosomatic Medicine.* Vol. 2. Edited by O. W. Hill. New York, Butterworths.

Bruch, H. (1977): Anorexia nervosa. In *Psychosomatic Medicine: Its Clinical Applications.* Edited by E. D. Wittkower and H. Warnes. Hagerstown, Md., Harper & Row.

Chambers, W. N. and Reiser, M. F. (1953): Emotional stress in the precipitation of congestive heart failure. *Psychosom. Med.* 15:38.

Crisp, A. H. (1977a): Diagnosis and outcome of anorexia nervosa: the St. George's view. *Proc. R. Soc. Med.* 70:464.

Crisp, A. H. (1977b): The differential diagnosis of anorexia nervosa. *Proc. R. Soc. Med.* 70:686.

Dimsdale, J. E. (1977): Emotional causes of sudden death. *Am. J. Psychiatry.* 134:1361.

Engel, G. L. (1955): Studies of ulcerative colitis: nature of psychologic processes. *Am. J. Med.* 19:231.

Engel, G. L. (1956): Studies of ulcerative colitis: the significance of headaches. *Psychosom. Med.* 18:334.

Engel, G. L. (1977): The need for a new medical model: a challenge for biomedicine. *Science.* 196:129.

French, T. M. and Alexander, F. (1941): *Psychogenic Factors in Bronchial Asthma.* Washington, D.C., National Research Council.

Friedman, M. and Rosenman, R. H. (1960): Overt behavior pattern in coronary disease. *J.A.M.A.* 173:1320.

Greene, W. A. and Miller, G. (1958): Psychological factors and reticuloendothelial disease. *Psychosom. Med.* 20:124.

Groen, J. J. (1976): Present status of the psychosomatic approach to bronchial asthma. In *Modern Trends in Psychosomatic Medicine.* Vol. 3. Edited by O. W. Hill. London, Butterworths.

Groen, H. H. (1976): Psychosomatic aspects of ischaemic (coronary) heart disease. In *Modern Trends in Psychosomatic Medicine.* Vol. 3. Edited by O. W. Hill. London, Butterworths.

Karush, A., Daniels, G. E., Flood, C., et al. (1977): *Psychotherapy in Chronic Ulcerative Colitis.* Philadelphia, Saunders.

LeShan, L. (1959): Psychological states as factors in the development of malignant disease: a critical review. *J. Nat. Cancer Inst.* 22:1.

Lipp, M. R., Looney, J. G., and Spitzer, R. L. (1977): Classifying psychophysiologic disorders: a new idea. *Psychosom. Med.* 39:285.

McDougall, H. (1974): The psychosoma and the psychoanalytic process. *Int. Rev. Psycho-Anal.* 1:437.

Mirsky, I. A. (1958): Physiologic, psychologic and social determinants in the etiology of duodenal ulcer. *Am. J. Dig. Dis.* 3:285.

Nemiah, J. D., Freyberger, H., and Sifneos, P. (1976): Alexithymia: a view of the psychosomatic process. In *Modern Trends in Psychosomatic Medicine.* Vol. 3. Edited by O. W. Hill. London, Butterworths.

O'Connor, J. F. (1970): A comprehensive approach to the treatment of ulcerative colitis. In *Modern Trends in Psychosomatic Medicine.* Edited by O. W. Hill. London, Butterworths.

Pinkerton, P. (1973): The enigma of asthma. *Psychosom. Med.* 35:461.

Schmale, A. H. and Iker, H. P. (1966): The affect of hopelessness and the development of cancer. *Psychosom. Med.* 28:714.

Schmale, A. H. (1972): Giving up as a final common pathway to changes in health. *Adv. Psychosom. Med.* 8:20.

Schonfield, J. (1975): Psychological and life-experience differences between Israeli women with benign and cancerous breast lesions. *J. Psychosom. Res.* 19:229.

Stavraky, K. M. (1968): Psychological factors in the outcome of human cancer. *J. Psychosom. Res.* 12:251.

Stein, M., and Luparello, T. J. (1970): Psychosomatic aspects of respiratory disorders. *Postgrad. Med.* 47:137.

Stein, M., Schiavi, R. C., and Camerino, M. (1976): Influence of brain and behavior on the immune system. *Science* 191:435.

Weiner, H. (1977): *Psychobiology and Human Disease.* New York, Elsevier.

Weiner, H., Thaler, M., and Reiser, M., et al. (1957): Etiology of duodenal ulcer: relation of specific psychological characteristics to rate of gastric secretion (serum pepsinogen). *Psychosom. Med.* 19:1.

Wolff, H. H. (1968): The psychodynamic approach to psychosomatic disorders: Contributions and limitations of psychoanalysis. *Br. J. Med. Psychol.* 41:343.

FURTHER READINGS

Freedman, A. M., Kaplan, H. I., and Sadock, B. H., eds. (1975): *Comprehensive Textbook of Psychiatry.* 2nd ed. Baltimore, Williams and Wilkins.
The chapter on Psychophysiological Disorders is a detailed discussion of selected psychosomatic disorders.

Lipowski, Z. J., ed. (1972): *Psychosocial Aspects of Physical Illness.* Basel, Karger.
A comprehensive review of psychosocial determinants of illness onset, psychological responses to illness, plus the patient and his environment.

Strain, J. H., and Grossman, S., eds. (1975): *Psychological Care of the Medically Ill: A Primer in Liaison Psychiatry.* New York, Appleton-Century Crofts.
A useful handbook which demonstrates the application of psychiatric and psychosomatic principles in the medical setting.

Weiner, H. (1977): *Psychobiology and Human Disease.* New York, Elsevier.
An extremely comprehensive and up-to-date review of six of the 'classical' psychosomatic disorders.

Wittkower, E. D. and Warnes, H., eds. (1977): *Psychosomatic Medicine: Its Clinical Applications.* Hagerstown, Md., Harper & Row.
A recent overview of psychosomatic principles, disorders and treatment.

CHAPTER 19

Pain

Robert Pos

Pain is the symptom that most often compels people to seek help from physicians, surgeons, and psychiatrists. The average psychiatrist hears complaints of pain from more than 60% of his patients who are ambulatory (Klee et al., 1959).

In 1811, Bell established the fact that there are sensory nerves and motor nerves, and Magendi confirmed this in 1822. In 1846, Weber began to differentiate the sensation of touch from the sensation of pain. Weber's work led to the specificity theory of pain, which is still taught in most medical schools. According to that theory, noxious stimuli produce crude sensations of pain, just as stimuli of light and sound produce crude visual and auditory sensations. Just as the intensity of a sound affects the intensity of a person's perception of the sound, so the intensity of an unpleasant stimulus (pain stimuli measured in dols) affects the intensity of the perception of pain. It is supposed that the number of dols of pain indicates the extent of the damage to tissue that exists in the painful part of the body. In other words, the amount of pain indicates the seriousness of the tissue damage, if not of the illness. The specificity theory suggests that pain is transmitted directly from certain peripheral pain receptors to a pain center in the brain. That

implication caused the popular belief that pain is always caused by damage to body tissue, or by malfunction of body tissue, and that removing such causes of pain by drugs or surgery should stop the pain.

BEYOND THE SPECIFICITY THEORY OF PAIN

Later research contradicted important aspects of the specificity theory. For example, research on the physiology of sensory input showed that only a fraction of the peripheral receptor excitation that stimulates the peripheral sensory nerves reaches the center of the nervous system. Sensory input from the peripheral sensory receptors has to pass sensory relays in the spinal cord, the thalamus, and the cerebral cortex. The total sensory input of all modalities, including the spino-thalamic pain modality, is carefully modulated at these different relays. Each relay is a "gate" allowing a portion of the stimulus to get through. In this way the brain continuously filters out particular patterns of information from the vast amount of total sensory input potentially available to it at any given moment. The regulation of this filtering process has to do with the physiology of attention. Research on the

157

psychophysiology of perception showed that paying attention to a perception intensifies the perception. If a person has a pain and pays attention to it, he increases the intensity of the pain. If he pays attention to something else, he diminishes or stops it. For example, some farmers used to bleed their horses by cutting a vein in their flank and they could do so without trouble if someone squeezed the horses' nostrils. Artificial stimuli in some parts of the body may counteract pain in other parts of the body. Melzack and Wall have suggested that many ancient medical practices were used because they produced counter-irritation and so diverted attention from other more serious sensations of pain. Among these were cupping, scarifying the skin, burning ("Moxa"), and perhaps also acupuncture.

Different people handle perceptions, including perceptions of pain, differently. Some people tend to intensify their perceptions, and some minimize them. Others seem to be average in this respect. Thus a person of the first type calls pain unbearable very soon, just as he overestimates the size of an object he perceives only by touch; whereas a person of the second type accepts more pain and also underestimates the size of an object that he touches (Petrie, 1967).

EXPERIMENTAL VERSUS CLINICAL PAIN

There is an important difference between pain that is induced experimentally (for example, by pricking the skin, by applying heat or cold to the skin, or by pressing hard on a part of the body) and so-called clinical pain (for example from cancer or postoperative wounds). Placebos help about 35% of people with clinical pain, but only 3.2% of the people who have pain that is induced by experiment. The more intense the feeling of clinical pain, the more such patients are helped by placebo (up to 40%) and the less intense the clinical pain, the smaller the effect of placebos (down to 26%). Since it is thought that placebos are effective psychologically but not biologically, the intensity and the occurrence of pain caused by illness has major psychological components, but not pain that is induced experimentally.

Narcotics such as morphine do not relieve pain that is induced experimentally, but they do relieve the pain that is caused by illness. People who have experimentally induced pain cannot distinguish large doses of morphine from large doses of normal saline solution. That fact suggested to Beecher (1965) that narcotics affect the pain that is caused by illness in its psychological components rather than in its physical cause or sensory conduction.

The results of Beecher's study reinforce the opinion that the subjectively experienced pain in illness has very important psychological dimensions. Beecher added further support to this point of view by demonstrating the placebo effect that a mammillary artery ligation may have on angina pectoris. Because the operation reduced patients' pain and their need for nitroglycerine, caused the patients' electrocardiograms to revert to a more nearly normal pattern, and increased the patients' ability to exercise, it became popular in North America. However, control studies convincingly demonstrated no difference between ligation and the placebo effect that it produced (Beecher, 1961).

Finally, Beecher compared the need for morphine of soldiers who were injured in war to the need of victims of civilian accidents. The psychological significance of a patient's wound affected his need for morphine. Twenty-five percent of the injured soldiers wanted morphine when it was offered to them, whereas more than 80% of the injured civilians wanted it. The soldiers saw their injuries as a way to safety and to survival, whereas the civilians saw their injuries as disasters (Beecher, 1956).

THE PSYCHOLOGICAL REACTION COMPONENT OF PAIN

Beecher's findings suggest that it is important to distinguish the perceptual and the psychological reaction components of pain. That is analogous to making a distinction between one's visual perception of something and the psychological reactions to the perception. For example, different people may react differently to seeing the same animal. A person's reaction to the animal would depend on his past experience.

Children are not born with established pain reactions. An infant who has a bleeding wound does not react to it as though it were painful. A child who is about 10 months old may bang his head against a wall as if his head were a foreign object (Schilder, 1960). Until a child learns that his body and his environment are separate he cannot distinguish between a negative emotional reaction that is related to his body (pain) and a negative reaction that is related to his environment (namely, anxiety). At that stage one sees undifferentiated "unpleasure" reactions (crying fits) that seem to be caused by the frustration of his biological needs. When the child's emotional reactions become differentiated into anxiety as triggered by his environment, and pain originating in the body, he has, in fact, achieved the psychological separation of his body and his environment.

Environmental and bodily (including spinothalamic) stimuli become associated with people, events, and the satisfaction and frustration of needs. Just as blind children will not develop meaningful responses to light stimuli, so animals that are not exposed to painful stimuli during their early development do not later develop normal reactions to pain stimuli (Hebb, 1949) and harm themselves since they do not avoid harmful objects. Some people have pain asymbolia, the absence of normal reactions to painful stimuli. Of course,

pain asymbolia has its dangers for the person who has it. He too may be burned or wounded without experiencing the alarm signals of pain. Spinothalamic stimuli, which are usually painful, become included in the configurations of other types of bodily and environmental sensory input and, as such, acquire meaning in terms of body image (localization as well as psychological-biological meaning). Much later, verbal reactions are added.

The preceding discussion of pain has pointed out that one should consider not only bodily stimuli, namely sensory signals, of actually or potentially harmful processes affecting the body, but also the presence of the psychological meaning of the pain perception to a person. This we refer to as the psychological pain reaction which is not present at birth but develops with life experience and maturation. This psychological pain reaction plays a major role in the way a person experiences his pain, especially its intensity. It also affects the way he behaves in response to the pain, including reactions of his autonomic nervous system. The psychological pain reaction is particularly important in clinical pain, and is less crucial in the perception of experimentally induced pain. The greater the pain caused by an illness, the greater the role of psychological pain reactions. This finding has clinical significance. Many physicians still try to stop pain by manipulating the body, including cutting pain conduction systems. Such surgical intervention is then supposed to stop the transmission of stimuli which cause the pain. But this kind of surgery does not consistently give good results (Melzack, 1973). For example, many patients are still crippled with pain in their backs after several orthopedic and/or neurosurgical operations. And the well-known phenomenon of the painful phantom-limb is often extremely resistant to somatic intervention.

In considering the psychological reac-

tion component of pain, two important issues must be given attention:

1. We are not born with a clear and
well-organized body image. It has to be
learned and it includes recognition of certain body experiences as painful. But the
spinothalamic pain stimuli do not occur in
isolation. They are part of the general sensory awareness of the affected body part
and the rest of the body. These complex
stimuli also contain information about the
environment. And in certain circumstances a stimulus that is in itself not
pain producing may produce pain, because of a previous association with a painful event. The painful part of the body then
represents the entire original situation in
which the pain was first experienced. This
kind of pain mechanism is often important
in some so-called conversion syndromes,
in which an emotional conflict is converted into pain in an area of the body. But
it may be important in many conditions
seen by the general practitioner (see Chap.
16). While these are not strictly conversion
syndromes, they speak of psychological
pain in somatic terms, including pelvic
pains, persistent pain following whiplash
or other injuries, pains in the tem-
poromandibular joint, and a variety of
headaches.

2. Both the early undifferentiated "unpleasure" responses of the infant (crying
fits) and, later, more differentiated pain
behavior affect the other people in the environment. They learn to respond and assist him in the relief of the painful state.
Gradually, life experience teaches the baby
that unpleasure responses and pain behavior lead to such social responses. By instrumental conditioning, pain experiences
and pain reactions may eventually and au-
tomatically (unconsciously) occur to bring
about the kind of social responses which
they originally provoked in order to fulfill
inner needs or to avoid frustrations, e.g. in
some asthmatic attacks which are often
first caused by allergens. Some parents respond with intense attention and concern.

In due course the child may become conditioned to have an asthma attack
whenever he wants that attention and concern. In similar fashion, pain in a body
part, and the pain behavior accompanying
it, may become coupled to the original social helping response. In such cases, the
pain may become a method of communicating emotional needs to others
without carrying medical information of
damage to the body (Szasz, 1957). Psychogenic, conditioned pain mechanisms produce subjective pain as real to the sufferer,
and as crippling, as pains that start on an
organic basis. And a protracted pain which
originated in an organic condition is frequently elaborated over time through one
or both of the described conditioned pain
mechanisms.

Unfortunately, when the physician goes
beyond "Where is the pain? What is it that
hurts?" and begins investigating the patient's psychological world, the patient
often feels accused of faking or imagining
his pain. Or, the physician may conclude
that "the pain is not real" following an
exhaustive but negative physical examination and investigation. In both cases a
stalemated doctor-patient relationship
may be the result. On the other hand, if
both the patient and the physician continue to view the pain according to the
specificity theory and fail to give importance to psychological factors, then the
physician may give the patient inappropriate narcotic medication, subject him to
endless investigation, further reinforcing
psychological factors, or surgical intervention. All of this may be without positive
results.

The group of patients with chronic pain
includes many people whose pain originally started through psychogenic, conditioned pain mechanisms with secondary, organic consequences: as a result of
their pain they may resort to drugs, or stop
using limbs, or assume damaging body
postures. However labeled, patients with
chronic pain are practically indistinguish-

able from one another on psychiatric examination (Woodforde and Merskey, 1972).

Once the physician has treated any of the organic aspects of pain that may threaten the patient's health, he must cope with the psychological aspects of the pain. He should try to understand these aspects of pain in terms of the patient's past, present, and future. It is in that light that he should make his decisions about taking any medical, surgical, psychotherapeutic, or behavior-modifying action.

REFERENCES

Beecher, H. K. (1956): Relationship of significance of wound to the pain experienced. *J.A.M.A.,* 161:1609.

Beecher, H. K. (1961): Surgery as placebo: a quantitative study of bias. *J.A.M.A.* 176:1102.

Beecher, H. K. (1965): Quantification of the subjective pain experience. In *Psychopathology of Perception.* Edited by P. H. Hoch and J. Zubin. New York, Grune & Stratton.

Melzack, R. (1974): Psychological concepts and methods for the control of pain. In *Advances in Neurology.* Vol. 4. Edited by J. J. Bonica. New York, Raven Press.

Petrie, A. (1967): *Individuality in Pain and Suffering.* Chicago, University of Chicago Press.

Pos, R. (1974): Psychological assessment of factors affecting pain. *Can. Med. Assoc. J.* 111:1213.

Schilder, P. (1960): The body image. In *Contributions to Developmental Neuropsychiatry.* Edited by L. Bender. New York, International Universities Press.

Szasz, T. S. (1957): *Pain and Pleasure: A Study of Bodily Function.* New York, Basic Books.

Woodforde, J. M. and Merskey, H. (1972): Some relationships between subjective measures of pain. *J. Psychosom. Res.* 16:172.

FURTHER READINGS

Bonica, J. J., ed. (1974): *Advances in Neurology.* Vol. 4. New York, Raven Press.

A review of pain treatment and research by 93 leading neurologists, neurosurgeons, anesthesiologists, pharmacologists, physiologists and psychiatrists.

Kapp, F. T. (1975): Psychogenic pain. In *Comprehensive Textbook of Psychiatry.* Edited by A. Freeman, H. Kaplan and B. Sadock. 2d ed., Baltimore, Williams & Wilkins.

A succinct review of psychological factors in pain syndromes.

CHAPTER 20

Sleep Disorders
Robert Pos

Most adults sleep for seven or eight hours each day; thus they spend about one-third of their lives in sleep. The person who does not sleep for a long time may suffer severe but reversible psychological disturbances that may be difficult to distinguish from schizophrenia. The sleepless person first becomes increasingly tired and sleepy. After about four days, perceptual functioning and the ability to pay attention to either the environment or his own mental processes become impaired. As a result, thoughts become fragmented, memory suffers, and emotions become labile. The person becomes disoriented, interprets events in a delusional way, and hallucinates, or confuses mental images and misperceptions (illusions) with reality. However, as soon as he is allowed to sleep without interruption, the mental disturbances disappear (Johnson, 1969).

During the 1950's, Aserinsky, Kleitman and Dement discovered that sleep was a complex phenomenon involving more than a simple loss of consciousness and slowing of brain waves. They found different physiological states alternating rhythmically during sleep (Dement and Kleitman, 1957). The activity of brain waves during sleep is cyclic. Each cycle is about ninety minutes long, and during each cycle, the brain-wave activity slows down (slow-wave sleep) and then returns to the waking level (fast-wave sleep) (Fig. 3).

During fast-wave sleep (shown by the dark areas in Fig. 3), electric tracings of the eyes show rapid eye movements (REM) and the muscle potentials flatten out. If the sleeper is awakened during this fast-wave sleep, he will often report typical nonlogical dreams (D-state). Although electric activity in the brain is the same during REM sleep as it is when the person is awake, it is more difficult to awaken a sleeper who is in REM sleep than one who is in slow-wave sleep ("paradoxic sleep," i.e., behaviorally "deep," electroencephalographically "light"). This is probably due to a general shutdown of the sensory relays that transmit input from the sleeper's body and environment, which in turn is related to loss of tonus in the voluntary musculature. In a sense, the brain appears to be in a state of relative functional isolation from the body and environment during REM sleep. And many physiological activities appear to function autonomously during REM sleep. For example, the sleeper's pulse, blood

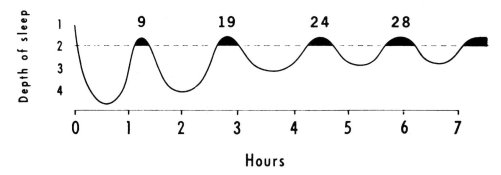

FIG. 3. Alternating periods of slow-wave sleep and fast-wave sleep. Dreaming and rapid eye
movements (REM) begin when the sleeper emerges from deep sleep to the level of electroencephalogram stage 1. The numbers over the dark areas show the length of successive
periods of dreaming REM periods). As sleep progresses, slow-wave sleep (non-REM periods)
becomes less deep and REM periods become longer. (Reproduced from Kleitman, N. (1966):
Patterns of dreaming. In *Psychobiology, the Biological Bases of Behavior: Readings from
Scientific American.* San Francisco and London, W. H. Freeman & Co.)

pressure, and respiration are irregular, with rebound phenomena within these irregularities. Also, the behavior of the sleeper's body is frequently unrelated to the content of the dream. For example, erection of the penis occurs and is not necessarily associated with sexual dreams. REM sleep goes together with a degree of physiological disorganization and is therefore stressful to the body (Pos, 1969). The corticosteroids—stress hormones—are most elevated during the last part of sleep, when REM sleep dominates. But the secretion of growth hormone (GH), which promotes synthesis of protein, occurs during slow-wave sleep, particularly during its first, longest, and deepest period. Several health problems may show up during the longest period of REM sleep, which occurs in the early morning, for example, cardiac decompensation, coronary occlusion, and attacks of migraine, ulcer pain, and asthma. There has been, and continues to be, much debate about the relative importance of sufficient amounts of REM sleep versus sufficient amounts of NREM sleep for normal mental functioning. The evidence favors NREM sleep. Perhaps Freud, who thought that dreaming protected the sleeper from waking up, was right.

SLEEP NEEDS AND ACTIVITY CHANGE DURING LIFE

At birth, the infant's brain activity occurs in sixty-minute cycles during which rest and activity alternate. Rest (sleep) occupies about two-thirds of the infant's time. The sleep is equally divided between NREM and REM sleep. With age—and the concomitant decrease in the metabolic rate—the rest-activity cycle slowly lengthens to a ninety-minute cycle. In adults, this cycle shows up in the NREM-REM cycle. During sleep, during waking, the cycle is also apparent in the rhythmic alternation of body activity and may, for example, be seen in the rhythmic alteration of gastric secretion in healthy adults who are kept in bed. Figure 4 shows the relationship between waking, REM sleep and NREM sleep throughout life.

Several biochemical-neurophysiological theories attempt to account for the adult's ninety-minute sleep cycle. The most popular theory, although it is not proven, is that of Jouvet (1972). Jouvet's theory proposes a feedback relationship between the median raphe area in the reticular formation of the pons (where NREM sleep may originate) and the locus ceruleus in the tegmentum of the pons

REM SLEEP/NREM SLEEP RELATIONSHIP
THROUGHOUT HUMAN LIFE

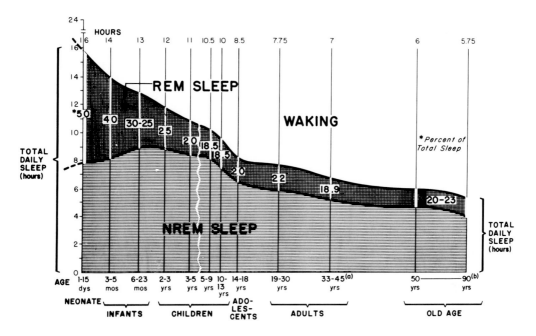

FIG. 4.   Graph showing changes (with age) in total amounts of daily REM sleep, and in percentage of REM sleep. Note sharp diminution of REM sleep in the early years. REM sleep falls from 8 hours at birth to less than 1 hour in old age. The amount of NREM sleep throughout life remains more constant, falling from 8 hours to 5 hours. In contrast to the steep decline of REM sleep, the quantity of NREM sleep is undiminished for many years. Although total daily REM sleep falls steadily during life, the percentage rises slightly in adolescence and early adulthood. This rise does not reflect an increase in amount; it is due to the fact that REM sleep does not diminish as quickly as total sleep. Data for the 33- to 45 and 50- to 90 year groups are taken from Strauch and Kales et al. (1967), Feinberg et al. (1967) and Kahn and Fisher (1969), respectively. (Revised by Roffwarg, Muzio and Dement since publication in *Science, 152*:604–619, 1966 and used with their permission.)

(where REM sleep may originate). It is thought that the median raphe produces serotonin and the locus ceruleus produces noradrenaline. The system operates in a ninety-minute cycle and drugs that interfere with either the median raphe or the locus ceruleus increase or decrease the relative amounts of NREM and REM sleep.

INSOMNIA

Since sleep deprivation can temporarily disorganize mental functioning, insomnia should be taken seriously. It is one of the problems most frequently encountered by the physician. The person with insomnia complains of trouble falling asleep or staying asleep, or he wakens too early, or a combination of those. To fall asleep and begin the NREM-REM cycle, one must first relax (relaxation increases alpha activity of the EEG). This is made easier by cutting down on external stimuli through silence and darkness, and reducing bodily stimuli by removing clothes that are too tight and lying still. Anything less than complete relaxation makes falling asleep difficult. Any preoccupation, whether worry, depression, anger, or even pleasurable excitement keeps the person awake because it arouses the brain. Pain also stimulates the brain, as does unaccustomed noise. Chemicals that stimulate the reticular-activating substance of the brain stem such as caffeine, amphetamines, or methylphenidate also prevent sleep.

Somewhat more difficult to detect, unless specifically looked for, are fears and anxieties of which the patient may not be aware, and which may prevent sleep. A patient may have a conscious or an unconscious sleep phobia. In such a case, the anticipation of falling asleep creates anxiety because the sleeper fears that he will become sick during sleep or that in his passive state he may be sexually assaulted. Or the patient may suffer from a dream phobia and stay awake to avoid frightening dreams. Another kind of psychological problem underlying insomnia may be seen in the child whose parents are upset because the child cannot sleep. Not falling asleep may be the child's unconscious way of upsetting the parents.

Once they have had some trouble falling asleep, many people begin to worry about insomnia. They anticipate an inability to fall asleep; and the anticipation functions as a self-fulfilling prophecy. The worry may be due to their assumption that there is something wrong with a person whose sleep is disturbed. They try hard to fall asleep so that they can function well the next day. Yet, their anxious efforts keep them awake.

People who keep themselves busy as a defense to block out disturbing thoughts and feelings often have trouble falling asleep. The silence and inactivity they experience when preparing for sleep or lying awake threatens them. They get up to do or eat something, or they waken the person with whom they are sleeping in order to make something happen.

The more a person anticipates being unable to sleep the more often he will ask the physician to prescribe sleeping pills. Most sleeping pills, including barbiturates and chloral hydrate, lose their effectiveness in a couple of weeks. Continuing the medication may help only because of its placebo effect. When the medication is stopped, the insomnia returns for psychological reasons, or the patient may experience wakefulness and agitation as the result of a "rebound effect."

Traveling from one time zone to another disturbs one's usual sleeping patterns. Adjustment to a new cycle of day and night may take a few days.

Difficulty in staying asleep during the night or waking in the early morning is often caused by waking up from REM sleep. The person may wake up from a disturbing dream without recalling the dream's content. Or, the shutdown reflex of REM sleep fails for some nonpsychological reason. Some medications may affect the occurrence and duration of REM sleep. Also, some forms of depression appear to reduce REM sleep. The person who wakes up in the very early morning out of the longest period of REM sleep may have had disturbed dreams during that period.

The people who worry about being unable to fall asleep in the first place also usually worry again when waking up during the night or the early morning. Their anxiety prevents the quick and smooth resumption of their NREM-REM cycle.

Insomnia is common in persons who have psychiatric disorders; as many as 80% of all psychiatric patients have insomnia. Depressed patients usually sleep less than normal. The total time of the REM sleep usually decreases, and the amount of their NREM sleep decreases both absolutely and relative to the amount of their REM sleep. As the patient's depression lifts, the amount of REM sleep first returns to normal. Next, the amount of NREM sleep returns to normal, and with this, the symptoms disappear (Hawkins and Mendels, 1966).

HYPERSOMNIA

A person who has hypersomnia sleeps more than nine hours each day. Usually, functioning is not impaired, although he may be slow to wake up, and confused when he does wake up. The physician in such a case should carefully assess the patient. The problem may be due to drugs, such as alcohol, barbiturates, tranquillizers, or antidepressants. Or, there may be metabolic cause, such as uremia, diabetes, hypoglycemia, the retention of carbon dioxide, or hepatic failure. Drowsiness may be related to neurological problems such as encephalitis, a vascular disturbance, a tumor close to the third ventricle, head injury, or increased intracranial pressure. The Pickwickian syndrome includes obesity, respiratory insufficiency, with the retention of carbon dioxide, and hypersomnia. The Kleine-Levin syndrome includes attacks of voracious eating and hypersomnia (the hypersomnia probably is caused by the overeating).

Although depression is usually accompanied by insomnia, it may be accompanied by hypersomnia which may be a psychological defense mechanism to avoid the painful state of being awake. Sullivan pointed out that some people generally use the defense of sleep when they face a stressful situation: he called it the reaction dynamism of somnolent withdrawal. In depressed patients this mechanism used during the day and insomnia at night leads to a reversal of their sleeping patterns.

DISORDERS OF NREM SLEEP: NIGHT TERROR, SLEEPWALKING, BEDWETTING

Gastaut and Broughton (1965) studied the episodic phenomena of night terror, sleepwalking, and bedwetting, and found that they occur during NREM sleep (slow-wave). Bedwetting occurs most frequently; it occurs in about 10% of children between four and five years old. It may occur together with sleepwalking. Sleepwalking itself has an incidence in the general population of up to 6% (Kales et al, 1975).

Contrary to popular belief, the person who is sleepwalking is not very well coordinated. He is confused, and he responds to environmental stimuli at a level that is lower than normal. Usually sleepwalking in children is a temporary problem. The children outgrow it, and it does not in itself indicate a psychological disturbance.

Night terror, also called pavor nocturnus (in children) and incubus (in adults), should not be confused with the bad dream or nightmare that may occur during REM sleep. The nightmare is only a dream, but is unpleasant and frightening. The content of the dream is well developed. The content of the dream and its physical expression, including reactions from the autonomic nervous system, are dissociated, so that any physical expression of fear during a nightmare is limited. This is to be expected from a dream during the REM state.

The sleeper often awakens from a nightmare. A night terror lasts about one or two minutes. It often occurs on the downcurve of the first period of NREM sleep. If the patient remembers the night terror, he usually remembers a single, frightening mental image such as a vision or a sound. The sleeper's psychological and behavioral reactions are consonant with his psychological experience. His reactions from the autonomic nervous system are notable—an increased heart rate, profuse sweating, and hyperventilation. The sleeper has a sense of doom or deep fright, and moans or screams. He does not easily and fully wake up from the night terror, and he may return to a peaceful sleep when it ends. If the sleeper is roused, he may not fully wake up (he may be in a state of clouded consciousness) and later he may not remember the episode at all. An electroencephalogram made during a night terror shows a waking alpha pattern. The EEG during a nightmare is typical of the REM state. In adults, but less so in children, night terrors often indicate major psychological disturbances.

DISORDERS OF REM-SLEEP: NARCOLEPSY AND SLEEP APNEA

Yoss and Daly (1960) described the so-called narcoleptic tetrad—narcolepsy, cataplexy, sleep paralysis and hypnagogic or hypnopompic hallucinations. Narcolepsy consists of sudden, irresistible attacks of sleep that last as long as fifteen minutes. Things that make healthy people drowsy such as eating, boredom, warmth and fatigue, may trigger an attack of narcolepsy in a susceptible person. The attack usually leaves the person refreshed. The person who has narcolepsy is often considered irresponsible or lazy. Many of these attacks of sleep that occur during the day and also the first phase of nocturnal sleep begin with REM sleep rather than NREM sleep (Rechtschaffen, 1969).

The most common symptom next to narcolepsy is cataplexy, a sudden, partial or complete loss of skeletal muscle tone. This may cause the person to have a serious accident or injury. The person may seem to be an alcoholic or epileptic. The attack is often provoked by intense, unexpected, or highly emotional stimulation. Laughing may trigger a cataleptic attack. Some investigators think that cataplexy attacks are related to the loss of muscle tone that occurs during REM sleep.

The third symptom of the narcoleptic tetrad is sleep paralysis. Sleep paralysis is a failure of motor control while the person is either going into or coming out of sleep. It is often accompanied by or associated with the fourth symptom of the narcoleptic tetrad—the occurrence of hallucinatory or illusionary experiences in the state between sleeping and waking. They are either hypnagogic (going into sleep) or hypnopompic (coming out of sleep). Hyp-

nagogic or hypnopompic hallucinations may also occur in people who do not have narcolepsy. They do not indicate a major psychiatric disorder.

The cause of narcolepsy is not known. In general, any person subjected to prolonged periods of sleep deprivation (doctors, shiftworkers, young mothers, etc.) are potential candidates for narcoleptic attacks. There are also genetic factors: relatives of narcoleptic patients are 200 times more likely to develop narcolepsy than others. Psychotherapeutic experience suggests that at least some people who have narcolepsy have, unwittingly, had a sleep phobia for many years.

Dextroamphetamine sulfate (Dexedrine) and methylphenidate (Ritalin) are often used to counteract the attacks of sleep, but a psychological investigation of the person with narcolepsy should be made. Recently, a drug synthesized from a brain substance, gamma-hydroxy-butyrate (GHB) has shown promise in the treatment of narcolepsy. If necessary, the person should undergo psychotherapy.

We have said that REM sleep is accompanied by a degree of physiological disorganization. REM sleep often includes short periods of apnea, particularly in healthy infants who are up to three months old. Steinschneider (1972) suggested a possible relationship between REM-apnea and crib death.

REFERENCES

Dement, W. and Kleitman, N. (1957): Cyclic variations in EEG during sleep and their relation to eye movements, body motility and dreaming. *Electroencephalog. Clin. Neurophysiol.* 9:673.

Gastaut, H. and Broughton, R. (1965): A clinical and polygraphic study of episodic phenomena during sleep. *Recent Adv. Biol. Psychiatry.* 7:197.

Hawkins, D. R. and Mendels, J. (1966): Sleep disturbance in depressive syndromes. *Am. J. Psychiatry.* 123:682.

Johnson, L. C. (1969): Psychological and physiological changes following total sleep deprivation. In *Sleep Physiology and Pathology.* Edited by A. Kales. Philadelphia, J. B. Lippincott.

Jouvet, M. (1972): The role of monoamines and acetylcholine-containing neurons in the regulation of the sleep waking cycle. *Ergeb. Physiol.* 64:166.

Pos, R. (1969): The biology of dreaming and the informational underload (sensory deprivation) theory of psychosis. *Canad. Psychiat. Ass. J.* 14:371.

Rechtschaffen, A. and Dement, W. C. (1969): Narcolepsy and hypersomnia. In *Sleep: Physiology and Pathology.* Edited by A. Kales. Philadelphia, J. B. Lippincott.

Steinschneider, A. (1972): Prolonged apnea and the sudden infant death syndrome: clinical and laboratory observations. *Pediatrics. 50:*646.

Yoss, R. E. and Daly, D. D. (1960): Narcolepsy. *Arch. Intern. Med. 106:*168.

FURTHER READINGS

Freud, S. (1953): The Interpretation of Dreams. In *The Standard Edition of the Complete Psychological Works of Sigmund Freud.* Vol. 4 and 5. London. Hogarth Press.

This is the classical psychoanalytic work on the psychological function, process and meaning of dreams.

Gastaut, H., Lugaresi, E., Berti Certoni, G., et al. (1968): *The Abnormalities of Sleep in Man.* Proceedings of the Reunion Europeene d' Information Electroencephalographique 15th Conference Held in Bologna, 1967. Bologna. A. Gaggi.

An international symposium reviewing the neurophysiological and neurochemical basis of sleep and discussing sleep disorders.

Hartmann, E. (1967): *The Biology of Dreaming.* Springfield, Ill., C. C Thomas.

A summary of sleep and dream research through 1967, concentrating on biological aspects.

Hartmann, E. ed. (1970): *Sleep and Dreaming.* Boston, Little, Brown.

A comprehensive review by well-known researchers and clinicians in the field of sleep and dream physiology and disorders, as well as psychoanalytic dream psychology.

21

Affective Disorders

Paul E. Garfinkel and Emmanuel Persad

Affect refers to a feeling tone, pleasurable or unpleasurable, that accompanies an idea. The term mood is used for sustained affects, although mood and affect may be used interchangeably. Affects include such feelings as grief, euphoria, anxiety and fear. Affective changes may vary from the normal mood swings of everyday life to persistent psychotic depressions. While there is a gradient between normal mood changes and pathological states, the distinction between the two is usually based on the intensity, duration and quality of mood, concomitant symptoms and the role of environmental influences. This chapter is concerned with depression and mania, often termed "The Affective Disorders."

As a feeling state, depression is a universal experience and refers to a sense of sadness. Depression becomes pathological when there is no identifiable loss associated with it (i.e. when it has risen "out of the blue") or when in response to an external situation its manifestations are excessive in intensity or duration. As psychopathology, depression may refer to a symptom or a group of syndromes. The symptom depression may occur in a variety of other illnesses. Affective symptoms seldom occur alone however; they are usu-

ally combined with somatic and psychosocial impairments, and when they form a particular cluster of signs and symptoms, one of the depressive syndromes is present.

An affective disorder is said to be *primary* when the depressive or manic syndrome occurs in an individual who has been previously well or whose only previous psychiatric illnesses were mania or depression. *Secondary* affective disorders occur in persons who have had other previous psychiatric (e.g. schizophrenia, obsessive-compulsive neurosis) or organic (e.g. influenza) illnesses. Primary affective disorders are defined as bipolar (manic-depressive) when mania occurs, whether depressions occur or not. Unipolar affective disorders involve depressions alone (Kendell, 1976).

HISTORY

Descriptions of affective disorder were noted in the Old Testament. In the first book of Samuel it is recorded that David's music made Saul "refreshed and well" that the "evil spirit departed from him" (1 Sam. 16:23). Similarly, Job faced the question of whether piety can withstand adversity. His response was evident in his behavior; although he met with repeated disaster, Job maintained his faith. During the test however, Job became depressed, reproached God and contemplated suicide.

Within medicine, Hippocrates was the first to write on the depressive syndrome. The term melancholia is usually attributed to him, as is the notion that it results from the influence of black bile on the brain. About five hundred years later, in the second century A.D., Areteaus recognized the association between mania and melancholia in some people; he also observed that mood disorders generally follow an episodic course. Like Hippocrates he attributed the course to a humoral imbalance (Knoff, 1975).

Current conceptions of affective disorders derive from the work of Kraepelin, at the end of the nineteenth century; he, in turn, was influenced by the writings of the French physician Falret. Falret described an episodic variety of depression with remissions and exacerbations, at times alternating with mania (la folie circulaire).

In 1896, Kraepelin made his major contribution by separating the functional psychoses into two groups, manic-depressive psychosis and dementia praecox (schizophrenia). The distinction was based on the outcome, with schizophrenia showing a chronic course and a bad prognosis. Kraepelin viewed manic-depressive psychosis as being independent of environmental influences with the cause related to constitutional factors (Kraepelin, 1919).

In 1917, Freud published *Mourning and Melancholia,* which outlined his theories on the psychodynamic genesis of depression by comparing it with normal grieving. Freud considered that melancholia resembles mourning because it occurs after a loss. Unlike mourning, however, melancholia occurs only in predisposed people and the melancholic may not have lost his loved object in reality but rather intrapsychically. That is, his emotional attachment

to it may have been broken off unconsciously because of hurt or disappointment. According to Freud, the normal person in mourning gradually withdraws his emotional attachment from the loved object. To the person in mourning, the world becomes poorer whereas one's self-regard is maintained. By contrast, in melancholia it is not the world that becomes empty, it is the person himself—he becomes full of self-directed anger and blame. To explain this self-directed anger Freud postulated that the melancholic does not loosen his emotional bonds with the unconsciously lost object. Rather, he identifies with the lost object. Therefore, the anger that the melancholic person directs against himself represents anger at the loved object.

From the 1920's descriptive psychiatrists began a prolonged controversy on the merits of subclassifying depressive illness into reactive and endogenous types. According to the proponents of that method of subclassifying (Gillespie and later Roth), a depression was *endogenous* when there was no clear environmental precipitant, when the patient did not respond to environmental influences, and when there was a typical clinical picture characterized by many vegetative signs of depression. Reactive depressions were said to lack these features. Others (Mapother, Lewis, and Kendell) viewed such a dichotomy to be artificial. They maintained that no valid or useful distinction can be drawn between the two, and that the differences that are observed are primarily differences in severity.

This system of subclassification has largely been discarded. Its major problem was that an etiological index—the presence or absence of precipitating psychosocial events—was used to classify depressions although the causes of the depressions were largely unknown. Moreover, the lack of psychosocial precipitants, thought to be characteristic of the endogenous depressive, often results from nonreporting although they are present. Depressive illnesses should be viewed as neither inherently psychosocial nor biological. Rather, they represent a final common pathway, the products of a variety of processes that may be described in many frames of reference. The heterogeneity of depressive disorders encountered in clinical practice can be understood as interactions among biological, psychological, and sociological factors (Akiskal and McKinney, 1975).

EPIDEMIOLOGY

Before studying the amounts and distribution of a disorder such as depression some consideration should be given to the methodological problems used. Statistics must be based on reliable diagnostic techniques; that is, there must be a particular set of indicators that can be said to contribute necessary and sufficient conditions for inferring the disease. Until recently the diagnosis of depression has not been uniform. Similarly, the method of case sampling from the population is important. Statistics from hospitals, although convenient, have limited utility. Field studies reveal more accurately the prevalence of a disease in the population. Whether the diagnosis is based on a questionnaire or a clinical interview (structured or unstructured) will also affect the results.

Prevalence refers to the number of existing cases of a disorder in the population at any one time. *Incidence* refers to the number of new cases of the disorder in the population per year. Annual first admissions to psychiatric hospitals for depression range from 2 to 29 per 100,000 for males. The corresponding figures for females are 4 to 50 per 100,000 (Fabrega, 1975). If outpatient facilities are also included, these figures triple. If information derived from general practitioners is included, the incidence is 10 times that of psychiatric admissions. The lifetime expectancy for anyone in the general population to be treated for depression has been estimated to be about 10%. Women treated for depression outnumber men treated by a ratio of at least 3:2. Affective disorders can begin at any age. It is generally acknowledged however, that the prevalence of depression is positively correlated with age. Bipolar disorders begin at an earlier age (the mean is about 30 years of age) than do unipolar depressions (the mean is the early 40's).

The incidence of bipolar illness has been commonly given as 3 to 4 per 1000. It is said to be less in Scandinavia and other parts of northern Europe. The Jews and Irish are said to have a higher than average incidence. In sharp contrast to schizophrenia, bipolar patients tend to come from middle and upper classes. Also unlike schizophrenic patients, those with bipolar illness are likely to be married.

ETIOLOGY

Genetic Factors

Several kinds of evidence may be used to support the idea that a disease of unknown etiology has a genetic basis. The first criterion suggesting a genetic background is the expectation that the risks for the same illness would be higher in family members of persons with the illness than in the general populations. The incidence of both unipolar and bipolar affective disorders are considerably increased in the families of patients. For example, Zerbin-Rudin evaluated the results of 25 investigations and noted the incidence of bipolar illness in parents, siblings, and children to be between 12 and 16%. In addition, the type of affective disorder tends to run true in families. Bipolar illness is common among relatives of bipolar patients.

Another finding that suggests a genetic factor is a greater concordance of the illness in monozygous than in dizygous twins. This has clearly been found to be the case with approximately 70% of monozygotic and 25% of dizygotic twins concordant for mood disorders.

A third finding supporting a genetic predisposition for mood disorder is the observation that other psychiatric syndromes occur more frequently in families of patients with affective disorders. Both alcoholism and sociopathy are overrepresented in the families of manic and depressive patients.

Further evidence that genetic factors are involved in some cases of bipolar mood disorder comes from linkage studies in which the distribution of an illness within families parallels that of a "genetic marker." Several families have been identified in which color blindness and bipolar illness were transmitted together (i.e. either both or neither were present in family members). Since color blindness is transmitted on the X-chromosome, this would suggest an X-linked mode of inheritance, at least for these few families. There have been other suggestions (Slater) that for some bipolar patients the mode of inheritance may be dependent on a single dominant gene with incomplete penetrance. There is less uniformity of opinion on unipolar illness, though some studies favor polygenic inheritance.

While these data strongly support a genetic component to the etiology of mood disorders, just what is inherited is a matter of speculation. Some have suggested it may be an alteration in neurohumoral control mechanism, others an ego weakness (Winokur, 1974).

Biological Factors

Biochemical explanations for depression date back to Hippocrates' description of a predominance of black bile as the cause of melancholia.

The possible role of altered metabolism of brain monoamine (MA) neurotransmitters (norepinephrine (NE), dopamine (DA), serotonin (5-HT)) in the etiology of some forms of depressive illness has become the dominant focus of biochemical research in affective disorders. (Chase and Murphy, 1973; Shopsin et al., 1974). This interest in MA's is a direct result of the recognition of the effectiveness of the tricyclic and monoamineoxidase inhibiting (MAOI) drugs as treatments for depression. These drugs, though acting via different mechanisms, tend to increase the amount of neurotransmitters available at synapses. These findings gave rise to the catecholamine/indoleamine hypothesis which stated that some types of depressive illness are related to a depletion of NE or 5-HT at nerve endings in the limbic system. The opposite is hypothesized for mania. The finding that reserpine, which depletes MA's from nerve cells, could cause depression supported this hypothesis. Lithium, an anti-manic agent, lowers the amount of NE at the synaptic cleft. Conversely electric shock and such mood stimulants as amphetamine and cocaine increase NE at the synapse.

More recently the MA hypotheses have been modified to include the possibility that the synaptic release of neurotransmitters may be normal but the post-synaptic receptor may be defective in its response. Further modifications have examined the interactions of brain MAs as possibly related to mood disorders; thus we have the cholinergic-adrenergic imbalance model (some depressions may show excessive cholinergic activity with mania excess adrenergic activity) and the permissive hypothesis (implicating imbalance between catechol and indole systems).

At present, each of these models is based on indirect psychopharmacological evidence and no direct proof exists to implicate altered MA's in mood disorders. In addition these models may not be mutually exclusive. It is possible that our methods of clinical description do not adequately separate depressive subtypes. Depression may be analogous to fever; that is, identical clinical syndromes may be associated with different biochemical systems. An example of a similar clinical picture with underlying differences in biochemistry and its importance for treatment relates to MHPG (3 Methoxy 4 Hydroxy Phenylglycol) excretion. MHPG is the major metabolite of NE from the brain. Patients with depressions tend to fall into two groups with regard to urinary MHPG excretion. There are several studies demonstrating that the level of urinary MHPG excretion may be predictive of which tricyclic drug will prove clinically useful for an individual. Further work is necessary, however, before such a biochemical classification of depressions can become clinically practical.

Psychosocial Factors

Freud's views on the psychological factors in depression were noted earlier. After Freud, Rado emphasized the psychological predisposition to depression. He stressed the precarious self-esteem of the depressive and his need for external gratification. He described the depressive as a person with intense narcissistic needs who reacts to loss by first rebelling angrily and then by self-punishment, with the hope of expiation in order to win back love. Melanie Klein, by contrast, elaborated the theory that the predisposition to depression depends on the quality of the mother-child relationship in the first year of life. If this relationship does not promote in the child a feeling that he is good and loved, he is never able to overcome his marked ambivalence towards close relationships and may be prone to recurrent depressions.

More recently, Bibring and others have directed less attention to Freud's self-directed aggression model of depression and more to the role of self-esteem. Depression basically represents a reduction or breakdown in self-esteem. In the psychoanalytic literature mania has generally been regarded as a defense against depression.

Bibring basically agreed with Rado in seeing that the predisposition to depression was a result of earlier childhood traumatic experiences which bring about a sense of helplessness and powerlessness. For Bibring depressions had a common basic structure, a loss of self-esteem due to situations in which one feels weak and helpless; situations in which one feels unworthy because of thoughts, feelings, or actions which one considers unacceptable; and situations in which one feels unloved by others who are considered important to him. Jacobson described several factors involved in the regulation of self-esteem: the superego (by virtue of feeling guilt), the self-critical ego functions (the more mature these are the more realistic one's goals), the ego ideal (the more within reach the more enhancing for self-esteem), the ego functions, and the self-representations (for example, a distorted body image will alter one's feelings of worth).

Clearly a number of factors are involved in the regulation of self-esteem. Of great importance are early parent-child interactions. As a child develops, an affectionate acceptance by his parents tends to produce a basic self-confidence in his worth. As the child continues to develop, his actual effectiveness and his confidence in himself, maintain and consolidate his self-worth. On the other hand, the child who has insufficient parental acceptance, too much parental devaluation and who feels ineffective in his early social activities will likely develop decreased self-esteem. As Jacobson emphasized, the superego, or internalized parental moral values, is also involved in the regulation of self-esteem. When these values are not lived up to in behavior, guilt is experienced, with a concomitant lessening of self-worth. Similarly, the more realistic one's ideals, the more possible it is to attain them, thereby strengthening one's sense of adequacy. The personality of the individual also plays a role in predisposition to depression. According to Chodoff and others, people who are excessively dependent on external or environmental factors for maintenance of a sense of self-worth become depressed more readily in the face of environmental precipitants.

From this, it is evident that the psychosocial precipitants to depression are quite variable. Depression can be precipitated by the loss of, or failure to obtain love; by engaging in behavior or experiencing feelings, such as sexual or aggressive feelings, that cause one to feel guilty or unworthy; or by a failure in the pursuit of realistic or unrealistic goals (Mendelson, 1974).

Separation and Depression

That separation from a loved object could lead to depression was first emphasized by Freud in 1917. Since then experimental psychologists, notably the Harlows, have demonstrated with primates that disrupting a significant attachment bond strongly affects primate behavior. In psychoanalytical terms, object loss refers to traumatic separation from significant objects of attachment. Since the meaning of a loss is highly subjective, it is often stated that in fantasy, trivial losses may actually function as real ones. The relationship between human depression and object loss is twofold: separation in adulthood may precipitate a depression; bereavement during childhood may predispose to the development of adult depressions.

Some evidence that separation may precipitate a depression is shown in the following findings:

At 1 month after loss of a spouse as many as 35% of persons develop symptoms resembling primary depressive illness. Parkes also found that psychiatric patients who had the onset of illness within six months of the death of a parent or spouse were at high risk for affective illness. However, loss is not specific for depression. There is a high incidence of separation preceding the onset of a variety of physical illnesses. Although the foregoing data suggest that separation figures prominently among the possible precipitating stresses of depressive illness, separation alone is generally not a sufficient cause of depression nor is it specific for depression (Brown, 1977).

CLINICAL ASPECTS OF DEPRESSION

Presentation

The presentation of depression is highly variable. In some people it abruptly follows an environmental precipitant while in others it appears to arise gradually. Many experience depression in psychological terms—as a state of sadness, with hopelessness, anger, and marked personal devaluation. The patient may present with self-reproach, guilt, and unworthiness; or he may first be seen following a suicide attempt. Others first note irritability and difficulty in relating to family and friends. Some people express depression in physical terms, complaining of anorexia, weight loss, loss of energy, insomnia, or constipation. Occasionally, excessive alcohol or drug use marks the individual's attempt at self-treatment.

Signs and Symptoms

The manifestations of depressive illness may be classified into affective, cognitive, vegetative, motor, and perceptual disturbances. Affectively, the core of depression is the sad, despairing mood with a sense of hopelessness and uselessness. Although sadness is the most notable affect, concomitant guilt, shame, and anxiety are common. Cognitively, there is a decrease in the patient's interest in himself and his world. He cares little for his appearance; family, hobbies, and friends are neglected. He may continue to work but lacking interest and enthusiasm finds it difficult to accomplish anything. Making even a minor decision may take hours. The patient's concentration becomes poor, so that even when reading or looking at television he finds his thoughts turning to his emotional and physical discomfort.

Frequently patients complain endlessly about aches and pains or they may focus on one or more of the autonomic nervous system symptoms associated with the depression. At times the psychotic depressive will have delusions about his body (e.g. "my stomach has rotted") or about himself ("I am the worst sinner in the world"; or "I am dead"). These delusions may be of a nihilistic nature, but persecutory delusions may also be seen ("they want to poison me, because I'm so bad"). In such severely depressed psychotic patients perceptual disturbances such as hallucinations may occur; these may be in any sensory modality. A sense of unreality, either in the self or environment, is quite frequent in depressed persons.

Physical symptoms may be prominent in the depressive syndrome. Many patients show loss of appetite and weight loss; occasionally the anorexia can be so marked that a superimposed delirium occurs. Some patients, however, turn to food for comfort and when depressed will overeat.

Insomnia is usually marked; the patient has trouble falling asleep and may spend hours in bed ruminating about his problems prior to sleep; fragmented sleep, with the patient awakening every few hours is also common. With severe depressions, early morning awakening (e.g. cannot get back to sleep after 4–5 a.m.) or total insomnia may be present. Other depressed patients may become hypersomnic, using sleep as a means of escape. Patients complain of fatigue and exhaustion and general lassitude. At times this lifts as the day progresses, together with the patient's mood (diurnal variation in mood). Loss of libido, impotence, and amenorrhea may occur and be the presenting complaints. Headaches, back and limb pain, and vague gastrointestinal complaints (hollowness in the pit of the stomach, belching, constipa-

tion) may lead the patient to an internist or surgeon and initially mask the underlying depression, which the patient will describe openly when appropriately interviewed.

The level of motor activity may be quite reduced. The "retarded" depressive appears glum, his posture slumped and his voice flat. He may sigh and cry when speaking. All thoughts and activity are slowed. At times they may be so severe that the patient appears stuporous (i.e. immobile and mute although conscious). Agitation may also occur in depression, particularly in the involutional period. This is evident by restlessness and hand wringing, at times with the patient unable to sit still.

The description of involutional melancholia as a specific type of depression dates back to Kraepelin. He felt that this was a particular type of depression distinct from manic-depressive illness in its relationship to environmental stress. Involutional melancholia occurs in a person of a particular age (40–60), who has no earlier history of mania or depression, whose clinical picture is characterized by hypochondriasis and agitation and whose premorbid personality was obsessive. Opinion is divided as to whether this disorder should be distinguished from the other affective illnesses. Likely, the reason it has endured so long as a distinct entity is its exceptionally good response to electro-convulsive therapy (ECT). There is little other reason to separate it from other unipolar depressions.

CLINICAL ASPECTS OF MANIA

The basic affect in mania is euphoria; in its pure form these patients feel happy and are free of worry. Commonly, while the mood is elated it is unstable and often the patient is quite irritable. He may be punning and teasing one moment and be suddenly transformed to vicious anger the next.

In addition to the mood change, the patient's speech, thinking and motor activity are increased. The patient's speech is difficult to interrupt (pressure of speech) and *clang* associations occur. He is constantly on the go and never seems to tire. He finds he has boundless energy and requires very little sleep. His thinking is easily distracted and increased in rate; his thought processes are difficult to follow both in logic and in rate (flight of ideas). Usually the patient feels exceptionally well and would not come to medical attention were it not for his changed behavior resulting in difficulties with his family, at work or with the law.

In contrast with the depressed patient, the manic is full of self-confidence. He is inconsiderate of others; no one is important to him. At times he may develop grandiose delusions (e.g. of a scheme in which he is the savior of the world). Usually these are more fleeting than in other functional psychoses. The patient's expansive mood, grandiosity and poor judgment often result in inappropriate behaviors; irresponsible spending, sexual promiscuity, and aggressive outbursts are commonly observed.

There are several gradations to the manic state. The hypomanic patient, while elated, maintains good contact with reality. In acute mania the disorder has progressed to the point where the individual is psychotic. Occasionally a superimposed organic brain syndrome may occur. This condition, delirious mania, is characterized by confusion and a clouded consciousness and generally is due to lack of sleep, lack of proper nutrition, and drug or alcohol use.

THE COURSE OF THE AFFECTIVE DISORDERS

Affective disorders are usually episodic (Angst et al., 1973). That is, periods of suffering alternate with periods of normal functioning. Most bipolar disorders are recurrent. It is rare to find a single episode of mania with no exacerbations. Although unipolar depressions are frequently recurrent, from 5 to 50% of patients can suffer from only a single episode (depending on the duration of the follow-up period). The number of episodes of affective disorder a patient has over a lifetime is highly variable. Some recent studies suggest the mean number of episodes in bipolar patients is about 8, in unipolar 5. Depressions are self-limiting and will spontaneously remit, with an average duration of 6 months if they are untreated. The "involutional" depressions generally last longer (2 to 7 years) without treatment. Manic episodes tend to last about 3 months, but the length varies greatly from person to person. The shift from mania to depression may be gradual or overnight. As the patient gets older, the intervals between attacks of bipolar illness tend to get shorter. The attacks themselves also tend to last longer. For other patients recurrences occur regularly (e.g. in the spring and fall) over the course of years.

COMPLICATIONS OF AFFECTIVE DISORDERS

While mood disorders are usually episodic, some long-term complications may arise.

Chronic Impairment Due to Depressive Illness. These depressed individuals are unable to function in their usual social roles over an extended period of time because of depressive symptoms. Reviews in this area have suggested that between 5 and 25% of depressed patients are chronically impaired.

Death. Although it is generally recognized that depressives are at greater risk of suicide than the general population, it is less well known that they are at greater risk for death by all causes; their age adjusted death rate is about twice that of the general population.

Suicide. Depression is an important contributing factor in suicide. Several studies have reported approximately half of all suicides were considered to be suffering from depressive syndromes.

DIAGNOSIS OF AFFECTIVE DISORDERS

The presence of an affective illness and its type are determined by several converging lines of enquiry. The clinical interview should elicit presenting signs and symptoms, the disorder's predisposing and precipitating factors, any familial mental illness, and the patient's current medications and physical illnesses. This information is augmented by the findings of a thorough physical examination and a collateral history—taken from someone who knows the patient well. Depending on the data obtained, laboratory and psychological testing may be required.

A number of other syndromes may resemble affective disorders but should be differentiated from them because of treatment and prognostic implications. These include:

Schizophrenia. Acute schizophrenias may mimic both mania and depression. Differentiation is based on the presence or absence of the thought processes and affective disturbances characteristic of schizophrenia. The presence of "Schneiderian first rank" symptoms of schizophrenia, the patient's premorbid personality, his family history, the course of the disorder, and the patient's level of functioning when his disorder is in remission all help in the differentiation.

Early Organic Brain Syndrome. The dementing illnesses may mimic the presentation of a retarded depression. Differentiation here is highly dependent on the results of the examination of the patient's mental status (intellectual functioning, memory, orientation) and on the results of psychological testing. Specific laboratory testing (electroencephalogram, brain scan, CAT scan, hematological studies) will usually determine an underlying cause of a dementia. Observation of the patient's

mood, vegetative signs of depression, and a personal and family history of depression also aid in the diagnosis.

Psychoneurotic Disorders. While anxiety is generally the predominant mood in the psychoneuroses, depressive symptoms may occur. The differentiation from primary affective disorder is based on the constellation of symptoms (e.g. obsessions, phobias, etc.) that precede the depressive picture and also is determined by observation of the natural history of the illness.

Secondary Affective Disorder. Once a diagnosis of a depressive syndrome has been made, differentiation of primary from secondary mood disorder becomes important in terms of treatment. The diagnosis is based on the presence or absence of physical signs and on the results of laboratory investigations. A depression secondary to the use of drugs (e.g. oral contraceptives, steroids, L-DOPA), metabolic disorders (hypothyroidism), infections (influenza, mononucleosis) and neoplastic disorders require treatment of the underlying illness in addition to therapy for the depression.

MANAGEMENT OF DEPRESSION

The management of depression must be based on a thorough understanding of the patient. A complete psychiatric history and a mental status examination provide an essential basis for proper diagnosis and meaningful treatment. Many depressed people come first to their family physician who, after making the diagnosis, may initiate treatment himself, or he may seek a second opinion from a psychiatrist prior to beginning treatment. Alternatively he may decide that the management of the patient would be best handled by a psychiatrist. In many cases referral to a psychiatrist is prompted by the question of whether the patient requires hospitalization or whether he can be effectively treated as an outpatient. In making this decision, the physician should consider several factors. These include an assessment of the severity of the depression, the suicidal risk present, the resources available to the patient and his family, and the need for further investigations. It is important to bear in mind that the symptoms of a depressive illness may render the patient incapable of making decisions himself. He may feel hopeless and may consider hospitalization a further insult to his already lowered self-esteem. The physician should help the patient view his treatment as in his best interests. This requires tact, understanding, and an ability to convey a sense of hope to a despairing human being. The physician himself is an important treatment tool.

Involuntary admission to the hospital may be considered necessary if the patient refuses treatment and if the physician thinks he is a serious danger to himself. Such a danger may be manifested by the patient's extreme neglect of basic needs, such as nutrition, and by active attempts at or ideas of suicide. Such a decision for involuntary committal cannot be lightly made.

A depressed patient's degree of risk for suicide must be assessed to determine whether the patient should be hospitalized and to help determine how his depression should be treated. In assessing the suicidal risk for a patient the physician should consider factors related to the present episode, family and social conditions, medical-psychiatric factors, and demographic factors.

General Measures. Often the person comes to his physician for help after he has tried to treat the depression himself. For example, he may have resorted to alcohol or other drugs to calm his agitation or anxiety; he may have tried non-prescription drugs for his sleep difficulties. He may have taken a vacation or altered his life situation but without experiencing any lasting improvement in his mood. The physician should provide the patient with advice on the necessity of an adequate diet and physical exercise, as well as properly supervised symptomatic treatment. This may include a sedative for sleeping and in severe cases a tranquilizer for agitation. A proper use of antidepressant pharmacotherapy however, will usually avoid the necessity of polypharmacy.

Somatic Therapies. ANTIDEPRESSANTS. It has been known for centuries that the use of certain drugs can alter one's mood. Antidepressants, however, differ from other drugs in that they effect pharmacological changes in a manner which results in not merely a transient mood change, but in a restitution of the depressed patient to his premorbid state. They do not cause mood elevation in non-depressed people.

The observation that patients treated with iproniazide for tuberculosis showed a lifting of their mood raised interest in this family of drugs in the early 1950's. At that time also, a search was underway for a more effective phenothiazine for the treatment of schizophrenia. That research resulted in the development of the tricyclics which have a structural resemblance to the phenothiazines, but seem to be more effective in depression than in schizophrenia. The first drug of this group was imipramine.

Two major classes of antidepressants are currently in use:

1. The tricyclics, such as imipramine, amitriptyline and closely related compounds.

2. The monoamineoxidase inhibitors such as tranylcypromine and phenelzine.

The two groups of antidepressants are discussed in Chapter 34. The use of stimulants such as methylphenidate and the amphetamines are to be avoided in the treatment of depression.

ELECTROCONVULSIVE THERAPY (ECT). Treating a severely depressed suicidal patient with medication outside of the hospital can be dangerous. The risk of suicide is ever present, and it may increase with the availability of medication. An overdose of an antidepressant can be fatal.

Patients who are severely depressed, and who are agitated and suicidal should be treated with electroconvulsive therapy

(ECT). ECT is effective and rapid. Its risks are minimal. For a detailed discussion of the uses of ECT see Chapter 34.

Psychotherapy. The psychotherapy of depression occurs even without being so labeled. For example, the careful attention the physician gives to the patient as the patient initially tells his story is of psychotherapeutic value. Psychotherapy can be supportive or uncovering. Supportive psychotherapy includes listening to the patient, counseling him, and assisting him in his attempts to cope with the limitations his illness imposes on him. It also includes helping the patient to understand the nature of his difficulties. For example, the patient is helped to understand that his weight loss or his loss of sexual drive do not denote physical illnesses, nor is his indecisiveness a reflection on his moral fortitude. Psychotherapy includes helping with the patient's family in educating them to understand better and to deal more effectively with the patient. Supportive psychotherapy, as indicated, is a necessary adjunct to the treatment of depression whether other treatment modalities include chemotherapy or ECT.

Uncovering psychotherapy is designed to alter the patient's internal mental set so that depression will not recur. Uncovering psychotherapy is appropriate in treating depressions that have a marked neurotic nature; in fact, such psychotherapy is then the primary treatment modality.

Recent studies have shown the continuing value of combined psychotherapy and pharmacotherapy after the patient has made an initial recovery. While pharmacotherapy is useful in preventing relapses, psychotherapy provides added gains in interpersonal and social functioning.

MANAGEMENT OF MANIA

Mania is one of the few psychiatric disorders in which a pharmacological agent produces complete remission and also prevents recurrences. The drug is lithium, and since it was first used by Cade in 1949,

an extensive literature has accumulated testifying to its effectiveness.

Like patients who are depressed, patients who are manic should be carefully investigated. The information gathered in the investigations should always be corroborated by someone who knows the patient well. Most manic or hypomanic patients experience a sense of extreme well-being and a lack of insight into their condition. Their impaired judgment may get them into serious difficulties and render them incompetent to manage their affairs. The physician must take immediate action to protect the patient. In most places, a facility such as the Public Trustee will assume responsibility for a patient's affairs on the recommendation of his physician.

The decision to admit a patient to hospital should be based on the severity of his illness, his willingness to comply with treatment and his physical condition. A manic patient may neglect himself and suffer from extreme states of exhaustion.

Like the treatment of depression, the treatment of mania can be discussed under the headings general measures, somatic therapies, and psychotherapy.

General Measures. The general measures of treating mania include making sure that the patient does not become dehydrated or exhausted and does not get into social difficulties because of his impaired judgement. The general practitioner should seek a psychiatric consultation for the patient as soon as possible although it may be necessary for him to initiate symptomatic treatment to control the patient or to provide him with much needed sleep and rest. Attention must be paid also to the patient's physical condition including the state of his nutrition.

Somatic therapies consist of pharmacotherapy and ECT. ECT is to be used only when medications have failed to control the manic state. The pharmacotherapy of mania includes the use of major tranquilizers and lithium. The drugs commonly used to control mania are listed in Table 4.

Table 4. Medications Commonly Used to Treat Mania

Generic Name	Brand Name	Daily Dosage
Chlorpromazine	Largactil Promosol	Varies widely—from 200–2000 mg
Thioridazine	Mellaril	Up to 800 mg
Haloperidol	Haldol	Up to 100 mg
Lithium	Lithane	Variable; depends on serum lithium level.

The considerations in the pharmacotherapy of mania include:

The choice of neuroleptic (major tranquilizer) or lithium depends on what the desired target effects are. In general the goals are both control of behavior and restoration of the patient's mood to normal. Although lithium is effective, when rapid behavioral control is desirable the use of a neuroleptic is usually warranted because neuroleptics work more rapidly than lithium.

The choice of a particular neuroleptic is based on the following:

1. the patient's past history of response to neuroleptics.
2. the physician's choice which should be based on his familiarity with several neuroleptics.
3. the side effects (such as hypotension or other autonomic side effects, and extrapyramidal side effects) which occur in varying degrees with different drugs.
4. the degree of sedation that is desirable for a particular patient.
5. the route of administration (if parenteral medication is used, more potent drugs, such as haloperidol, are preferable).
6. the cost.

The dosage of the drug must be individualized for each patient. The dosage is influenced by the patient's size, his age and general health, the target effects, the degree of the patient's manic excitement, and his previous response to drug treatment. Initially, for the severely excited patient hourly drug administration may be required until he is settled.

The route of administration, parenteral or oral, is determined by considering the patient's compliance with treatment and the degree of his mania.

The adverse side effects of the neuroleptic may limit the size of the daily dose. These occur in varying degrees with most drugs. Common adverse side effects include drowsiness, dryness of the mouth, constipation, extrapyramidal signs and hypotension. These are discussed in greater detail in Chapter 34.

Lithium was used in the 1940s as a salt substitute for people on low sodium diets, but with disastrous results. In 1949 Cade, in Australia, reported on its use in the treatment of mania. Since then many workers have confirmed both its effectiveness as an antimanic agent and its efficacy in prophylaxis. Specific details of lithium and its use are described in Chapter 34.

Psychotherapy. The psychological approach to the manic patient involves a firm, yet supportive manner with an emphasis on control of his behavior, setting appropriate limits, encouraging reality testing and avoiding excess environmental stimulation.

Outcome. The treatment of a manic or hypomanic episode is usually successful with a complete remission occurring within 2–3 weeks. When the patient recovers, it must be decided whether he should take lithium for prophylaxis. As a general rule, if there is no doubt about the diagnosis and there are no physical contraindications, the patient should be advised to take lithium indefinitely. That decision is less difficult if the patient has a family history of affective disorder, and if the patient himself had previous episodes of mania or depression. The decision is more difficult if the patient is relatively young and if it is his first episode.

Affective disorders constitute a large part of any medical practice. Besides the personal suffering involved in affective disorders, suicide remains a significant complicating factor. Studies of suicide in England revealed that most of the patients had consulted their family physicians within a few weeks of attempting suicide. In North America suicide is one of the 10 leading causes of death. More than 90% of the people who commit suicide have a history of psychiatric illness and most of these people have affective disorders. Yet affective illnesses can be treated successfully. Prompt diagnosis and effective management of affective disorders are a major health concern.

REFERENCES

Akiskal, H. S. and McKinney, W. T. Jr. (1975): Overview of recent research in depression. *Arch. Gen. Psychiatry.* 32:285.

Angst, J., et al. (1973): The course of monopolar depression and bipolar psychoses. *Psychiat. Neurol. Neurochir.* 76:489.

Chase, T. N. and Murphy, D. L. (1973): Serotonin and central nervous system function. *Ann. Rev. Pharmacol.* 13:181.

Fabrega, H. Jr. (1975): Social factors in depression. In *Depression and Human Existence.* Edited by E. J. Anthony and T. Benedek. Boston, Little Brown.

Freud, S. (1953): Mourning and melancholia. In *The Standard Edition of the Works of Sigmund Freud.* Vol 14. London, Hogarth Press.

Kendell, R. E. (1976): The classification of depression: a review of contemporary confusion. *Br. J. Psychiatry.* 129:15.

Knoff, W. F. (1975): Depression: a historical overview. *Am. J. Psychoanal.* 35:41.

Kraepelin, E. (1919): *Dementia Praecox and Paraphrenia.* Edinburgh, E. & S. Livingstone.

Mendelson, M. (1974): *Psychoanalytic Concepts of Depression.* 2nd ed. New York, Spectrum.

Shopsin, B., et al. (1974): Catecholamines and affective disorders revised: a critical assessment. *J. Nerv. Ment. Dis.* 158:369.

Winokur, G. (1974): The division of depressive illness into depressive spectrum disease and pure depressive disease. *Int. Pharmacopsychiatry* 9:5.

FURTHER READINGS

Brown, G. W., Harris, T. and Copeland, J. R. (1977): Depression and loss. *Brit. J. Psychiatry.* 130:1.

Lehmann, H. E. (1966): On the phenomenology of the depressive illnesses. *Can. Psychiat. Assoc. J.* 11:S3.

Lindemann, E. (1944): Symptomatology and management of acute grief. *Am. J. Psychiatry.* 101:141.

CHAPTER **22**

Paranoid Disorders

Alexander Bonkalo

The ancient Greek word 'paranoia' meant, literally, that the mind was "beside itself," and it referred to several varieties of mental derangement. Today, the adjective paranoid also has several shades of meaning. In its broadest sense it refers to delusional thinking in all its forms, as in paranoid schizophrenia. In a narrower sense it refers to a mistrusting, hostile mode of thinking. At its core, paranoid refers to a manner of thought in which the person is prone to *project* outward his intrapsychic difficulties, tending to put blame on others, or on circumstances while denying his own faults and unsolvable problems. Generally, the paranoid person looks for external explanations for his internal difficulties, shortcomings, weaknesses, and subconscious conflicts. The subconscious conflicts are derived primarily from the repression of socially unacceptable expressions of his aggressive and sexual needs. The paranoid syndrome ranges from mildly abnormal to outright psychotic forms, with no definite dividing lines. Morbidly paranoid individuals are egocentric, hypersensitive, and rigid in thought and attitude. They tend to overreact if they are criticized yet they themselves are excessively critical of others.

They are extremely suspicious, they are excessively alert to the possibility of some form of ill will emanating from others, they see the world around them as hostile, and they tend to attribute special meaning or evil motives to everyday events. The extreme suspiciousness and deep-seated hostility, however, are often well camouflaged in paranoid persons; furthermore, their thinking remains well organized. Thus, paranoid persons may seem, on the surface, to be well-enough adjusted, undisturbed, and polite. Nevertheless, they may become conspicuous by being rigidly scrupulous, highly principled, self-righteous, humorless in a cold, obtuse fashion, and irrationally stubborn. They also tend to be unduly domineering; they feel compelled to maintain authority and control in almost any situation, as this attitude enables them to safeguard their "rights" and their "security." For the same reason, they tend to be consistently watchful, tense, and prepared. Most paranoid persons are socially isolated, secretive, and quarrelsome, mainly because they are unable to fully understand their environment or to be sensitive to the thoughts and motivations of others. They cannot see the other side of an argument, and they cannot compromise. Though paranoid people are consistent in their basic characteristics, each paranoid person develops his own protective shell. Some are shy, defensively withdrawn, and mind their own business; others are abrasive, aggressive, openly suspicious, and hostile. However, most paranoid people, whether they have personality disorders or are well-controlled psychotics, remain essentially balanced. They may function reasonably well for years, even a lifetime. Nevertheless, they are brittle in their adjustment, and they are liable to suffer emotional breakdowns. Moreover, the paranoid person is a hazard to his environment because he may endanger the emotional balance of others by interfering in their affairs or by being rigid, overly critical, and often outright disruptive.

At a psychotic level, paranoid thinking manifests itself in *ideas of reference* and in frank *delusions*. In ideas of reference the person believes, irrationally, that certain aspects of the environment are directed at him or that certain outside events are purposefully arranged to have a personal bearing on him—one patient was convinced that a radio talk on monsters was directed at him and ridiculed him for certain physical defects. Paranoid delusions are firmly maintained false ideas in which the subject is convinced that he is being persecuted in some form or other, that he is the center of attention in a grandiose scheme, that he is the victim of a powerful force, or that he is the target of some malicious plot of conspiracy. He may falsely identify or suspect one person in particular, or he may blame a more or less well-defined group (named "paranoid pseudo community" by Cameron) as the perpetrators of hostile actions. Like other delusions, paranoid delusions are fully personalized, and emotionally highly charged. They are foremost in the patient's mind, shaping his actions and life-style.

Paranoid psychoses are mental disorders in which the central abnormality is the presence of delusion. Disturbances in perception, mood, thought and behavior are derived from the delusion. Consequently, the paranoid person's mental functions and general behavior are essentially in harmony with his delusional thinking. Paranoid psychoses are usually classified as *paranoia*, a tightly organized syndrome, and *psychotic paranoid disorder* or *paranoid state*, which includes all other kinds of psychotic paranoid conditions.

PARANOIA

Paranoia in its pure presentation is a rare syndrome. The person is dominated by a uniform, coherent, delusional system that is complex and elaborate; it develops gradually and logically from a misinterpreted idea or event. The parts of the personality that are not directly involved in the delusional system remain reasonably intact. Memory is well preserved, although its content may become retrospectively adjusted in accord with the delusion. The person's thinking and general behavior remain formally intact and well organized. He has no hallucinations or illusions. His emotional responses are in harmony with the delusional content, as is his entire mental and behavioral attitude. Paranoia is usually chronic, and it resists treatment.

PSYCHOTIC PARANOID DISORDER

The term, *psychotic paranoid disorder,* (*paranoid state, chronic paranoid psychosis*) refers to a mixed group of conditions other than paranoia. Delusions in these conditions do not form a single or uniform system; instead they are multiple, sometimes heterogeneous, and often diffusely interwoven with the personality. Hallucinations and illusions may occur, and if they do, they are in accord with the content of the delusions. The formal aspects of the patient's personality and the structure of his thinking remain intact. Indeed, the absence of personality fragmentation and the absence of formal thought disorder are the chief findings that distinguish genuine paranoid conditions from schizophrenia. Nevertheless, some psychiatric classification systems challenge the validity of this nosological dichotomy and they include all forms of paranoid psychosis under the heading of schizophrenia.

Apart from those classification principles, differences in their predisposing and precipitating factors allow the paranoid psychoses to be arranged into clinical forms, such as *shared paranoid psychosis* and *involutional paraphrenia*. Furthermore, paranoid features are common symptomatic manifestations of depression, certain toxic conditions (e.g. amphetamine addiction), and organic mental disorders.

SHARED PARANOID PSYCHOSIS

Shared paranoid psychosis is a paranoid illness in which two or more individuals influence each other in such a way that they manifest essentially similar delusions (depending on the number of people involved, the disorder is known as *folie à deux* and *folie à beaucoup*). The transmission of psychosis from one person to another requires the presence of special factors. This condition may occur only between individuals who have a long-standing, dominant-dependent emotional relationship and who live together or communicate with each other regularly in relative social isolation. Moreover, they have constitutional or psychodynamic dispositions that facilitate the development of delusion. The key to treating them is to separate them. That, in itself, often leads to the recovery of the recipient or recipients of the delusion; the donor, however, who is the dominant person in the partnership, always requires full therapeutic attention.

INVOLUTIONAL PARAPHRENIA

Involutional paraphrenia is a paranoid illness that begins in a person in late middle age or in senescence. The disorder manifests itself in delusions, often florid or bizarre and, usually, hallucinations and illusions. However, unlike in schizophrenia, in involutional paraphrenia the patient does not have a formal thought disorder nor does his personality disintegrate. Neither is definite dementia demonstrable. If it were, involutional paraphrenia could be considered organic mental disorder. Lack of communication due to social isolation or to deafness are strong contributory factors in the development of involutional paraphrenia. In treatment, the cautious use of tranquilizers in keeping with the patient's age, supportive psychotherapy, and socialization is beneficial. Full recovery is rare.

PARANOID CONDITIONS GROUPED ACCORDING TO DELUSIONS

For clinical convenience, paranoid syndromes may be grouped according to the content of the delusions independently from their form, such as paranoia, psychotic paranoid disorder and so forth. Conditions in which the predominant delusions are of a persecutory character are relatively common. The person is convinced that he is maliciously and purposefully deceived and exploited. He may cause endless discontent, and initiate quarrels and litigation. He may feel "trapped," and he may either escape or attack. His escape techniques, which can involve actual moving away or merely devices for secrecy and camouflage, may be foolish or disruptive, but they are usually harmless. The alternative, however, an aggressive response in the form of an attack, is an ominous and potentially dangerous outcome of paranoid panic. The person manifesting paranoid grandiosity (megalomania) has a relatively rare but severe, fixed, and persistent form of paranoid reaction. The delusional content may center on power, wealth, or technical and intellectual innovations. The person manifesting delusional jealousy is convinced, irrationally, that his or her partner is sexually unfaithful. Such a person may assemble blatantly irrational data that "prove" the partner's unfaithfulness. Alcohol abuse is often a precipitating or complicating factor. Lonely individuals, primarily elderly women who live alone, may have erotic delusions that involve an unsuspecting person in their environment or a public figure. The delusions are usually projections of the patient's own frustrated sexual desires. In the syndrome characterized by hypochondriacal delusions, the person firmly believes that he is suffering from a specific chronic illness. His complaints have no proven medical basis, although at the patient's insistence many unnecessary clinical examinations may have been done. The hypochondriacal delusions may represent a deep-seated need to suffer, that is prompted by subconscious feelings of guilt; the delusions may be displacements of other kinds of intensive anxiety, or they may be subconscious manifestations of aggression acted out toward one's self or one's environment.

TREATMENT

In the treatment of paranoid disorders the first consideration is the prevention of possible danger and the elimination of environmental factors that contribute to the patient's delusions. Hospitalization may be necessary, but outpatient therapy is the treatment of choice, because the paranoid person may respond with extreme irrational hostility to the restriction of his freedom that hospitalization would bring. The first therapeutic objective is to reduce anxiety. The use of the major tranquilizers is usually mandatory. At the same time, the physician must establish a non-threatening psychotherapeutic relationship with the patient. The paranoid person should feel free to unload his anxieties and hostilities. When a comfortable relationship has been established between the pa-

tient and the physician, they should be able to discuss the patient's problem. But, the therapist should not reinforce the patient's delusions by seeming to agree with him, nor should he attempt to reason forcefully with the patient. It should be kept in mind that the patient has already been subjected to both friendly and argumentative reasoning from others. The therapist should offer a new setting for the patient, one in which he can find trust and acceptance, rather than a wall of rejective, patronizing or confrontative disbelief. The therapy offers a forum for the mutual exploration of ideas, which may lead to a total or partial resolution of the patient's irrational problems. However, the reduction of tension and the establishment of the patient's ability to live with the delusions is frequently the only possible therapeutic compromise.

FURTHER READINGS

Paranoid Disorders

Cameron, N. (1959): Paranoid conditions and paranoia. In *Amer. Handbook of Psychiat.* Edited by S. Arieti. New York, Basic Books.
Kaplan, H. I. and Sadock, B. J. (1971): The status of the paranoid today: his diagnosis, prognosis and treatment. *Psychiat. Quart.* 45:528.
Swanson, D. W., Bohnert, P. J. and Smith, J. A. (1970): *The Paranoid*, Boston, Little, Brown.

The Concept "Paranoid"

Kovab, L. (1966): A reconsideration of paranoia. *Psychiatry*, 29:289.
Noyes, R. Jr., Clancy, J. and Travis, T. A. (1974): The paranoid personality. *Postgrad. Med.* 55:141.
Salzman, L. (1960): Paranoid states: theory and therapy. *Arch. Gen. Psychiat.* 2:679.
Schwartz, D. A. (1964): A review of the "paranoid" concept. *Arch. Gen. Psychiat.* 8:349.

Other Specific Aspects

Kay, D. W. K. (1963): Late paraphrenia and its bearing on the aetiology of schizophrenia. *Acta Psychiat. Scand.* 39:159.
Retterstol, N. (1968): Paranoid psychoses with hypochondriac delusions as the main delusion. *Acta Psychiat. Scand.* 44:334.
Shepherd, M. (1961): Morbid jealousy: some clinical and social aspects of a psychiatric symptom. *J. Ment. Sci.* 107:687.

23

Schizophrenic Disorders

Henry B. Kedward and Mary V. Seeman

EPIDEMIOLOGY

The distribution of schizophrenia is difficult to determine and estimates can only be regarded as approximate. Different rates cited for schizophrenia in different places may be less a function of actual differences in the distribution of the disorder than a reflection of differences in casefinding methods, diagnostic practices, or the anomalous structure of the population studied. When allowances have been made for such factors, the general view among epidemiologists is that the distribution of schizophrenia is similar in populations throughout the world; no societies are completely free of it, and there is insufficient evidence to conclude that schizophrenia is the product of urbanization or rapid social development. There is wide agreement on the seriousness of schizophrenia as a health problem. It has been estimated that until recent years one-third of all hospital (not only psychiatric hospital) beds in Canada for example, and one-half of all hospital beds in the United Kingdom were occupied by long-staying psychiatric patients. Furthermore, the seriousness of the disease is determined by its early onset and chronic course, which may result in lifelong disability and loss of productive capacity.

Estimates of the incidence of schizophrenia in the general population in Western societies range from 50 per 100,000 people per year to more than 250 per 100,000 people per year (Freedman, et al., 1972). Calculations of the lifetime prevalence in the general population that were derived from surveys of major communities range from 0.75 to 2.75% (Hagnell, 1966).

Hospital Admission Figures

Despite a lack of uniformity in hospital reporting, it was formerly assumed that first admission figures would accurately reflect the true incidence of schizophrenia. It was thought that everyone with schizophrenia would be treated in the hospital at some time because the disorder is so severe. However, it has been demonstrated (Lemkau, et al., 1943) that between 15 and 25% of people with schizophrenia never enter the hospital, and that that percentage may have increased with the expansion of community psychiatry.

The calculation of rates is, of course, subject to many errors. Nevertheless, the estimate that one person in 100 will develop schizophrenia at some time in his life is a reasonably conservative one.

Demographic and Social Factors

Sex. Men tend to be hospitalized for schizophrenia somewhat more often than women are, although that may be due to differences in how psychiatric agencies view the roles, social expectations, and treatment needs of men and women.

Age. Schizophrenia most often begins in young adulthood; the highest age-specific rate for first admission to the hospital is consistently found in people 25 to 34 years of age.

Marital Status. Most schizophrenic patients are single, although women less often than men. Schizophrenia probably predisposes the person toward single life, and the lack of a spouse and family may be a significant factor in the longer hospital stays of single patients.

Occupation and Social Class. A clustering of schizophrenia in the lowest socioeconomic groups has been frequently reported. Originally it was attributed to the harsh life at the bottom of the social scale. That view gave way to the idea of social "drift," which suggested that schizophrenic patients slip down the social scale as their mental competence declines, move to poorer sections of the city to lead solitary lives in rooming houses, and perform undemanding, menial work or live the marginal existence of the unemployed. A study that related the socioeconomic status of the schizophrenic patient to that of his father at the time of the patient's birth supported the idea of social drift (Goldberg and Morrison, 1963).

Migration. A common finding is that migrants have a higher rate of schizophrenia than indigenous populations do. It is not clear whether some preschizophrenic condition prediposes a person toward migration or whether the stresses of emigration precipitate schizophrenic breakdown.

ETIOLOGY

The causes of schizophrenia are unknown. Many theories exist as to whether schizophrenia is the product of an inborn constitutional weakness or predisposition, or whether it arises in response to stresses in the person's environment. According to different views, the disposition may be physical or psychological, and the environmental stresses may include destructive childbearing patterns, fevers, pregnancy, traumatic life events, migration, poverty, and disturbances of interpersonal communications. There is scarcely an organ in the body or an element in human social life that has not at some time been discussed as important in the genesis of schizophrenia. Many theories are persuasive, but no single factor has been demonstrated to be a necessary and sufficient cause for schizophrenia. A growing body of opinion tends toward the multiple causation, or interactionist view that schizophrenia develops in a vulnerable, genetically predisposed person who is subjected to environmental stresses of a particular type with which he is unable to cope.

Biological Theories

Constitutional. The proponents of constitutional theories of schizophrenia have ranged wide in their search for a specific cause. The main avenues of research have been genetics, neurophysiology, and biochemistry. Early work on a possible biological basis for schizophrenia uncovered evidence of multiple defects in almost all the body systems of schizophrenics, but the findings were subsequently attributed to deficiencies in methodology. Research findings based on autopsy material from schizophrenics that showed neurological degeneration or other anomalies often failed to take into account such factors as the patient's age and the cause of his death, his diet, and his living conditions during the years he was hospitalized. Furthermore, it was usually impossible to determine whether the physiological or metabolic anomaly that was identified preceded or followed the development of the disease.

Genetic. The role of genetic factors in

schizophrenia has been examined critically. It has been demonstrated that the people who are related to a person with schizophrenia are at higher risk for the disorder, the risk ranging from 3% for second-degree relatives, 7 to 15% for siblings and the children of one schizophrenic parent, and 40% for the children of two schizophrenics. However, most schizophrenics are not born to schizophrenic parents. Concordance rates in dizygotic twins (i.e., both twins are schizophrenic) are in the range of 10 to 15%, whereas the concordance rates for monozygotic twins are about three times higher. The risk of the relatives of schizophrenics appears to vary with the severity of the proband's (subject's) illness and the number of other relatives affected.

A number of well-designed adoption studies have attempted to determine the relative importance of genetic and environmental factors. Among their findings are that children of schizophrenics placed for nonfamilial adoption develop schizophrenia at higher rates than do people in general and that higher rates of schizophrenia are found among the biological but not the adoptive parents of schizophrenic adopted children. Identical twins reared apart from childhood are concordant for schizophrenia to the same degree as those reared together, and children adopted into homes in which a parent becomes schizophrenic do not have increased rates.

Some genetic studies have considerably broadened the concept of schizophrenia to include a spectrum of schizophrenic disorders of varying severity. The spectrum includes people who may have shared the schizophrenic gene pool but who received an insufficient amount of genetic material to produce a florid phenotype. Research is in progress that prospectively follows the development of those at high risk for schizophrenia, i.e., the children of schizophrenic parents. This research aims to uncover possible etiologic factors.

It has not been established how schizophrenia is transmitted genetically. The data do not fit a simple Mendelian pattern of inheritance; they are more suggestive of a polygenic basis.

Neurological. A large body of research has examined the hypothesis that a physical (probably a neurological) abnormality or lesion is the basis for schizophrenia. Evidence has been accumulated from a variety of sources: neurological, psychological and electroencephalographic investigations of living patients, histopathological examination of autopsy and biopsy material, especially lobotomized brain tissue, and examination of case histories for evidence of neurological damage. A number of studies reported a higher than expected frequency of complications of pregnancy and delivery (and thus an increased risk of central nervous system damage) at the birth of people who later became schizophrenic. Diffuse, nonspecific neurological abnormalities, atypical electroencephalographic tracings and subnormal intelligence have all been reported in schizophrenia although their relationship to schizophrenia remains obscure. Damage arising from infectious and inflammatory processes (e.g., tuberculosis) has also been investigated without encouraging results. Much of the research may be considered disappointing only if viewed as a search for universally present causal factors. Lovett Doust suggested that schizophrenic symptoms occur frequently in response to a variety of diseases. He proposed a diagnostic distinction between primary schizophrenia and schizophrenia secondary to organic disease.

Biochemical. Many biochemical theories of the causes of schizophrenia seemed promising initially but remain unsubstantiated. A variety of metabolic and endocrine abnormalities have been suggested; they include errors in protein metabolism, abnormal nitrogen retention, a deficiency of serotonin, elevated levels of ceruloplasmin, and the presence in the blood of an anomalous protein constituent, taraxcin, which is thought to produce alterations in metabolic pathways. Several of those lines of research derive from the model psychosis theory. The model psychosis theory holds that, since hallucinogenic drugs produce psychotic, schizophrenia-like states, schizophrenia may be the product of an endogenous hallucinogen that originates in an endocrine anomaly or metabolic error, such as the abnormal methylation of metabolites. The chemical structure of serotonin (5HT), a chemical transmitter in the nervous system that is important in the control of thought and affect, is similar to the chemical structure of the hallucinogens LSD and psilocybin, drugs that block the serotonin synapses and produce schizophrenia-like alterations in feeling and behavior.

One of the major hypotheses currently being investigated is the dopamine hypothesis. Hornykiewicz (1966) demonstrated a deficiency of dopamine secondary to degeneration of the nigrostriatal pathways in Parkinson's disease. Since the phenothiazine drugs that have antipsychotic properties when used to treat schizophrenia often have side effects similar to those of Parkinson's disease, it seemed possible that dopamine could be implicated in schizophrenia. Studies of the phenothiazines—their mode of action, structure, and blood levels necessary for therapeutic effectiveness—have encouraged further research. The neuroleptics used in the treatment of schizophrenia, block dopamine synapses. This is suggestive of excessive activity of the dopamine system in schizophrenic disorders. Investigation of the dopamine receptors in the brain is a promising field of enquiry.

Psychosocial Theories

The hypothesis that schizophrenia is environmental rather than constitutional in origin has been examined in a number of different ways. Evidence obtained from epidemiological surveys has suggested to some that social factors, such as social disorganization or threatening life events, may be critically important in the genesis of schizophrenia. It may be that those factors are secondary rather than causative (see the previously mentioned drift theory). The stress of isolation has been posited as the key causative element and threatening life events involving personal isolation, such as emigration, bereavement, or the ending of a significant relationship, have been observed as precipitating factors in schizophrenic breakdown of the acute reactive type. A different cause has been postulated for process schizophrenia, which is the insidious deterioration of a person psychologically predisposed to schizophrenia. Seclusive, introverted, and unable to enter into satisfying social relationships, the person with process schizophrenia becomes progressively unable to cope with the demands of adult life and he finally breaks down under stress. A substantial body of opinion considers family pathology (Lidz and Lidz, 1949), destructive child-rearing patterns, and the subjection of the child to emotionally ambiguous modes of communication, the psychodynamic precipitants of schizophrenia. A common finding was that of the "schizophrenogenic" mother—dominant, cold, and fundamentally rejecting yet overpossessive—and a passive, ineffectual father (although aggressive, sadistic fathers were also observed). Although there may be open "marital schism," a facade of good relations, or "pseudomutuality" may be maintained, giving rise to ambiguous modes of communication, such as the "double bind" (Bateson, 1956). In the double-bind communication, the mother sends warm positive messages to the child while covertly rejecting him. One of the conflicting messages may be verbal, the other nonverbal, e.g., the mother praises her child but at the same time, in her behavior, indicates disapproval and contempt. Unable to interpret her messages, unable to make himself acceptable to her, and unable to escape, the child becomes locked into a destructive relationship with his mother, that is characterized by a pervasive and inhibiting anxiety. It is postulated that the child gradually withdraws from reality until he is finally overwhelmed by the stresses of adolescence and the impending demands of adult life.

Psychoanalytic theories consider the critical factor to be the failure of the person's ego boundaries and sex-role identification to develop. According to Arieti (1967), the schizophrenic's life passes through four phases. During the first phase, the negative emotions and hostility of the family compel him to take part as little as possible in the unpleasant external reality. The second phase of compensation is one with some hope for adjustment to life and is achieved by defenses against deep involvement. Here is seen the basis for the schizoid personality, which Arieti summarized as a "patched up self-image." The majority of people subjected to the stresses of these family conditions do not deteriorate further. The third phase, for those who later become schizophrenic, occurs when the defenses cease to be adequate and this is commonly at the age of puberty. The fourth stage is the descent into psychosis with diminution of contact with external reality. In psychodynamic terms, there is an "assumption of regressive forms."

Research into the genesis of schizophrenia has uncovered evidence of a number of significant associations but no conclusive evidence of causation. Thus the end state of schizophrenia—severe ego disturbance, perceptual disorganization, and behavioral changes—may arise from an inborn factor or an environmental trauma or a combination of the two. When the person who is genetically predisposed and psychologically vulnerable to schizophrenia is subjected to a pathological child-rearing process, he may develop a maladaptive response to stress. A neurophysiological anomaly, biochemical imbalance or a threatening life event may be equally significant in that, as has been suggested, schizophrenia may be not a single disorder, but a syndrome consisting of discrete disorders with varying causes that find their common expression in the symptoms of schizophrenia.

DIAGNOSING A FIRST EPISODE OF SCHIZOPHRENIA

When a patient who presents in a psychotic state has had a previous episode of illness, diagnosis is made relatively less difficult by:

1. Information about the quality and severity of the first episode,
2. Information about the patient's response to past treatment,
3. Information about the quality of the patient's life between episodes.

By contrast, a first illness presents a challenging diagnostic problem.

If one can speak of a typical presentation for a first episode, it is a person in his late teens or early twenties, brought to the doctor at the urging of someone other than himself. Most often, the accompanying person is a parent; sometimes, in a case involving eccentric behavior, a policeman.

Chief Complaint. The patient's complaints may be vague. He most frequently talks about body and mind concerns, but he may absolutely deny that anything is wrong. Sometimes there are magical-religious overtones to the presenting complaint or persecutory feelings expressed in a bewildered, unsystematic fashion. Examples of presenting complaints are: "My thighs are too thin for my chest;" "Someone put a spell on me and I've lost my erections;" "Three and three makes six so I have to find my six missions in life;" "Sometimes I'm God, sometimes I'm the Devil."

Evaluation of the complaint will depend upon:

1. The *suddenness* of its appearance (remembering that it is not infrequent for young people in general to be preoccupied with their bodies or with religious concerns);

2. How unnatural it appears to those with whom the patient lives (it may be a cultural norm);
3. How *globally* the conviction or fear or preoccupation is affecting the patient's life; and
4. How *firm* is his conviction that his mistaken impression, or perceptual distortion is unquestionably real.

In schizophrenia, collaborative evidence from parents or others will suggest that the preoccupations or the behaviors that they lead to are *new* for the patient, outside of the cultural norm, affect *all* of the patient's life, and that the patient cannot be talked out of his beliefs.

History of the Present Illness. This may be difficult to obtain from the patient. There may or may not be several of the symptoms presented in Table 5. There is often an avoidance of people, sleep disturbance, failure at school, on the job and in interpersonal relations all going back several weeks or months. Sometimes there may seem to be a precipitant such as a severe illness, the birth of a baby, going away to college, the beginning of a love relationship or approaching exams, but it is not always clear whether the disturbed feelings, thoughts and behaviors had already begun and were perhaps responsible for what appears as the trigger. Importantly, all areas of living are disturbed. Functional physical enquiry reveals many problems. There are difficulties with family, with friends, with love relationships, with schooling and employment. Often there are accompanying difficulties in thinking and concentration.

Table 5. Common Presenting Complaints in Schizophrenia

Mind not working
Part of body not working
Feeling under attack
Feeling hypnotized
Feeling special
Feeling of chaos, bewilderment
Voices in the head

Past Illnesses. There may be a surprising lack of past psychiatric difficulty in schizophrenia. In some cases, parents will say they have worried about this particular child for some time because he has been sensitive or withdrawn, but often that is not the case. Past psychiatric difficulties may have already marked the onset of incipient schizophrenia.

Family History. There is a hereditary component to schizophrenia and where there is a positive family history, this is very helpful in diagnosis. Usually, an exact diagnosis of a relative is impossible to obtain, but the history of lifelong psychiatric difficulties with concomitant problems in living (i.e. never married, unemployed, isolated) heightens the likelihood that the illness in the relative was schizophrenia. The treatment history of the relative may be a clue to diagnosis, but it must be kept in mind that psychiatric treatments have changed dramatically in the last twenty years.

Personal History. Despite decades of searching, nothing specific has been found about the early life of the schizophrenic-to-be child that is helpful in arriving at a diagnosis. In studies of identical twins discordant for schizophrenia, it has been found that the smaller birth-weight twin, the twin that is sicklier in infancy is more likely than the other to develop the illness. Clinically, it often seems as if the young adult with schizophrenia is characterized by parents as having been a particularly "good," obedient, compliant child, less rebellious than his siblings.

As for many adolescents, puberty is a stormy time for the schizophrenic-to-be and it is usual to elicit many interpersonal and sexual problems at this time of life as well as dependence-independence struggles vis-a-vis parents. This is, of course, not diagnostic by any means. In contrast to normal adolescent problems, however, these conflicts never get resolved in schizophrenia.

Mental Status. Findings on mental status vary. They may be minimal to florid.

The young person usually appears distracted and disorganized and unable to maintain eye contact. There may be something bizarre about his dress or his behavior.

In acute schizophrenia the *affect* is mainly that of fear and distrust. There may be a palpable hostility and fury. Sometimes the patient is docile and passive, sometimes apathetic, often ambivalent (mixed feelings). Depressive or excited affects may be present as well. The patient's affect appears not to match the examiner's. In response to the examiner's questions, there may be unexpected giggling or seemingly unprovoked tears. This is the inappropriate affect often described in schizophrenia (Table 6).

Flow of thought is difficult to follow. The patient appears to be responding to inner cues (autism) as much, if not more, than to the interview situation. This leads to an associational defect, which may take the form of tangential thinking, punning, clang associations, or neologism formation. This response seems to be triggered by the form or sound of certain words, rather than by their meaning—e.g. "Are you feeling blue?" "I am the Prince of Wales!" (—i.e. "I have *blue* blood"). In addition, the patient does not seem able to stay on the examiner's level of abstraction. He may over-abstract (e.g. "How are you feeling today?" "Feelings are ephemeral, they mean nothing in the cosmic consciousness.") or he may be over-concrete ("What brought you into the hospital?" "First the #3 bus and then I waited thirty minutes for a street car and walked the rest of the way."). These difficulties are highlighted when the patient is asked to attempt tasks of similarities, differences or

Table 6. Bleuler's Criteria (Primary Symptoms of Schizophrenia)

Autism
Ambivalence
Associational defect
Affective inappropriateness

proverb interpretation. "What is the same about an apple and an orange?" "They both have skins" (concrete) or "Nothing, oranges did not cause the fall of mankind." Proverb interpretation is usually concrete: "A stitch in time saves nine," "If you sew up a hole right away it won't get bigger," or idiosyncratic: "God gave us Time, we must beware." It must be remembered that intellectually retarded or brain-damaged people also give concrete answers to proverbs. Also, the ability or inability to interpret a proverb "correctly" is a test of intelligence and not only of schizophrenic thinking.

Thought content in schizophrenia is characterized by delusions—i.e. firmly held erroneous convictions. These may be paranoid in nature. For example, the patient is preoccupied with and convinced of the fact that someone is following him or threatening him or simply watching over him. The watching over is frequently ominous, but may be benign. The delusions may be grandiose. For instance, the patient is convinced that he has been selected for a special mission, that he is the reincarnation of God, that he has special powers. The delusions may be somatic: bizarre transformations occurring within one's body. A person may feel "out of" his body (depersonalized). Delusions may be nihilistic: the world coming to an end, the approach of death. These and other types of delusions occur in schizophrenia as they do in other psychotic disorders. Grandiose and sometimes paranoid delusions occur in mania and somatic and nihilistic ones are seen in depressions. What characterizes schizophrenic delusions is often their bizarre quality, although one must be careful because bizarreness is culture-bound. For instance, the conviction that a love-potion administered by a gypsy caused impotence may not be a schizophrenic paranoid delusion, but a depressive equivalent in people coming from other cultures.

A second characteristic of schizophrenic delusions is that they are frequently supported by perceptual distortions, which form the unarguable evidence behind the delusion.—i.e. "I know the T.V. sportscaster is talking about me because I *heard* him whisper my name." These perceptual distortions may be merely illusions such as may occur in states of anxiety or fatigue, or frank hallucinations. In schizophrenia, the hallucinations are usually auditory, hence the clinical association of "hearing voices" with schizophrenia. Other common thought content criteria are shown in Table 7. Visual and tactile hallucinations also occur, but less commonly. Their presence is an indication to rule out organic pathology.

Another characteristic of the delusions and hallucinations of schizophrenia is that they are pervasive. Hearing voices may be reported by people with histrionic personalities but, with them, the voices appear incidental and do not seem to affect the daily course of their life. The delusions and hallucinations of schizophrenia, on the other hand, play a very significant role in the mental functioning of the schizophrenic and may profoundly affect his life. Eccentricities of behavior in schizophrenia can normally be traced back to delusional beliefs reinforced by hallucinations.

The *sensorium* may be intact in acute schizophrenia. On the other hand, the patient may arrive in a state of panic after days of insomnia and dehydration. Under those circumstances he will be disoriented

Table 7. Schneiderian First Rank Symptoms (Thought Content Criteria)

Thought blocking

Thought broadcasting

Thought insertion

Thought withdrawal

Control by an external agency

Delusional interpretation of somatic hallucination

Delusional perception: special significance read into an ordinary perception

Voices commenting on thoughts, feelings, behaviors

Voices repeating or anticipating thoughts

---

and delirious. It is this form of presentation that mimics an acute toxic psychosis or a drug-induced psychosis, especially an amphetamine psychosis. Judgement, in those instances, will be correspondingly disturbed and the patient will have no insight into the fact that he is ill.

Differential Diagnosis. Characteristic symptoms appearing for the first time in a person in his late teens with a family history of schizophrenia, especially where those symptoms affect every facet of living, pose no problem in diagnosis. The problem is that there is usually no family history, symptomatology is mixed and precipitating factors are unclear. Drug-induced psychosis and other forms of acute brain pathology must be ruled out. High anxiety and histrionic personality can sometimes prove confusing especially where too much weight is placed on the presence of "pathognomonic symptoms" and not enough on the pervasiveness of illness and the total breakdown of functioning. Acute mania is often confused with acute schizophrenia and only the subsequent course of illness can distinguish the two. Depression may be present in schizophrenia and the signs and symptoms of depression, including preoccupation with suicide, may loom so large that the schizophrenic elements are overlooked. Severe obsessive-compulsive illness may produce circumstantial and concrete thought disturbance and eccentric rituals that may be confused with schizophrenia. The obsessional person who can not touch a door knob without first wiping it does it with full knowledge that his behavior is odd, but cannot help himself. The schizophrenic performing the same ritual will usually say that he is being commanded to do it or that someone else is doing it through him or that it is not germs, but radioactive protons that he is wiping off. He sees the behavior as mandatory and therefore not odd. Being "out of touch with reality" or "lacking insight" are therefore important elements in diagnosing schizophrenia although one can readily appreciate that unless one can totally share another's experience, "reality" is difficult to define.

Categories. As has been mentioned, schizophrenia is probably not a unitary disease and there have been many attempts at subdividing the illness into *categories*. All of these categories are more or less overlapping and are not particularly useful as far as treatment decisions go. Schizophrenia may be divided into:

GOOD VERSUS POOR PROGNOSIS SCHIZOPHRENIA. Good prognosis schizophrenia has a later age of onset, there is no family history of the disease, there is a good premorbid personality and the illness is acute, there are many affective signs (depressive, anxious, euphoric, hostile feelings), there is quick response to treatment and few if any symptoms remain after the acute attack. Good prognosis schizophrenia (also called reactive schizophrenia as opposed to process schizophrenia) means that the relapses will be few and that good functioning will be maintained in between relapses. It used to be thought that this kind of schizophrenia did not require maintenance neuroleptic medication, but at this stage in our knowledge, requirement for maintenance neuroleptics cannot be predicted on the basis of the aforementioned factors.

PARANOID SCHIZOPHRENIA VERSUS NON-PARANOID—I.E., SIMPLE CATATONIC, HEBEPHRENIC, UNDIFFERENTIATED SCHIZOPHRENIAS. A patient who presents with well-systematized paranoid delusions has a better prognosis than one who cannot evolve such an "explanation" for what has gone wrong. The categories simple, catatonic, etc. refer to modes of presentation of the illness. A person with "simple" schizophrenia seems to skip over the acute phase and presents with chronic features (see later). Catatonic presentation refers to behavioral features. The patient who is mute or excited and hyperactive and who does not share his thoughts is referred to as catatonic.

Hebephrenic presentation emphasizes the inappropriate giggling and labile, shallow affect that sometimes overshadows other features. Undifferentiated schizophrenia means a mixed picture with no predominating feature. Where a paranoid system is the main aspect of the illness, the patient is usually intelligent and verbal and has been able to "explain" somatic and perceptual distortions as well as difficulties in living by attributing them to the malevolence of a powerful agency (the "authorities," the "communists") and thus psychologically coming to terms with personal failings. The better prognosis in this form of schizophrenia does not refer to symptom remission, since the paranoid symptoms stay and expand over time, but to the fact that re-hospitalizations are usually avoided and that, where the delusion can be relatively encapsulated, the patient can carry on with life, albeit in an isolated manner. Paranoid illness beginning late in life can be confused with, but is not, schizophrenia (see Chapter 22).

ACUTE VERSUS CHRONIC SCHIZOPHRENIA. Acute schizophrenia is what was described under "first episode schizophrenia." Characteristically, similar episodes recur throughout a lifetime, more frequently for some than for others. In between episodes, the acute symptoms wane either spontaneously or else in response to treatment but other symptoms, the so-called "negative" symptoms of schizophrenia, emerge. These are apathy, social withdrawal, lack of energy, lack of interest, lack of motivation, lack of ambition, lack of emotional warmth. Where there have never been acute symptoms, this form of the illness is referred to as "simple" schizophrenia. Where acute symptoms have occurred in the past but are no longer present, this form of the illness is called "chronic." Usually some degree of acute symptoms remains as well and this may be referred to as "residual" schizophrenia. Although negative symptoms may in some people be a temporary aftermath to an acute illness or a form of post-schizophrenic depression or, in some instances, a side effect of neuroleptics, in most cases these symptoms remain indefinitely, do not respond to treatment and augur ill in the sense that they lead to an unfulfilled, impoverished life.

SCHIZO-AFFECTIVE SCHIZOPHRENIA. Where affective and cognitive symptoms occur in equal proportion and where the illness tends to be cyclical with good periods of functioning in between, it is called schizo-affective. This form of illness responds to lithium salts given in conjunction with neuroleptics. In between episodes the patient tends to be free of negative symptoms but is depression-prone and is at higher risk of suicide.

TREATMENT OF SCHIZOPHRENIA AS A LIFETIME ILLNESS

Principles of Treatment of Acute Schizophrenia

The initial episode usually requires hospitalization and the immediate institution of psychosocial supports for patient and family. Hospitalization may need to be involuntary at first, i.e. implemented against the patient's will if his behavior presents a risk to his or others' safety. Treatment imposed against a person's will begins the therapeutic relationship on a negative footing and creates further strains within a family. Even when a patient voluntarily accepts treatment the nature of the illness makes any interpersonal closeness difficult and frightening. Initial efforts at therapy will frequently be experienced as interfering or attacking. A firm, unequivocal insistence on early hospitalization shortens the agony and allows treatment to begin promptly.

The acute episode will require treatment with neuroleptics. Whereas psychopharmacology is dealt with in Chapter 34, several principles of drug therapy of schizophrenia are important to stress here.

1. In general, all neuroleptics work if given in adequate doses. The choice of drug will depend on the physician's experience, a history of previous positive drug response if it exists, and a clinical evaluation of which side effects a particular individual is likely to tolerate best. Side effects produce body sensations, which are often incorporated into a patient's delusional system. The high-dose drugs (100 mg per dose) have predominantly sedative, endocrine and cardiovascular side effects. Where a patient has a delusion of changing gender or is plagued with being "done to," i.e. "passivity phenomena," these drugs are best avoided. The low-dose drugs (2 to 5 mg per dose) produce predominantly extrapyramidal side effects, namely muscle constriction, tensions, tremors, and restlessness. Patients who feel under attack are stressed further by the curtailment of their freedom of movement.

2. There is as yet no neuroleptic without unwanted side effect. Many of these unwanted effects are dose dependent. A gradually and slowly increasing dose often produces fewer side effects, but rapid neuroleptization can usually be accomplished without undue problems. Much discomfort can be obviated by the judicious use of anti-parkinson drugs, explanation and reassurance. Patient's complaints about side effects must be listened to and taken seriously.

3. Individuals have widely different plasma concentrations after equivalent doses. Since plasma concentration determinations cannot yet be routinely done, doses must be individually tailored to the patient.

4. A reasonable strategy of treatment is to select a target symptom and titrate neuroleptic dose to it. Once this symptom has responded to treatment, a second target symptom may be selected. After the acute phase, the patient will be able to collaborate with the physician in the selection of target symptoms.

5. When selecting target symptoms, it is

important to remember the usual schedule of symptom response to neuroleptics. Combativeness, hyperactivity, excitement, agitation, mutism, or extreme suspiciousness disappear within five days if the dose of drugs is adequate. Intramuscular drugs may be required during this period if the patient's behavior is disorganized and a threat to his own or others' safety. Given adequate dosage, perceptual distortions and primary delusions stop within two weeks. Associational defects and affective incongruities may take two months to disappear. Secondary delusions (explanation of past events) may never be given up. As the acute stage clears, depression frequently sets in. It must be recognized and treated psychotherapeutically.

6. Improvement due to neuroleptics is most rapid in the first eight weeks but continues for approximately six months.

Explanation and reassurance are needed in large doses in the initial period for family members as well as for the patient. The nature of the illness and its probable course must be repeatedly explained. Families need a chance to air their concerns, guilts, and requests for direction. This is a good time to dispel myths and fears about the disease and to lay the foundation for prolonged post-hospital treatment.

During the first two weeks the patient keeps himself at a distance from others and seems to need to remove himself from social stimuli. After that begins a lengthy period of redeveloping trust in others and increasing confidence in himself. To be successful, interpersonal exposure must be slow and gradual.

There are advantages and disadvantages to a long first hospitalization. A long period in hospital can ensure optimal treatment and can also impress upon the patient and family the seriousness of the disorder. The patient is protected from returning too quickly to school or job and suffering another failure. He is prevented from too early forced interaction with par-

ents and friends. However, a long hospitalization interferes with school, job and outside relationships. Transition from hospital to home must be made carefully. Visits and weekends at home may bridge this gap. An in-between period in a day hospital or in a community residential setting (halfway house) is very helpful. The transition between hospital doctor and family doctor must be well planned with good communication between the two. Reintroduction into education, occupational and social responsibilities must be slow, gradual but persistent.

Principles of Treatment after the Acute Phase

Drug Therapy. If they do not receive medication, 60 to 70% of patients relapse within one year. This figure is reduced to 30% if a person is medicated (Hogarty et al., 1974). These findings have been confirmed many times although it must be remembered that large-scale studies are done on large samples of people and not on individuals. In the individual case, with careful supervision, the physician should be able to sort out the various factors that may be contributing to relapse. Is the drug being taken? Is the dose inadequate? Are individual metabolic factors creating a low plasma concentration? Are the stresses of living too great? Is this a more severe form of the illness? Are social supports deficient? Is the family environment too emotional?

As a general rule drug therapy should be maintained for at least two years after an acute illness, supervised by frequent visits to the physician. This is true even after the patient has become asymptomatic and has re-integrated into his pre-illness existence. During the critical period of finishing one's education, establishing oneself in a career, committing oneself to another person, it is particularly important to prevent relapse. Since there are risks to health with indefinite continuation of neuroleptics, attempts at weaning and drug holidays should be instituted after the critical period.

The maintenance drug dose need be only minimal to prevent relapse. The equivalent of 25–100 mg. h.s. chlorpromazine is usually sufficient. After six months the dose should always be low enough to avoid side effects. If symptoms reappear, the dose is adjusted upwards. Long-acting (1 to 3 weeks) injectable medication is available for people who do not take oral medication reliably.

Psychotherapy. The nature of the therapeutic relationship with a schizophrenic patient is different than with a neurotic patient. The doctor must be an "ambassador of reality" (Fromm-Reichmann, 1954) and be prepared to allow himself to serve as a model or "auxiliary ego" for the patient. The doctor should be seen as a real human being who feels, fails, tries, perseveres, considers options, acts, reacts and is able to maintain control of any given situation. The schizophrenic patient benefits more from stable, consistent models of appropriate behavior than from directives or interpretations.

Principles of Treatment and Rehabilitation for Chronic Schizophrenia

After several schizophrenic relapses, treatment focus must shift from the prevention and quick control of acute episodes to the more difficult goal of improving the quality of life during periods of remission (Seeman, 1979). Only 20% of schizophrenics who have had two or more acute illnesses are successfully employed. Although interpersonal success is more difficult to measure than employment success, it is safe to estimate that a far smaller percentage lead an interpersonally satisfying life. Treatment facilities for the chronic schizophrenic must include a social support system able to provide the following:

1. Around-the-clock *availability* of therapeutic personnel who know the pa-

tient and can intercede in crisis. It is best not to try to treat the chronic schizophrenic alone since changes of doctor are difficult to adjust to (Burnham, 1965). A therapeutic team should be available to listen, help the patient with tasks of living, bring relatives together, talk to an employer, arrange for emergency housing, income, food or clothing. Crisis intervention may mean modifying pharmacotherapy or providing an emergency hospital bed.

2. Liaison services with *residential facilities* that are inexpensive but not demoralizing (Kedward et al., 1974). Patients' economic status often forces them to live in squalid and degrading surroundings. Appropriate residences may be supervised settings, foster home placements, communal living arrangements, government-supported housing projects or private rooming houses run by interested, cooperative landlords.

3. Liaison with *vocational* rehabilitation services. Available employment is often ill-paid and demeaning. Appropriate services include preparation-for-work training, on-the-job training, retraining grants, sheltered workshops, communal work opportunities and open communication lines to interested and cooperative employers.

4. *Group* activities. The patient needs to know he is not alone in his disability. Patient organizations, discussion groups, communal projects of all sorts, recreational opportunities for patient groups, social groups, activity groups build solidarity between people and increase individual self-esteem. Professional staff needs to be skilled in group techniques to provide social skill learning, athletics, socializing, role playing, assertiveness training, learning of grooming and nutrition skills, and job motivation. Groups are useful for relatives' concerns, medication problems, group psychotherapy, marital and parenting problems and learning about schizophrenia.

5. *Individual* counselling is necessary,

perhaps intermittently, as the patient progresses through difficult life stages.

6. *Family* counselling. There must be an open line of communication to the patient's family. The family must be encouraged to be involved to some degree with the patient and, at the same time, not to take over decision-making entirely. Formal family therapy, may be useful from time to time to relieve guilt, allow the expression of mutual frustration and resolve conflicting needs.

7. Patients need to be encouraged in *creative pursuits* in which they are often skillful. This includes instrumental and vocal music, poetry and prose writing, food preparation, gardening, handicrafts, painting, sculpting, and many other artistic endeavors.

8. Periodically, "new treatments" for schizophrenia are heralded—e.g. diet, vitamins, dialysis, antiviral agents. The physician needs to keep abreast of new developments and to caution his patients against abandoning what works, if only to a degree, in favor of something which may not work at all.

PROGNOSIS

Currently, a diagnosis of schizophrenia implies a difficult life, punctuated by psychiatric hospitalizations. Acute relapses can, however, be prevented. Hospitalizations, when necessary, can be kept short so as to minimize interference with the tasks of living. Remissions, unfortunately, may be imperfect and may be plagued by the negative symptoms of apathy and isolation. These symptoms do not respond to neuroleptic medications and may, in fact, be made worse by them.

PREVENTION

Since we do not know what causes the disease, we do not know how to prevent it. Genetic couselling is warranted (Tsuang,

1978) as is familial intervention to help prevent relapse (Brown et al., 1972). As we better understand the ways in which neuroleptics remove some symptoms, but not others, we will be able to develop more effective preventive measures and perhaps, too, understand the pathogenesis of the illnesses we call schizophrenia.

REFERENCES

Arieti, S. (1967): New view on the psychodynamics of schizophrenia. *Am. J. Psychiatry.* 124:453.

Bateson, G., Jackson, D. D., Haley, J. et al. (1956): Toward a theory of schizophrenia. *Behav. Sci.* 1:251.

Brown, G. W., Birley, J. L. T., and Wing, J. K. (1972): Influence of family life on the course of schizophrenic disorders: A replication. *Br. J. Psychiatry:* 121:241.

Burnham, D. L. (1965): Separation anxiety: a factor in the object relations of schizophrenic patients. *Arch. Gen. Psychiatry.* 13:346.

Freedman, A. M., Kaplan, H. I. and Sadock, B. J. (1975): *Comprehensive Textbook of Psychiatry.* 2nd ed. Baltimore, Williams & Wilkins.

Fromm-Reichmann, F. (1954): Psychotherapy of schizophrenia. *Am. J. Psychiatry.* III:410.

Goldberg, E. M. and Morrison, S. L. (1963): Schizophrenia and social class. *Br. J. Psychiatry.* 109:785.

Hagnell, O. (1966): *The Prospective Study of the Incidence of Mental Disorder.* Stockholm, Svenska Bokforlget.

Hogarty, G. E., Goldberg, S. C., and Schooler, M. R., et al. (1974): Drug and sociotherapy in the aftercare of schizophrenic patients: two year relapse rates. *Arch. Gen. Psychiatry.* 31:603.

Hornykiewicz, O. (1966): Dopamine (3 hydroxytyramine) and brain function. *Pharmacol. Rev.* 18:925.

Kedward, H. B., Eastwood, M. R., Allodi, F., et al. (1974): The evaluation of chronic psychiatric care. *Can. Med. Assoc. Journal.* 110:519.

Lemkau, P. V., Tietze, C., and Cooper, M. (1943): Survey of statistical studies on prevalence and incidence of mental disorder in sample populations. *Public Health Rep.* 58:1909.

Lidz, R. N. and Lidz, T. (1949): The family environment of schizophrenic patients. *Amer. J. Psychiatry.* 106:332.

Lovett Doust, J. The causes of schizophrenia. Publication pending. Toronto. University of Toronto Press.

Seeman, M. V. (1979): Management of the schizophrenic patient. *Can. Med. Assoc. Journal* 120:1097.

Tsuang, M. T. (1978): Genetic counselling for psychiatric patients and their families. *Am. J. Psychiatry.* 135:1465.

FURTHER READINGS

Arieti, S. (1974): *The Interpretation of Schizophrenia.* 2nd ed. New York, Basic Books.

This is the second edition of Arieti's classical synthesis of the psychological understanding and treatment of schizophrenia. Arieti's view of schizophrenia is not shared by everyone but since he had edited the current bible of American psychiatry, the six-volume *American Handbook of Psychiatry*, and has himself contributed many of the chapters dealing with schizophrenia, his view is probably the one best known to North American psychiatrists.

Feinsilver, D. B. and Gunderson, J. G. (1971): Psychotherapy for schizophrenics—is it indicated? A review of the relevant literature. *Schizophrenia Bulletin.* 6:11.

This paper reviews controlled outcome studies of individual psychotherapy in schizophrenia without being biased in either direction of the drug vs. psychotherapy controversy. The *Schizophrenia Bulletin*, a quarterly published by the National Institute of Health in Bethesda, is an excellent up-to-date source of current thinking about schizophrenia.

Lee, T., Seeman, P., Tourtellotte, W. W., Farley, I. J., et al. (1978): Binding of 3H-neuroleptics and 3H-apomorphine in schizophrenic brains. *Nature* 274:897.

This paper suggests that in schizophrenia certain brain regions possess more than the usual amount of dopamine receptor sites.

Sanders, D. H. (1972): Innovative environments in the community: a life for the chronic patient. *Schizophrenia Bulletin.* 6:49.

This paper reviews several approaches to the difficult problem of the rehabilitation of the chronically ill schizophrenic patient.

Searles, H. (1965): *Collected Papers on Schizophrenia and Related Subjects.* New York, International Universities Press.

This is a collection of essays on the emotional impact of intensive psychotherapy with very ill schizophrenic patients, not only on the patient but also on the therapist.

Seeman, P., Lee, T., Chau-Wong, M., et al. (1976): Antipsychotic drug doses and neuroleptic/dopamine receptors. *Nature.* 261:717.

This paper describes the recently discovered neuroleptic receptor which provides the basis for predicting the antipsychotic dosage of all neuroleptics.

CHAPTER 24

Personality Disorders

J. Donald Atcheson and Gordon E. Warme

Every patient, whether or not defined as having a psychiatric problem, has an habitual style of behavior which he brings to bear on his illness, the physician, and the world in general. This style of behavior is said to constitute *personality* which can be defined as *an individual's enduring patterns of physical and mental activities and attitudes, both conscious and unconscious, particularly actions and attitudes toward other persons.*

The word personality is used in other ways as well. For example personality may refer to social skill or adroitness, or to personal identity, i.e. one's personal experience of who one is. The *persona* is the mask worn by the characters in Greek theatre and the personality may, therefore, also refer to the facade which one presents to the world.

Character, in psychiatric usage, has come to be indistinguishable from personality. The original Greek refers to an instrument for marking and suggests that character is imprinted on an individual; an idea which has both popular and scientific support. Also a person may be considered "a character" and following from this individuals are said to act "in character" or "out of character." Finally the word can be

used to mean moral strength. It is extremely important to remember that the personality of a patient profoundly affects the way in which he manifests his illness and how he behaves toward the physician and the treatment. For example, we all know that histrionic persons exaggerate the significance of minor somatic sensations, while other patients tend to deny even very significant physical and psychological handicaps.

An individual's personality becomes a psychiatric issue when his characteristic behavioral style leads to significant persistent impairment of day to day functioning. He is then said to suffer from a *personality disorder*. This impairment may be noticed and defined as significant by the individual himself, or this perception of impairment may be made by other persons. Typically, persons whose personality organization is relatively mature (reality oriented, self-regulating) notice their own dysfunctional status. Those whose personality organization is immature (infantile, archaic) typically deny problems and are defined as disordered by their families or by society at large. Relatively mature persons with deviant functioning may be thought of as having "high level" personality disorders whereas immature persons are said to have "low level" personality disorders.

For example, the diagnosis of histrionic personality gives us a certain amount of important descriptive information about the way in which that patient approaches the world. However, it does not tell us how severe and disabling that histrionic style is. It was once thought that such histrionic persons were mature and sophisticated in their reality orientation, hence good candidates for intensive psychotherapeutic intervention. Practice did not confirm this and it is now known that many histrionic individuals cannot tolerate the demands of intensive psychotherapy or psychoanalysis, and require a reality oriented and directive form of psychotherapy. This latter group of patients would be said to suffer from a low-level histrionic personality disorder. At times they have been less flatteringly referred to as "bad hysterics."

Individuals who exhibit certain personality types tend to be mature and high level in their functioning although this is not invariant. Compulsive, obsessional, histrionic and depressive persons *tend* to function well. Narcissistic, dependent, avoidant and impulsive persons *tend* to have low level functioning. We would refer to paranoid, schizoid and antisocial individuals as low-level personality disorders.

EPIDEMIOLOGY

The incidence of personality disorders is extremely difficult to determine. At the turn of the century, psychiatrists did not consider an individual's personality to be a medical issue and even today one hesitates to call a personality disorder an illness although we may think of it as a deformity. There has been a major expansion of the definition of psychiatric disorder, and attention to defects in personality organization constitutes a considerable proportion of this expansion. This is particularly apparent in psychiatric office practice and in other forms of medical practice. The reasons are twofold. First, the definition itself has been altered, particularly since the recognition that psychotherapeutic work may permit people to change their personality styles. Second, the practice of consultation-liaison psychiatry has increased our awareness of the psychosomatic (i.e. personality and somatic) aspects of all forms of medical practice. However, the lack of rigor in the diagnosis of personality disorder makes unwise precise statements regarding incidence. Those studies that have been reported, all refer to populations in special clinical settings, and say little about over-all incidence. In private office practice one sees individuals with generally adequate functioning, i.e. high level personality functioning. In a forensic clinic one would see the opposite.

It has been argued that societal changes have altered the incidence and nature of the personality disorders that are seen. For example much has been written regarding "anomie," and the absence of ritualized guidelines.

"[In our culture] emphasis is placed upon certain goals without regard to institutionally prescribed means (little concern is paid to institutional norms) . . . . The central question . . . is, which of the available procedures is most efficient in netting culturally approved value? The most efficient procedure to achieve success becomes the preferred behavior whether it is legitimate or not. As such a process continues, a society becomes increasingly unstable and develops what Durkheim termed anomie (normlessness). Merton considers contemporary American culture to approximate this model. This might help account for the increased incidence and prevalence of personality disorders. As the American society becomes deinstitutionalized . . . external controls and sanctions, whether in the family or community, will become more difficult to internalize. . . . this is a core defect in personality pathology. Merton's types of deviance may be correlated with types of personality disorders—ritualism and obsessive-compulsive type; retreatism and addictive, schizoid, and asthenic types; rebellion and paranoid, explosive, and antisocial types. Thus, Merton states, the social structure produces a strain toward anomie and deviant behavior. The pressure of such a social order is upon outdoing one's competitors."

(Albert 1974)

ETIOLOGY

Personality development is the product of interactions or transactions of the human organism and the psychophysical-social world. Genetic information provides the raw material of personality, e.g. the temperamental differences apparent at birth. As the individual moves from the complete dependency of infancy to maturity, this raw material is molded into characteristic patterns of behaving and thinking. It is the molding of the genetic givens that eventuates in the integrated array of roles, traits, values, self-images, abilities, and emotional patterns which lead to homeostasis within the complex biological, socio-cultural environment.

When we categorize an individual as exhibiting a personality disorder, it is implied that his characteristic patterns of adjustment are not appropriate. To isolate factors which contribute to maladaptive patterns of behavior we need to fully appreciate the importance of early phases of the human life cycle. Following birth, and in early infancy, the sensory input and the emotional milieu will be of exquisite importance in determining future personality. An understanding of the developmental environment with its complex interplay of psychodynamic interrelationships between parent and child is crucial in order to have even a partial theoretical explanation of the eventual personality characteristics.

The developmental environment in the early phases of existence is primarily provided by adult parenting figures. This unique developmental environment is the soil from which the equally unique individual emerges. Many studies support the idea that future personality function is in large part a product of early identifications with the parents. They provide the sensory and cognitive information which form the basis of culturally significant values and roles.

Other factors may play a significant role in the development of personality disorders. A person with a sound genetic inheritance who develops in an adequate environment may still experience significant physical and emotional traumata at critical periods in his developmental cycle. These traumata affect future personality functioning. Disabling illnesses, brain damage, and cosmetic flaws may result in deviant rather than reality oriented self-images.

There may be many possible reasons for parental privation and deprivation and they may come into play at varying times during the developmental process. Separation from parents and the attendant loss of security may be a serious contributing cause of future personality disorder (Rutter, 1972).

The etiology of personality disorders can therefore be considered under three major headings:

1. Genetic and constitutional factors.
2. Development and environmental factors.
3. Situational or traumatic factors.

It is the interaction of these elements in the life cycle which creates the ultimate unique personality organization of an individual. Defects in all or any of these factors may lead to malfunction or personality disorder.

As numerous types of personality disorders are recognized, it is obvious that the origin of the disorder in a particular case has a number of contributing interacting factors. And a careful assessment of personal history is essential for understanding a particular case: why, for example, one individual has a self-image of inadequacy, and responds to this interpretation of self with paranoid ideation and defenses, while another individual demonstrates impulsive behavior.

CLASSIFICATION (AMERICAN PSYCHIATRIC ASSOCIATION, 1977)

A system of classification of any group of human disorders may be formulated on either the basis of a description of presenting signs and symptoms, or upon an awareness of etiological factors commonly found in a given syndrome. In those conditions in which specific etiological factors can be identified and found to be statistically meaningful, specific therapies can be directed toward specific causes, e.g. in the personality disorders which may follow brain damage or other disorders of the central nervous system, the relationship between this damage and subsequent changes in the characteristic patterns of the individual is clearly recognized.

In other types of personality disorder, for example those described as antisocial, very clear relationships have been found with emotional deprivation during early childhood. These persons fail to achieve a sense of moral or cultural values and are referred to as personality disorders, antisocial type. The term psychopathic personality has frequently been applied to this group (Cleckly, 1976).

There is perhaps some justification for separating these patients into two syndromes, i.e. personality disorder, antisocial type, and psychopathic personality, although this is not reflected in all classifications. People with antisocial personalities frequently have histories of inadequate early environmments. There are other individuals, the so-called psychopathic personalities, who appear to have been reared in a secure and appropriate awareness of the effect of their behavior on

others. They, too, may be described as having failed to develop a conscience, or super-ego. In this group there is a significantly elevated incidence of electroencephalographic abnormalities. They totally fail to profit from experience in terms of modifying their antisocial behavior. They demonstrate a need for immediate gratification of their wishes and are baffled and infuriated when others do not cooperate with them (Robins, 1966).

Most other types of personality disorders are described in terms of the characteristic patterns of behavior. The most clearly defined classification of personality disorders is to be found in the *Diagnostic Statistical Manual of Mental Disorders*, 3rd edition, prepared by the Task Force of Nomenclature and Statistics of the American Psychiatric Association (DSM III).

Personality disorders are defined as deeply ingrained, inadequate patterns of behavior and thought, of sufficient severity to cause impairment in adaptive functioning, or subjective distress. They represent persistent character traits, that is, the characteristic way of relating to the environment in a specific style and are exhibited in a wide range of important social and personal contacts.

This classification presents each type of personality disorder under very specific headings:

1. Essential features
2. Associated features
3. Impairment
4. Differential diagnosis
5. Operational criteria

The following types of personality disorder are described:

Paranoid personality disorder. Essential features are avoidance of accepting deserved blame and an unwarranted view of others as malevolent. The latter is expressed as suspiciousness, hypersensitivity, and mistrust. They feel easily slighted and take offense. There is a general state of hyper-vigilance manifested by continual scanning of the environment for signs of threat.

Asocial personality disorder (Schizoid). Individuals demonstrating this type of personality disorder present a behavior pattern of shyness, over-sensitivity, seclusiveness, and rejection of close or competitive relationships. They are characteristically lonely and uninvolved with others and are not distressed by social distance. They usually demonstrate no desire for greater social involvement.

Schizotypal personality disorder (Latent borderline schizophrenia). There is no single feature which is invariably present in these patients. However, they manifest eccentricities of thought, perception, communication, and behavior; but the pathology is never severe enough to meet the criteria for schizophrenia. They frequently demonstrate paranoid ideation. Essential disorders may include illusions, depersonalization, or derealization. Frequently, but not invariably, they are socially isolated and their constructed or inappropriate affect interferes with rapport in face to face interactions with other people.

Histrionic personality disorder (hysterical personality). Essential features are attention-seeking, histrionic and demanding interpersonal relationships, and affect which is overly reactive and expressed intensely. They are often perceived by others as lacking genuineness and behaving as if a role were being acted out. They are often referred to by others as being "shallow" in terms of depth of feeling.

Narcissistic personality disorder. Essential features of this condition are interpersonal difficulties caused by an inflated sense of self-worth and indifference to the welfare of others. Deficits in their achievements are justified and sustained by a boastful arrogance. They are often socially irresponsible and will present expansive fantasies.

Antisocial personality disorders (with predominant sociopathic or asocial manifestations). Essential features relate to the recognition that antisocial behavior in many areas begins before the age of 15, typically from earlier school years or before, and persists into adulthood. In adulthood there is invariably a marked impaired capacity to sustain lasting, close, warm, and responsible relationships with family, friends, or sexual partners, and to sustain good job performance over a period of years.

Unstable personality disorder (borderline personality organization). Although no single features are invariably present, patients with this disorder are characterized by instability in a variety of areas, including interpersonal relationships, behavior, mood, and self-image. Profound identity disturbance may be manifested by uncertainty about several issues related to identity such as self-image, gender identity, long term goals, or values. They may have trouble being alone and experience chronic feelings of emptiness or boredom. There are often many features of schizotypal personality disorder.

Avoidant personality disorders. Essential features are excessive social inhibitions and shyness, a tendency to withdraw from opportunities for developing close relationships and a fearful expectation that they will be belittled and humiliated. Although they demonstrate a desire for affection and acceptance, they have a negative self-image which prevents the completion of satisfactory relationships. They are frequently lonely and very isolated.

Dependent personality disorders. Essential features of this personality type are excessive dependency, a lack of initiative and competitiveness, and avoidance of self-assertion. The patient cannot tolerate isolation, and actively seeks companionship in order to get other persons to assume responsibilities for tasks that most individuals are able to complete on their own.

Compulsive personality disorder (Anankastic personality disorder). Essential features are excessive emotional control and concern with conformity and adherence to internalized standards. There is a great need for organization and efficiency, and simple, every day relationships are made conventional, formal, and serious. This pattern often prevents unstructured relaxation. Individuals of this type tend to be perfectionists and to focus on meticulous detail, and to be extremely upset by deviations from known routine. They place high expectations on their capacity to work and to be productive to the exclusion of pleasures and interpersonal relationships.

DIAGNOSIS

Personality diagnosis, strictly speaking, is separate from the diagnosis of psychiatric syndromes (see DSM III and the concept of diagnosis on five axes). However, for practical purposes, the diagnosis of personality disorder must be distinguished from psychosis, from psychoneurosis and from organic brain syndrome.

Psychotic illnesses are characterized by a relatively enduring defect in reality testing. They may be obvious as in acute psychotic episodes or in other regressive states. However psychosis may be difficult to detect in paranoid persons who have no thought disorder, either clinically or on psychological testing. Persons with low level personality organizations may show evidence of thought disorder, particularly on projective psychological testing with the Rorschach test, and under conditions of stress. However, they are not psychotic because their reality testing remains intact, or can be re-established within a few hours or days, and by skillful clinical interviewing. This is seen in its most typical form in the self-limited "micropsychotic" episodes of the so-called "borderline" syndrome.

Psychoneurotic illness is experienced as ego-alien and in this way may be differentiated from personality disorder. Persons with deviant personality functioning think their behavior is appropriate and acceptable and take offence when their deviant behavior is discussed, whereas patients with neuroses complain about and are offended by their phobias, anxieties, obsessions, etc.

Brain syndromes may lead to a change in personality functioning (Goldstein, 1952). Some authors have described distinctive personality styles in patients with epilepsy, multiple sclerosis, and other organic brain syndromes. The evidence for this is uncertain.

TREATMENT

Certain patients with personality disorders develop a gradually increasing awareness that their characteristic style of living is self-defeating and they, therefore, wish to make changes in themselves. These patients, of their own accord, seek treatment.

Many other persons with personality disorders never request psychiatric treatment of their own accord. To them, their behavioral styles are perfectly ego syntonic even though others might define their behavior as deviant. This second group of patients generally come to psychiatric attention in two circumstances. First, other people may exert pressure on the individual in question and persuade or coerce him into obtaining treatment. If he can really be convinced that his behavioral patterns are maladaptive, then treatment becomes feasible. Secondly, patients with personality disorders may, under pressure, decompensate and develop painful symptoms which cause them to seek treatment. The following case vignette of a man with a compulsive personality who developed severe neurotic symptoms under stress, will illustrate the latter instance.

Mr. R., a 35 year old executive, was highly organized and efficient. In his personal life he was extremely tidy and demanded of himself and his family that the home be immaculately clean, tidy, and organized. Although his perfectionism and demanding behavior were unpleasant for all concerned, he prided himself on the clock-work efficiency of his and his family's daily routine. Following a promotion in his work, the patient began feeling distressed. Having become responsible for the administration of a complex and constantly changing business unit, he found, to his distress, that he could not maintain things in a perfectly organized pattern. Uncertainty and unpredictability were inevitable in the unit for which he was responsible. Increasingly he became incapable of making decisions, developed anxiety, and insomnia, and ultimately had to consult a psychiatrist.

The specific treatment for the various personality disorders depends largely on the level of functioning of the patient. Relatively mature patients are treated psychotherapeutically. Patients with major impairments must be treated with support and/or re-educational efforts.

At one time it would have been said that persons with high level personality disorders must be offered formal psychoanalytic treatment. Were this easily available this would still be true. However, it seems that intensive psychotherapeutic intervention may lead to real personality change and psychoanalysis can be reserved for patients who will derive additional educational benefits from the treatment.

Patients with more severe personality disorders have also been treated psychoanalytically. This is, however, an heroic undertaking, and in the current state of our knowledge must, in most cases, be considered a research effort. Additionally, few of these patients have a desire for fundamental change and therefore rarely make a serious effort towards changing themselves psychotherapeutically.

Most individuals with severe personality disorders must be treated supportively. They suffer absolute defects in certain aspects of their functioning and the physician must assume this function for the patient. Examples of psychological deficits commonly seen are impaired anxiety tolerance, inability to use good judgment, lack of control over impulses, and so on. The physician takes over these functions of the patient via drugs, reassurance, exhortation, and explanation. However, this does not mean that the physician cannot use more traditional psychotherapeutic methods. Indeed, insofar as the patient is able, the physician ought to make psychotherapeutic demands in order to effect some personality changes. According to this rationale supportive treatment may, after a period of months or years, develop into a more classical psychotherapeutic situation with ambitious goals of major personality change.

A further group of such personality disordered patients exists. These persons are so disabled that they cannot function independently or are apprehended by social or law enforcement agencies. These patients must be treated in partial or total institutional settings. Generally total institutions are less desirable except when absolutely necessary. Patients in partial institutions fare better, largely because they are obliged to remain responsible for a larger measure of their own functioning. Institutional treatment is, ideally, a massive, psychologically sophisticated re-educational manuever. Such efforts tax the morale of the personnel and countertransference problems are frequent. Usually the institutions best suited for such work are those with a particular interest in the treatment of patients with severe personality disorders. General psychiatric inpatient units are particularly taxed by such patients. No pharmacological or other somatic treatment plays a definitive role in the treatment of these patients. Drug therapy is most commonly prescribed by frustrated physicians who are unable or unwilling to undertake more definitive treatment.

REFERENCES

Albert, J.S. (1974): Sociocultural determinants of personality pathology. In *Personality Disorders.*

Edited by J. R. Lion. Baltimore, Williams and Wilkins.

American Psychiatric Association. (1968): *Diagnostic and Statistical Manual of Mental Disorder*, 2nd ed. (DSM II). Washington, D.C., American Psychiatric Association.

Cleckly, H. (1976): *The Mask of Sanity*, 5th ed. St. Louis, C. V. Mosby.

Goldstein, K. (1952): The effect of brain damage on the personality. *Psychiatry. 15*:245.

Robins, L.N. (1966): *Deviant Children Grown Up*. Baltimore, Williams and Wilkins.

Rutter, M. (1972): Maternal deprivation reconsidered. *J. Psychosomat. Res. 16*:241.

FURTHER READINGS

Bowlby, J. (1944): Forty-four juvenile thieves. *Int. J. Psychoanal. 25*:19.

Bovet, L. (1951): *Psychiatric Aspects of Juvenile Delinquency*. Westport, Conn., Greenwood.

Kernberg, O. (1970): Psychoanalytic classification of character pathology. *J. Amer. Psychoanal. Assoc. 18*:800.

Leon, R.J. (1974): *Personality disorders—Diagnosis and Management*. Baltimore, Williams and Wilkins.

Parsons, T. (1964): *Social Structure and Personality*. New York, Free Press.

CHAPTER 25

Disorders of Sexual Behavior

Kurt Freund and Betty W. Steiner

Many people consult physicians about problems directly or indirectly related to sex, problems that affect their erotic response to others, or their capacity to engage satisfactorily in intercourse.

For the sake of convenience, behavioral sexologists separate sexual problems into those directly involved in intercourse, in which the patient manifests "sexual adequacy or inadequacy" (Masters and Johnson) and those related to erotic or sexual interaction other than intercourse (the domain of erotic preferences).

SEXUAL INADEQUACY IN MEN

According to Masters and Johnson, impotence is the condition of being unable to insert the penis into the vagina or to keep it there for a reasonable period of time. Premature ejaculation is a lack of control of the ejaculatory process for a sufficient period of time to satisfy the woman, in at least 50% of attempts at intercourse. Ejaculatory incompetence is the man's inability to ejaculate while his penis is in the vagina.

The conditions of having an abnormally weak or abnormally strong sexual appetite are called hyposexuality and hypersexuality, respectively.

Dyspareunia, which can affect men and women, is defined as genital, abdominal, or pelvic pain on intercourse that seriously interferes with the sex life. The cause of male dyspareunia is most often a physical one, for example, urethritis, prostatitis, or phimosis.

Causation of Sexual Inadequacy

Classification of cases of sexual inadequacy according to their causes is difficult. At present the most common differentiation is between "psychological" (experiential) and "organic" causes.

Psychological causes of sexual inadequacy are usually thought to be related to particular interpersonal patterns that were important in the person's early life, for instance a puritanical upbringing, an unwholesome parent-child relationship, an overt or disguised incest situation, or some other type of circumstance thought to be detrimental to one's psychosexual adjustment. Assessing the structure of such situations—and their impact—is a highly controversial matter.

The notion of *concurrent* psychological causes of erectile difficulties and premature ejaculation seems to be better founded. The main categories are *perfor-*

mance anxiety which often seems to form a superstructure over other psychological problems or non-psychological causes; or *anomalies in erotic preferences*, where the erotic (arousal) value of the physically mature female or of the usual situation of sexual interaction is abnormally low. In these cases also, a superstructure of performance anxiety often seems to be present. Psychiatric illness, particularly depressions, are usually accompanied by decreased sex drive or other sexual inadequacies. However it is not at all certain whether, for example in manic depressive illness, the decreased sex drive level of a depressive phase or the hypersexuality of a manic phase are caused by the manic or depressive mood or by the underlying physiological disorder.

In *situational impotence*, i.e. in cases where the disturbance occurs only in particular situations and not in others, the psychological component is usually thought to be the sole causative agent. In the majority of such cases coming to our attention, the patients indicated there was no disturbance when patients masturbated themselves, but there was impotence at attempted intercourse. However, it often becomes apparent later on that the gap between these two situations in regard to erectile functioning was not as wide as at first reported. Among the infrequent extreme cases where there is no difficulty in automasturbation but where there is impotence in intercourse there is usually an anomalous erotic preference. The patient is much better able to fantasize the preferred type of partner or interaction in automasturbation than in intercourse.

Organic causes of sexual inadequacies may seem to be more reliable and technically simpler to diagnose than experiential causes. However, that too has its difficulties because there are still too many unknowns in the physiology of the sexual system.

Among the better known organic causes of sexual inadequacy in the male are diseases of, or traumatic damage to, the vascular and nervous systems. Because of the high flow rate necessary to keep the corpora cavernosa filled for the required period of time, erectile impotence can occur long before gross impairment of the vascular system is diagnosed. Methods for assessing penile vascular insufficiency are available but will have to be modified before they can be routinely used with large numbers of patients. Vascular impotence can also be caused by extensive bleeding from a pelvic fracture followed by thromboses in the local vascular bed, or by vascular anomalies.

Arteriosclerotic interference with erectile capacity, like other arteriosclerotic symptoms, tends to fluctuate for a long period of time before becoming constant. Such fluctuation is often erroneously perceived as an indicator that the erectile problem is psychological and not organic. On the other hand, performance anxiety and depressive mood, particularly after a coronary infarction or a stroke, can sometimes be the main cause of sexual inadequacy.

In diabetic neuropathy, as in arteriosclerosis, erectile impotence may be the first diagnosed symptom. In contrast to arteriosclerosis however, diabetic neuropathy also seems to lead early on to extinction of the ejaculatory reflex. But sometimes diabetic impotence is due to the concomitant arteriosclerotic changes and is not caused by neuropathy. Other neuropathies, whether caused by poisons like lead or mercury, metabolic diseases, gross insufficiency of certain vitamins, or by infections, can also interfere with normal sexual functioning.

Damage to the superior hypogastric sympathetic plexus (the "presacral nerve") during aortoiliac surgery carried out to restore blood flow to the legs and penis, or during extended intestinal reconstruction, interferes mainly with the ejaculatory reflex. Other kinds of surgery, e.g. dissection of the muscles of the neck of the bladder (sphincterotomy) in para-plegics, or prostatectomy by the perineal route, can lead primarily to impairment of the erectile reflex.

Impairment of the spinal cord, whether traumatic or through various diseases, often causes sexual inadequacy, for in-stance in multiple sclerosis, where erectile impotence is sometimes one of the first symptoms to come to the physician's atten-tion. Interference of spinal cord lesions, whatever their cause, depends on their lo-cation and extent.

The erectile reflex is activated either by touch in the genital region or "psychologi-cally," i.e. through other kinds of stimuli (mainly optical, olfactory, acoustic) in-cluding fantasies. Touch, temperature, or pain applied to the genital region are con-ducted by the pudendal nerves to the sac-ral part of the cord, to be processed there by a center which sends impulses through the parasympathetic sacral rami erigentes to the blood vessels involved in erection.

A complete transverse lesion in the thoracic part of the spinal cord abolishes penile tumescence response to psycholog-ical stimulation, as well as the feeling of orgasm which normally accompanies ejaculation. The spinal ejaculatory center is located in the lumbar region and it is very likely that both centers are connected. The afferent impulses, particularly those from the glans penis, are conducted to this center via pudendal nerves, and the effer-ent stimuli reach the striped and smooth musculature involved in the ejaculatory reflex via communicating rami and presac-ral nerves.

The least well explored part of the re-productive system is that located in the brain. Experimentation on animals has shown involvement of septum, substantia preoptica, and hypothalamus, including the median forebrain bundle. There is also some direct involvement of other parts of the brain, e.g. the amygdala. In primates, pathways from and to erectile and ejaculatory centers of the spinal cord have

been mapped. These latter centers have been shown to be sensitive to testosterone, and the same is true for some of the regions of the reproductive system located in the brain, particularly the area preoptica.

A comprehensive list of the main dis-eases which cause sexual inadequacies can be found in Masters and Johnson (1970), among them diseases or other kinds of im-pairment of the endocrine glands. It ap-pears that virtually normal sex life is some-times possible on abnormally low testos-terone levels, but we do not know for how long. In humans and in most vertebrate species, removal of both gonads (castra-tion) eventually always abolishes erectile and ejaculatory reflexes, and lowers sexual interest. As expected, this also holds for grossly insufficient gonadotropin release by the pituitary or—on a third level—for insufficient secretion of LH-releasing hormone of the hypothalamus. The behav-ioral and/or psychological effects of the various sex hormone metabolites have not yet been very well explored, particularly changes in hormonal sensitivity of the var-ious kinds of cell receptors involved.

Interference with erectile or ejaculatory capability has been observed after pro-longed use of various routinely prescribed drugs, mainly the phenothiazines—and in particular Thioridazine (Mellaril). Loss of ejaculatory capability results first, fol-lowed by erectile difficulties and lowering of sex drive, and there is a tendency toward retrograde ejaculation (backwards, into the bladder). Ismeline (guanethidine sulfate) has a similar effect but, with this latter drug, a decrease of erectile capability would appear to be particularly frequent. This pertains also to a second antihyper-tonic, Reserpine, which primarily affects erectile capability, and to the "anxiolytic" agent Diazepam. Interference with sexual function has also been noted with tricyclic antidepressants, monoamine oxidase in-hibitors, and amphetamines.

Serotonin-depleting drugs such as L-Dopa and Apomorphine have an aphrodisiac effect, but for this effect to occur there has to be an adequate level of such androgens which by themselves also activate sexual behavior. Where the level of such androgens is too low, no aphrodisiac effect is observed. On the basis of these findings, Gessa and Tagliamonte (1975) advanced the hypothesis that androgens prime a neuronal system which initiates or maintains sexual behavior, and that this system is inhibited by another system in which serotonin is the critical compound.

Alcohol, when abused in large quantities for a number of years, is the principal non-medically used drug responsible for the largest number of cases of impairment of sexual function. Such impairment may persist even after years of sobriety. Heroin leads to ejaculatory incompetence and later to erectile impotence. Methadone has a similar but less pronounced effect.

SEXUAL INADEQUACY IN WOMEN

The work of Kinsey and his associates (1953) was the first comprehensive evaluation of sexual behavior in women. The Kinsey group found that the frequency with which a woman had an orgasm during heterosexual intercourse was directly related to her ability to achieve orgasm by masturbation.

Masters and Johnson conducted the first systematic study of the physiology of the female orgasm. They divided the sexual-response cycle into four phases. During the first phase, the excitement phase, the woman experiences erection of the nipples, tachycardia, elevation of blood pressure, erection of the clitoris, and vaginal lubrication. In addition, she may develop a maculopapular rash.

The second phase, the plateau phase, is characterized by a further increase in breast size, increased vasocongestion with engorgement of the labia majora and minora, a well-developed "sex flush," and hyperventilation. In addition, in most women the introitus of the vagina becomes extremely sensitive. Masters and Johnson suggested that all women are capable of orgasm once they reach the plateau phase.

In the third phase, the orgasmic phase, the woman experiences involuntary contractions of the pelvic and abdominal muscles. In addition, the uterus is elevated into the false pelvis and the width and depth of the vaginal barrel increases further, creating a seminal receptacle, the "seminal pool."

The mechanism by which orgasm is achieved is not known, but it is known that the clitoris is always involved when there is considerable sexual arousal and that the clitoris is the trigger that discharges the woman's sexual tension.

Primary anorgasmia is the complete and lifelong inability to achieve orgasm no matter what method of sexual arousal is used, including masturbation. Secondary anorgasmia is the inability to achieve orgasm in a woman who had formerly achieved it.

Vaginismus is the involuntary contraction of the lower third of the vagina during intercourse. Masters and Johnson identified the following as factors that are associated with both vaginismus and anorgasmia: religious orthodoxy, inadequate psychosexual identification with the female role, masturbatory inadequacy; and other psychogenic factors, such as homosexuality, or a psychological trauma such as rape or incest. A low sex drive, together with organic factors such as dyspareunia, are also considered to be factors associated with anorgasmia.

The causes of dyspareunia in women are vaginal causes, such as vaginal infections, lack of vaginal lubrication which may be caused by inadequate sexual arousal, and vaginal sensitivity to chemical contraceptives; pelvic causes, such as tears and lacerations of the broad ligament, endometriosis, pelvic infections, and postsurgical problems such as tight suturing after an episiotomy; and psychological causes, such as fear, inhibitions or anxiety, unreal expectations about intercourse, or lack of affection for the partner.

THERAPY FOR MEN AND WOMEN

The sex therapy developed by Masters and Johnson has been remarkably effective. It is based on conveying relevant information, and uses relatively direct behavior modification techniques. The information was gathered mainly by direct observations of people having intercourse, and by interviews with very sexually experienced women about their own sexual responses. The couple are taught certain remedial procedures such as the Semans technique (see below) which is to alleviate premature ejaculation, and they are encouraged to enhance mutual communication, particularly about their sexual wishes and sensations.

Sex therapy tackles only the psychological component of sexual inadequacies and it is very likely that, at least in the male, there are many non-psychological causes which are not yet appropriately diagnosed. However, as already stated, the psychological component often participates substantially even in the basically non-psychological cases.

The paragraphs that follow discuss only a few selected features of sex therapy. Readers who wish more detailed information are referred to Masters and Johnson.

The couple being treated are told to refrain from intercourse for several days. During this "sensate focus phase" the couple are encouraged to engage in petting and "pleasuring." Each partner is encouraged to caress the other for 30 to 60 minutes. The partners take turns pleasuring each other. One partner guides the other to show what he or she likes in terms of pressure and location. Sexual play for its own sake, i.e. not as a prelude to intercourse, is emphasized.

Treatment of impotence. In treating problems in erection, the goal is to achieve a situation in which the "demand compo-nent" is held as low as possible in order to alleviate the man's performance anxiety (the Frankl technique). In the realm of pharmacology there is still not enough known to warrant an indication of general guidelines of such treatment of impotence. When thorough investigations of penile circulation become more widespread, arterial bypass operations may also become more common. Little therapeutic use has been made even of options where the relevant realm is well known, as for instance in cases of impairment of central neural structure or the cauda equina, and an intact vascular system. In such conditions electrostimulation of peripheral nerves could be employed.

Treatment of premature ejaculation. Masters and Johnson improved and extended Semans' technique for controlling premature ejaculation. The woman stimulates the man's erect penis manually until he feels he is about to ejaculate. At that point she stops stimulating him and applies pressure to the base of the glans (the "squeeze technique") until the erection subsides. Then she again starts to stimulate the penis. The procedure is repeated several times, and later manual stimulation is replaced by intravaginal containment. In cases in which premature ejaculation preceded or accompanies impotence, the respective treatment methods are combined.

There are great discrepancies between authors (e.g. Masters and Johnson, and Cooper, 1969) in reported outcome of sex therapy. A likely explanation is the differences in defining prematurity, in defining therapeutic effect, and in selection of couples according to an undefined extent of mutual cooperativeness. It would seem that where premature ejaculation is not mainly due to insufficient intercourse and/or lack of information in respect to the female partner's needs, therapeutic effects are overestimated. This would appear to hamper pharmacological developments and other "organic" approaches (e.g. tackling of the innervation of the seminal vesicles by local treatments).

Treatment of ejaculatory incompetence. The behavior therapeutic procedures employed in the treatment of ejaculatory incompetence are similar to those used for impotence. The aim in both cases is the same, to relieve anxiety. Not too rarely this affliction is situational and caused by an anomalous erotic preference.

Treatment of orgasmic dysfunction. After development of a reasonably intensive and prolonged phase of stimulation and vaginal containment, women who are still anorgasmic are told that they should first try to achieve orgasm by any means whatsoever. Thus if manual or oral stimulation of the vulva by the partner does not bring the woman to orgasm, it is recommended that she masturbate manually and, if necessary, by applying a vibrator. One of the aims of this approach is to prove to the woman that she is capable of achieving orgasm. According to Kaplan, almost all women with primary anorgasmia can be brought to climax by clitoral stimulation; and most orgasmically inhibited women can achieve climax in the presence of their husbands. However, only about 50% of Kaplan's patients who were anorgasmic were able during treatment to reach climax during intercourse.

Treatment of vaginismus. To treat the patient with vaginismus, a gynecologist demonstrates to her and her partner how the vagina contracts during a pelvic examination. The couple are then given a set of Hager's dilators, which are graduated in size. The woman is told to insert the smallest dilator, well lubricated, into her vagina and to keep it there for two to three minutes. After the woman can insert and contain the largest dilator for hours (preferably overnight), the man is told to insert the dilators into her vagina, and the woman is told to contain them. To alleviate anxiety, which may interfere with sexual response, the patient may be treated with Wolpe's desensitization therapy. In this therapy the relaxation technique is used to reduce anxiety, and it is combined with a series of imaginary situations that are graded according to how much anxiety they evoke in the woman.

ANOMALOUS EROTIC OR SEXUAL PREFERENCES

Norms for erotic preferences, though not clearly delineated, are sufficiently well known for gross anomalies to be recognized. The following is a brief review of such anomalies.

Anomalies as to Preferred Body Shape

Homosexuality, pedophilia and hebephilia are anomalies in erotic preference as to preferred body shape of the partner.

Homosexuality. This is a sustained erotic preference for persons of one's own sex, when potential partners of both sexes are available and are comparable as to other attributes which contribute to erotic attractiveness. In this definition the term sex denotes identifiable male or female body shape, particularly of genitals.

The definition of bisexuality is also based on preferred body shape. The smaller the person's erotic preference for the body shape of either sex over that of the other, the greater her/his degree of bisexuality proper. The person whose erotic inclination for body shapes of men and women are about the same is fully bisexual.

Estimates of the prevalence of homosexuality vary considerably. According to Kinsey and his associates (1948) about 13% of the white male population in the United States respond predominantly, but not exclusively, in a homosexual way for at least a 3-year period between the ages of 16 and 55. The percentage is extremely high and it raises the suspicion that it may be an artifact of Kinsey's sampling methods. A more realistic estimate of the incidence of homosexuality—one based on the statements of a number of authors who have treated homosexuals extensively—is 3%, but exact data are not available.

Pedophilia. This is defined as sustained erotic preference for children as contrasted to an erotic inclination toward physically mature persons. A further refinement of pedophilia is hebephilia which is an erotic preference for pubescents. Almost nothing is known about the incidence of pedophilia or hebephilia. Both are rare in women.

Often the adults who make sexual advances to children or pubescents actually prefer people with mature body shapes as sexual partners but, because they are handicapped either socially or by age, they are not able to attract suitable partners. Similarly, in many such intrafamilial cases, the adult is not really pedophilic but approaches only children with whom he has a very close relationship.

Gerontophilia. The erotic preference for the body shape of an old person, is either extremely rare or it goes almost unnoticed. In most cases in which young people interact sexually with old people, the circumstances are such that one doubts that a true reciprocal erotic attraction is present. Quite simply, money and power rather than sex may be the attraction.

Cross Gender Identity

Some homosexual persons who have an erotic preference for partners with mature body shape display mannerisms and attitudes that are typical of members of the opposite gender, and prefer the role of the other gender in sexual interactions. This deviation from the norm is a gender identity disturbance and, if it is very conspicuous, we could call it cross gender identity; however, the gender identity of many homosexual persons appears to be congruent with the heterosexual norm. There are two modes of cross gender identity: transvestism and transsexualism.

Transvestism. This takes place only in

heterosexual persons and almost exclusively in males. In situations in which he is sexually aroused the transvestite erotically prefers to imagine himself as a person of the opposite gender. In situations in which there is virtually no sexual arousal, there is no cross gender identity. Transvestite men usually masturbate dressed in women's underwear, often in front of a mirror. There is almost always fetishism for some article of female clothing. The incidence of transvestism is not known.

Transsexualism. This is the desire to be socially accepted as a person of the opposite gender. The transsexual desire does *not* disappear when there is virtually no sexual arousal. According to Hoenig transsexualism is not simply an erotic anomaly but affects the person's entire self-perception. The incidence of transsexualism is about one in thirty or forty thousand people.

Additional Anomalies

A strong erotic preference for inanimate objects is defined as fetishism. In their tactile qualities, fetish objects usually resemble skin or body hair (silk, nylon, velvet, rubber, fur) and the shapes of parts of the body (shoes, boots, gloves) or they may represent parts of the body in other ways (pieces of clothing, particularly garments worn directly over the skin, such as underwear). Parts of the body themselves (hands, feet, arms) may have such an abnormally high sexual arousal value for some people that they feel little erotic interest in a potential partner's other attributes. Also, particular situations or behavioral patterns of potential partners may acquire the characteristics of fetishes. Combinations of fetishism with masochism or sadism are relatively frequent.

Unlike transvestism, in simple fetishism there is often a strong erotic preference for a garment that has been worn, rather than a new garment, and sometimes the smell of such a garment is capable of producing strong erotic arousal. The preference for garments that have been worn may explain why many people with such fetishes prefer to steal the garments rather than buy them.

Necrophilia, pygmalionism, zoophilia. In some anomalies of sexual preference, the normal shape of the human body is the most preferred erotic stimulus, but it must be a body that is incapable of spontaneous movement, such as a dead body or a statue. The erotic preference for corpses is called necrophilia; the erotic preference for statues is called pygmalionism. Zoophilia is an erotic preference for animals. These rather exotic anomalies are believed to be rare.

Anomalies in Phasing of Courtship Behavior

Normal erotic or sexual interaction can be seen as proceeding in *four phases*: location and/or choice of a suitable partner; pretactile interaction—looking, smiling, posturing, and talking to the prospective partner; tactile interaction; and sexual intercourse.

In ethologic terms, erotic or sexual approach behavior up to, but excluding intercourse is denoted courtship behavior. The following anomalies are the main types of *conspicuous distortion* of the usual *phase sequence* of courtship behavior.

Voyeurism. This is an exaggerated desire to look stealthily at a member of the opposite sex either in some stage of undress, or having intercourse, or urinating and so on. Voyeurism can be seen as an exaggerated and distorted first phase of normal courtship behavior, with the remaining phases only abortively present or nonexistent.

Exhibitionism. This is a conspicuous erotic preference for exposing one's genitals, or less frequently, other parts of the body, from a distance and, according to Mohr and his associates, taking the onlooker by surprise. Exhibitionism can be

seen as an exaggeration and distortion of the second phase of normal courtship behavior.

Toucheurism. This anomaly is an unusually strong erotic preference for touching the breasts or the genitals of an unknown woman, taking her by surprise.

Frotteurism. This is the unusually strong erotic preference for approaching an unsuspecting female stranger from the rear and pressing or rubbing the penis against her buttocks. Both toucheurism and frotteurism can be understood as abnormal representatives of the third phase of courtship behavior.

The pathological rape pattern. This is characterized by a man's strong erotic preference for having intercourse with a woman not known to him, and with practically no preceding erotic interaction. The anomaly usually manifests itself in forced intercourse or forced fellatio. In the pathological rape pattern, courtship behavior is present only very abortively or not at all. The pathological rape pattern has little to do with rape as a surrogate activity, in which the man would prefer, but is not able, to have intercourse with a willing partner whom he finds acceptable. Often, two or more of the anomalies just described occur in the same person, and some people show a pattern which is a combination of all these anomalies in phasing of courtship behavior.

Sadism

Krafft-Ebing defined sadism as "the experience of pleasurable sexual sensations (including orgasm) produced by acts of cruelty, or bodily punishment, carried out by oneself or witnessed in others, be they animals or human beings. It may also consist of a desire to humiliate, hurt, wound, or even destroy others in order thereby to create sexual pleasure in one's self."

In medical usage the meaning of the term sadism has been narrowed to indicate sexual activities that are physically dangerous. Therefore it might be useful to modify Krafft-Ebing's broad definition accordingly. Since Krafft-Ebing's term "desire to humiliate" indicates a person's preference for being extremely dominant and for having his erotic partner be extremely submissive, the term *erotic hyperdominance* would convey Krafft-Ebing's broader concept of sadism. The term sadism could then be confined to those cases in which there is an erotic desire to cause physical harm or physical suffering to another person or an animal. Apart from that, dangerous sadism and nondangerous (or mild) sadism should be differentiated. In dangerous sadism the person's erotic behavior has a predatory aspect. He may mutilate or kill his sexual objects and even eat the corpses (sadistic necrophilia). The term dangerous sadism would also include those cases in which such a patient wishes to assault the partner, or to mete out other potentially dangerous punishment to the partner.

Nondangerous sadism is shown by the person who seeks only to punish the partner symbolically, for example, by lightly spanking the partner's buttocks, lightly slapping the partner, withholding favors from the partner, or making the partner obey trivial commands or do other things that indicate that the patient is in "full command;" for example, tying the partner to a chair or a bed, or tying the partner's hands or feet. In the majority of cases such practices would seem to be a nuisance to the partner rather than a real danger.

Other forms of nondangerous sadism are the erotically motivated defiling of other people with feces, urine, mud, and the like, or erotically motivated cutting of a strand of hair from the head of an unsuspecting victim (usually referred to as hair despoiling).

Abortive sadism (Krafft-Ebing's term) also seems to be nondangerous. The term refers to those cases in which a person has the erotic preference for being a spectator to the maltreatment of another, rather than for being a participant in the maltreatment. Some such individuals prefer to watch animals being maltreated.

The most common *nonsadistic hyperdominance pattern* (listed by Krafft-Ebing under his broad category of sadism) is an erotic preference for degrading a potential partner, or for socially degraded persons as partners, for instance prostitutes.

Destruction-bent eroticism, another important syndrome related to sadism, is the inclination toward achieving a strong erotic arousal by destroying things, particularly occupied or unoccupied living quarters. Sexually motivated arson is the most common manifestation of destruction-bent eroticism.

Masochism

Masochism is defined by Krafft-Ebing as an individual "being controlled by the idea of being completely and unconditionally subject to the will of another person, ... of being treated by this person as by a master, of being humiliated and abused." Some masochistic men punish themselves severely while masturbating. They may strangulate themselves by performing pseudo-hangings, or they may place occlusive devices, such as hoods or plastic bags, over the mouth and nose. Such practices have led to accidental death.

REFERENCES

Kaplan, J.S. (1974): *The New Sex Therapy: Active Treatment of Sexual Dysfunctions.* New York, Brunner/Mazel.

Kinsey, A.C., Pomeroy, W.B., Martin, C.E., et al. (1953): *Sexual Behavior in the Human Female.* Philadelphia, W. B. Saunders.

Masters, W.H. and Johnson, V.E. (1970): *Human Sexual Inadequacy.* Boston, Little, Brown.

Masters, W.H. and Johnson, V.E. (1976): Principles of the new sex therapy. *Am. J. Psychiatry. 133*:548.

Mohr, J.E., Turner, R.E., and Jerry, M.B. (1964): *Pedophilia and Exhibitionism.* Toronto, University of Toronto Press.

Wolpe, J. and Lazarus, A.A. (1966): *Behavior Therapy Techniques: A Guide to the Treatment of Neuroses.* Oxford, Pergamon Press.

Zeitlin, A.B., Cottrell, T.L. and Lloyd, F.A. (1957): Sexology of the paraplegic male. *Fertility and Sterility.* 8:337.

FURTHER READINGS

Freund, K., Langevin, R., Satterberg, J., et al. (1977): Extension of the gender identity scale for males. *Arch. Sex. Behav.* 6:507.

Hoenig, J. and Kenna, J.C. (1974): The nosological position of transsexualism. *Arch. Sex. Behav.* 3:273.

Krafft-Ebing, R. (1950): *Psychopathia Sexualis: A Medico-Forensic Study.* (Reprint of 1886 ed.) New York, Pioneer Pub.

26

Drug Use Disorders

Richard P. Swinson

Dependence on alcohol and other drugs was defined by a WHO Expert Committee (1969) to be "a state, psychic and sometimes physical, resulting from the interaction between a living organism and a drug, characterized by behavioral and other responses that always include a compulsion to take the drug on a continuous or periodic basis in order to experience its psychic effects and sometimes to avoid the discomfort of its absence."

This wordy definition was introduced in order to clarify the terminology in use since words such as abuse, addiction, and dependence, which do not mean the same thing, are sometimes used interchangeably.

Drug abuse is a phrase with very wide meaning covering any non-medical use of prescription drugs or the excess use of socially sanctioned drugs such as alcohol. Drug abuse is also commonly used in referring to LSD or cannabis usage where habituation and tolerance are not commonly encountered. Drug addiction is defined as a state of periodic or chronic intoxication produced by the repeated consumption of a drug. Its characteristics include:

1. An overpowering desire or need to continue taking the drug and to obtain it by any means.

2. A tendency to increase the dose, though some people may remain indefinitely on a stationary dose.

3. A psychological and physical dependence on the effects of the drug.

4. The appearance of a characteristic abstinence syndrome in a subject from whom the drug is withdrawn.

5. An effect detrimental to the individual and society.

Drug habituation is a condition resulting from the continued consumption of a drug. Its characteristics include:

1. A desire to continue taking the drug for the sense of improved well-being which it engenders.

2. Little or no tendency to increase the dose.

3. Some degree of psychological dependence on the effect of the drug but absence of physical dependence and hence of an abstinence syndrome.

4. Detrimental effects, if any, primarily on the individual himself (WHO, 1964).

Addiction has been thus defined as being largely physical and as involving tolerance to the drug consumed. Habituation has been seen as being totally psychological. The problem with this dichotomy is that the distinction between the two is far from clear in practice. While the favored term for drug related problems is "dependence of drug X type" it is still appropriate to use the term addiction when discussing drug problems involving a social and public health risk as well as a risk to the individual.

CLASSIFICATION OF MAJOR PSYCHOTROPIC DRUGS (From the Final Report of the LeDain Commission of Inquiry into the Nonmedical Use of Drugs, 1973).

The range of drugs which are abused is very wide, so wide that someone, somewhere has abused everything available in the pharmacological field and many apparently unlikely substances in addition. Eight main groups were delineated by the LeDain Commission:

1. Sedative-Hypnotics
   Alcohol
   Barbiturates
   Minor tranquillizers
   Others, e.g. methaqualone, methyprylon
2. Stimulants
   Amphetamine
   Amphetamine-like compounds, e.g. cocaine, diethylpropion, methylphenidate, phenmetrazine
   Others, e.g. caffeine, khat, nicotine
3. Psychedelic-hallucinogens
   Cannabinoids
   Datura-Belladonna alkaloids
   Indole tryptophan derivatives, e.g. DMT, LSD, psilocybin
   Phenethylamines, e.g. MDA, mescaline, PMA, STP
   Others, e.g. P.C.P.
4. Opiate narcotics
   Natural, e.g. codeine, morphine, opium
   Semi-synthetic, e.g. heroin, hydromorphone
   Synthetic, e.g. pethidine, methadone, propoxyphene

5. Volatile substances
   Active compounds, e.g. amylnitrite, ether, nitrous oxide
   Common substances, e.g. glue, paint thinner, gasoline
6. Non-narcotic analgesics
   Salicylates
   Para-aminophenol derivatives, e.g. acetaminophen, phenacetin
7. Antidepressants
   Monoamine oxidase inhibitors, e.g. phenelzine, tranylcypromine
   Tricyclics, e.g. Amitriptyline, Imipramine
8. Major tranquillizers
   Butyrophenones, e.g. haloperidol
   Phenothiazines, e.g. chlorpromazine
   Rauwolfia alkaloids, e.g. reserpine
   Thioxanthenes, e.g. chlorprothixene

The last two groups present little problem in terms of drug abuse and will not be considered further here.

DRUG ABUSE SYNDROMES

The areas of alcoholism and drug abuse exemplify the multifactorial etiology of may psychiatric disorders and the multidimensional approach necessary for successful therapy.

Etiology

The factors implicated in the etiology of substance abuse can be briefly summarised as follows: individual variables, social variables, and substance variables.

Individual Variables. Although multiple, these can be summarized under the headings of biological and psychological variables. In terms of biological factors there is evidence that the offspring of alcoholics are at much greater risk of developing alcoholism than are the offspring of nonalcoholics. This holds true even when the children of alcoholics are adopted out of the alcoholic family and reared in a nonalcoholic environment. It appears that alcoholism is, at least in male alcoholics, a partially genetically determined disorder. Further supporting evidence for this conclusion is available from the work of the familial nature of affective disorders, the likely genetic component involved, and the association of affective disorders with alcoholism. Similar evidence is not available at the present time for substances other than alcohol.

Psychological factors have been examined in exhaustive detail in these areas. Formulations have been derived in psychoanalytic terms which have stressed fixation at very early (oral) levels of development, and in learning theory terms which have concentrated on the anxiety reducing properties of many drugs. Psychometric surveys using the M.M.P.I. and other psychological tests have also been employed in searching for the "alcoholic" or "drug-abusing" personality.

It has not been shown to be possible to delineate such a personality structure, particularly when one looks in a *prospective* manner at people at risk. The search is basically an illogical task and should properly be abandoned. There are, however, some personality characteristics which occur commonly in alcoholics and drug abusers. The personality traits found tend to fall into two groups, the dysthymic, tense, depressed, anxious, inhibited type, or the psychopathic, angry, impulsive, antisocial type.

Social Variables. The factors classified under social variables occur at any level of social organization from the level of the immediate family to the national or even international level.

FAMILY. Children reared in a stable environment which provides for physical and psychological development tend to grow up into fairly healthy adults. Variations from this ideal lead, as evidenced throughout this book, to all manner of ills including substance abuse.

The most severe disruption of normal family functioning comes about by way of parental deprivation and thus it is not surprising to find that both alcoholics and drug abusers have commonly (up to 50%) suffered the loss of at least one parent during childhood. Prospective studies of the development of alcoholism have been carried out which have shown that the occurrence of dependency conflicts and role confusion in families tends to predict the onset of alcoholism in the sons of such families. Broadly the factors in the parents leading to dependency conflicts and role confusion were maternal ambivalence, escapism or sexual deviance and paternal antagonism or denigration of the mother by the father. Conflict with grandparents about child rearing was also a significant factor.

Obviously role models are of extreme importance to a developing child and behaviors displayed by the parents will be observed, learned, rehearsed covertly or overtly and, finally, exhibited as part of the child's repertoire. There is evidence that mothers who frequently take tablets have children who do the same. It is important, therefore, not to use medication indiscriminately to help deal with patients' complaints since this may influence the likelihood of the children of the patients taking tablets at times of stress.

PEER GROUP. As the child loosens some attachments with the core family, he becomes increasingly influenced by outsiders, commonly his own peer group. The core family experience determines to whom the child gravitates as he experiments with his freedom.

A peer group which values experimentation with alcohol and drugs may well attract and provide a focus for an adolescent who is feeling rejected by his family and unsure of his role. In some groups drug taking, or other behavior which is generally considered as socially undesirable, may be a requisite part of remaining in the group and of confirming an identity. When someone who is attached to such a group seeks help in order to cease drug taking it is usually necessary to separate the person from the group prior to rehabilitation or the chances of success become slim.

SOCIETY IN GENERAL. Societies regulate their members in many ways. Some of these are explicit in the form of legal sanctions, while others are implicit in terms of appropriate social class behaviors. Other regulations are in a state of flux, as with behaviors determined by gender. Alcoholism and drug abuse vary in prevalence and incidence from society to society and across groups within societies. Low rates are generally found in stable societies, strongly religious groups, societies where alcohol and drug taking has a largely ceremonial function and in middle socio-economic classes. Women in general drink less than men and so have about one quarter the incidence of problems with alcohol. There is some evidence that middle-aged women abuse prescribed medications more commonly than do men. Whether this is a substitute activity in the place of alcohol intake or whether it is due to the, largely male, medical profession over-prescribing psychoactive drugs to women is not clear. A combination of causes no doubt operates.

When one considers those forms of drug abuse which are seen as being very deviant, e.g. opiate abuse, then males outnumber females by a considerable margin.

Legal sanctions do have an effect on substance consumption although the effect may be transient. Prohibition of alcohol or heroin, as in the U.S.A., no doubt reduced the problems for a time but created many others in terms of criminalising the supply, consumption and possession of the prohibited substance. There is a complex relationship between criminal behavior and alcohol or drug abuse. Substance abusers are overrepresented among criminals, particularly recidivist populations, and conversely criminal acts are often entered into by substance abusers either to obtain funds to maintain their habit or as an example of generally deviant behavior.

Taxation laws have some place in determining the prevalence of alcoholism since alcohol consumption goes down as alcoholic beverages become more expensive.

Specific Syndromes

It is not possible in the confines of this section to consider in detail the ways in which alcoholism and drug dependence present and the way in which the syndromes develop. The interested reader is encouraged to read an article by the National Council on Alcoholism on the diagnosis of alcoholism, which gives considerable detail of the behavioral, psychological, social, and medical ways in which alcoholism may present. An account of alcoholism and drug dependence in general is available in Swinson and Eaves (1978).

Drugs of dependence, as all psychoactive agents, produce many specific effects which may present clinically. Primarily psychological changes can occur in the cognitive area which appear as lowering of consciousness, vagueness, loss of concentration, memory defects and disorientation, when depressant drugs such as alcohol and barbiturates are consumed. Affective changes can vary from deep depression with alcohol to excitement with amphetamines and anxiety with hallucinogenic agents or in delirium. Disorders of perception occur acutely with the hallucinogens and cannabis and chronically with alcohol, cocaine or amphetamine abuse.

Disorders of thought involving content, stream, possession and form of thought can occur if alcohol, cocaine or amphetamines are taken over long periods.

Behavioral changes tend to be widespread and may be alarming to the patient and to those involved with him. These range from such actions as hiding the supply of the drug to the acting out of some behavior suggested by hallucinatory voices.

Medical complications arise as a result of direct action of the drugs, e.g. liver damage, alcoholic cardiomyopathy, respiratory depression with opiates, or as a secondary phenomenon. These are legion and include sepsis from contaminated injections, peripheral neuropathy from malnutrition and physical injury from accidents.

DIAGNOSIS OF ALCOHOLISM

Feighner and his colleagues (1972) have selected a number of behavioral characteristics and symptoms from the wide range of symptoms which occur in alcoholism and divided them into the four groups below. The occurrence of symptoms in three of the four groups is sufficient for the diagnosis to be made.

Group 1
  Any manifestation of withdrawal—tremulousness, convulsions, hallucinations or delirium.
  History of medical complications.
  Alcoholic blackouts.
  Alcoholic binges of 48 hours or longer.
Group 2
  The inability to stop drinking despite the wish to stop.
  Self imposed restrictions on drinking.
  Drinking before breakfast.
  Drinking non-beverage alcohol.
Group 3
  Arrests for drinking.
  Traffic difficulties due to drinking.
  Work problems due to drinking.
  Fighting due to drinking.
Group 4
  Patient thinks he drinks too much.
  Family objects to the patient's drinking.
  Loss of friends because of drinking.
  Other people object to the patient's drinking.
  Guilt feelings about drinking.

Syndromes in association with alcoholism. The following syndromes are generally associated with alcoholism.

DRUNKENNESS. Though drunkenness is often fairly easy to diagnose, the diagnosis should not be made on the basis of a cursory examination. Head injuries and the ingestion of other substances may well complicate the picture. Hypoglycemia is an important differential diagnosis.

WITHDRAWAL EFFECTS. These are commonly experienced in the morning, after a previous day's drinking, in the form of "the shakes" which are both visible and felt by the patient in his stomach. The symptom is commonly relieved by further intake of alcohol.

If further alcohol is not available or if there is an intercurrent infection, usually pneumonia, then the withdrawal state is likely to progress to a more serious condition. The delirium of withdrawal may be heralded by a gradual lowering of consciousness or by the sudden onset of grand mal seizures. Fortunately the less dramatic onset is more common and consists of increasing anxiety, restlessness, disorientation, weakness, nausea, and insomnia. Hallucinations, or more frequently illusions, are common and may be terrifying in nature. Sedative, anticonvulsant medication such as Diazepam is required together with calm reassurance in a situation of moderate sensory input. Repeated orienting information is helpful. Since the seizure threshold is lowered during withdrawal, it is best to avoid the use of major tranquillizers, which have been shown to be epileptogenic.

DISORDERS OF MEMORY. Memory defects occur in alcoholism in a number of ways. Palimpsests are short, transient defects occurring at times of high blood alcohol levels. This symptom can occur in non-alcoholics but the repeated experience of "black outs" suggests that the person's alcohol intake is excessive. The Korsakoff syndrome commonly arises out of a withdrawal state. It is characterized by short term memory loss together with an acute or subacute organic brain dysfunction. Patients may then lie, often very convincingly, to fill in the gaps in their experience caused by memory loss. This lying is called confabulation. The basic defect consists of hemorrhagic lesions in the dorsomedial thalamic nuclei and the mammillary bodies associated with thiamine deficiency.

Wernicke's encephalopathy may be superimposed upon the above picture. Oculomotor dysfunctions and ataxia occur in conjunction with the dysmnesic syndrome.

An uncommon result of a period of delirium tremens is the onset of a twilight state in which consciousness is slightly lowered. This state may persist for weeks and be evident mainly at night in the form of disorientation, restlessness and illusions.

In chronic alcoholism dementia may develop with progressive failure of memory, and other cognitive and psychological functions. Although male alcoholics outnumber females with the disorder, there are in absolute numbers more females than males with brain disorders secondary to alcoholism.

OTHER PHYSICAL SYNDROMES. Space does not allow a review of all the physical effects of alcohol abuse. Suffice it to say that widespread effects are common and include gastric ulceration, liver damage, pancreatitis, cardiomyopathy, peripheral neuropathy, cerebellar degeneration, carcinoma of the upper gastrointestinal tract and bronchus. There is also evidence that alcohol can cause fetal damage.

PSYCHOLOGICAL EFFECTS. Alcohol in excess causes depression of mood and suicide is a common concomitant of alcoholism. Aggression against others may also be released by alcohol or other dysinhibitors such as minor tranquillizers.

Just as other physical disorders can arise out of delirium tremens so can psychological syndromes. The commonest of these is alcoholic hallucinosis. In this state the patient experiences the sudden onset of hallucinatory voices which are often threatening and so determine the patient's affect. Thought disorder does not occur. Occa-

sionally this state persists for years but it usually clears up in less than four weeks.

"Delusions of jealousy" or, more properly, delusions of infidelity occur in both sexes of alcoholics. They are more commonly reported in males who accuse their wives of repeated infidelity. They may go to extreme lengths looking for proof of their delusion. This state is frequently intractable even if the alcoholic stops drinking. The spouses of such people may be at risk and murder, although rare, does occur.

DIAGNOSIS OF DRUG DEPENDENCE

According to the criteria offered by Feighner et al. the occurrence of any one of the following is sufficient for the diagnosis of drug dependence: history of withdrawal symptoms; hospitalization for drug abuse or its complications; indiscriminate prolonged abuse of CNS active drugs.

Syndromes in association with drugs other than ethyl alcohol. Because of the confines of space only the more important syndromes will be described. It should be noted that drug dependent people commonly abuse more than one substance and very bizarre clinical pictures may occur.

SEDATIVE-HYPNOTICS. The barbiturates will be used to illustrate this group of drugs. The effects, side effects and dangers of barbiturates are so great that their use should be reserved only for the treatment of epilepsy and withdrawal effects. No conscientious doctor should consider them as part of his regular repertoire of drugs and certainly no repeat prescription of barbiturates need ever be issued.

The main danger to the barbiturate addict, apart from death by overdosage, lies in the withdrawal syndrome. After a honeymoon period of lightening consciousness the addict, unless treated, will enter into status epilepticus if the daily dose has been 1,000 mgm of amylobarbital, or equivalent. This is only five times the therapeutic dosage! There is a considerable mortality rate from this state.

In treating a barbiturate addict it is necessary to establish the patient on an initial dosage approximating his previous daily dose and then to reduce the dose by 10% per day. Another anticonvulsant, such as phenytoin, should be administered concurrently. Ideally EEG monitoring should be employed on a daily basis.

STIMULANTS. Amphetamines and cocaine have very similar actions and produce similar clinical pictures.

Acute administration of amphetamines produces a lessening of fatigue, increased wakefulness and may lead to a subjective feeling of confidence, security and enhanced ability. Although most subjects comment favorably upon the effects, some people experience increased tension, restlessness, inability to concentrate and difficulty in thinking.

The antidepressant and anorexiant properties for which amphetamines were prescribed in the past are very short lived, demonstrating how quickly tolerance develops to these substances.

Overdosage can cause acute excitement, restlessness and overactivity. Death is reported with sufficient dosage. The main syndrome of psychiatric interest is the onset of a delusional (paranoid) syndrome with the chronic intake of stimulants. This may be complicated by tactile hallucinations but thought form disorders do not occur. The psychosis responds to major tranquillizers.

PSYCHEDELIC-HALLUCINOGENS. Cannabis produces its actions by way of a group of chemicals known as tetrahydrocannabinoids (THC). Cannabis is absorbed from the respiratory tract on inhalation and 40–50% of the THC content of a marijuana cigarette can be absorbed in this manner.

The physical effects consist of increased heart rate, increase in blood pressure, dilation of the blood vessels of the conjunctiva and dilatation of the pupils. Occasionally vomiting and vertigo occur.

The psychological effects are complex and variable. People who have had little or no experience with the drug experience unpleasant emotions. A dreamy state with loss of reality follows. Distortions occur in the perception of time, space and body image. Depersonalization, illusions and hallucinations may also be experienced.

LSD effects are produced by minute amounts of the compound (50 to 100 micrograms) and have their onset about 15 minutes after oral consumption.

The physical effects consist of increase in muscle tension, headache, sweating, a rise in blood pressure and nausea. The psychological changes are widespread. The mood varies through the whole range of emotion and changes very rapidly.

Thought processes are disturbed in rate, form and content with the production of symptomatology very similar to that in schizophrenia. Visual perceptual disturbances are common. Objects appear to change in shape, size, color, shade or intensity.

In an acute drug-induced hallucinatory state it is important not to administer major tranquillizers. Many street drugs are contaminated by atropine and other substances and the addition of major tranquillizers can precipitate a life threatening atropine crisis. This can be reversed by physostigmine. Generally, if medication has to be given in this situation to calm someone then Diazepam is the safest. Long term effects are seen in the form of "flashbacks." These are hallucinatory episodes occurring spontaneously weeks or months after the last ingestion of a psychedelic drug. Other long term effects, such as the amotivational syndrome or brain damage due to cannabis, are still debatable.

OPIATE NARCOTICS. With this group of substances the withdrawal syndrome presents problems. The onset of the syndrome with heroin occurs within four or five hours. There is craving, anxiety, lachrymation and rhinorrhea. Insomnia, nausea, vomiting and diarrhea occur later and can lead to dehydration and collapse. Spontaneous erections and profuse menorrhagia can also occur. Treatment consists of drug replacement by methadone and then gradual withdrawal.

Psychotic states are not seen with these agents. The main problems, apart from withdrawal, are due to nonsterile injection technique, contaminated drugs, accidental overdosage, malnutrition, suicide, and murder. The risk of dying for a heroin addict is about 30 times as high as for a nonaddict of the same age.

VOLATILE SUBSTANCES. These rapidly acting substances cause acute intoxication. They may also cause death from cardiac arrhythmias. Other serious effects are hepatic and renal damage, brain damage and sometimes irreversible changes to the hemopoietic system.

Treatment of Alcoholism

The treatment of acute withdrawal has been discussed above. The long term treatment of alcoholism is usually intended to produce life long abstinence in the alcoholic. Some attempts have been reported to allow the alcoholic to return to social drinking but these are poorly researched and are often seized upon by alcoholics as excuses to resume drinking. These reports will not be considered here.

The first step in treatment is to dry out the patient. This may be done as an outpatient, or as an inpatient in a general hospital, general psychiatric unit or a special addiction unit. After withdrawing the patient from alcohol Antabuse (disulfiram) is frequently prescribed to prevent the patient from responding to his impulsive urges to drink. Disulfiram produces an unpleasant physical response of tightness in the chest, increased heart rate and flushing, if the patient drinks alcohol. It takes

three or four days of regular use of the drug to establish this effect, and as many days of non-use for the Antabuse-alcohol reaction to disappear. Patients should be carefully instructed in the use and possible side-effects of the drug.

Psychotherapy, individual or group, should continue for at least twelve months following the drying out phase. The alcoholic can also obtain help from attendance at Alcoholics Anonymous. Due to the effects of alcoholism on the family the spouse and children should also be involved in the treatment process. Such a treatment program is likely to produce abstinence at the end of the first year in 30 to 40% of patients.

Treatment of Drug Dependence

As in the treatment of alcoholism the first step is to withdraw the drug of dependence. The same process of long term psychotherapy is also indicated.

REFERENCES

National Council on Alcoholism. Criteria Committee (1972): Criteria for the diagnosis of alcoholism. *Ann. Int. Med.* 77:249.

Feighner, J.P., Robuis, E., Guze, S.B., et al. (1972): Diagnostic criteria for use in psychiatric research. *Arch. Gen. Psychiat.* 26:57.

Swinson, R.P. and Eaves, D. (1978): *Alcoholism and Addiction.* Plymouth, U.K., Macdonald & Evans.

FURTHER READINGS

Kalant, H. and Kalant, O.T. (1971): *Drugs, Society and Personal Choice.* Toronto, Paperjacks.
Introductory text in the field of drug dependence, which is written very clearly and succinctly. Information is presented without bias.

Kessel, N. and Walton, H. (1965): *Alcoholism.* London, Penguin.
This is a short readable book dealing with all aspects of alcoholism and is well suited for undergraduate reading.

CHAPTER 27

Organic Disorders (Intracerebral)

Alexander Bonkalo and Alistair Munro

This chapter deals with the intracerebral causes of organic brain disorder, and the following chapter deals with extracerebral causes. We should emphasize that this distinction is somewhat artificial, since the end-states are essentially the same, but we believe it is helpful to the reader to make the differentiation.

Organic mental disorders result from demonstrable physical disorders affecting the brain. The grossly organic origin of such mental disorders is proven by the presence of a significant time relationship between the mental disorder and the physical pathology, as well as by the parallelism in their longitudinal courses. An organic mental disorder may be the result of structural damage to the brain tissue, such as in senile dementia, or the result of abnormal functioning of the central nervous system that has occurred in response to a physical illness, such as in febrile delirium. The emerging psychiatric syndrome is determined largely by how the physical disorder is distributed anatomically in the brain, as well as by the rate of its progression, timing, and duration. In other words, the patient's psychiatric condition depends primarily on how disruptive the disorder is and only secondarily on its specific quality. Furthermore, the or-

ganic psychiatric syndrome is shaped by the person's characteristics, his differential vulnerability, his age, and his personality. Depending on the nature of the physical disorder, the organic mental disorder may be acute, subacute, or chronic, static or progressive, and completely or partly reversible or irreversible.

CLINICAL PRESENTATION

That a mental disorder is primarily intracerebral in origin may be assumed or suspected when a characteristic group of symptoms usually referred to as the organic psychiatric syndrome is present. The symptoms may include impairment of consciousness, thought, and attention; confusion; disorientation; memory disorder; and shallowness or inappropriateness and lability of affect. Also, the person may exhibit individual psychological symptoms that arise out of his personality. Those symptoms, which occasionally mask the organic mental disorder, may be stress responses to the illness or they may be release phenomena of hitherto inhibited or suppressed psychological mechanisms. Thus the person's mental state may be dominated by exaggerations of his premorbid personality traits, by neurotic responses, or even by outright psychotic symptoms, with depressive, paranoid, or schizophrenic manifestations.

Organic brain syndromes can be conveniently divided into: acute or subacute organic brain syndromes, which are primarily functional and are more or less transitory and reversible; and chronic organic brain syndromes, which are usually caused by diffuse or localized structural changes.

These conditions are irreversible although sometimes they can be arrested.

ACUTE ORGANIC BRAIN SYNDROME

The acute organic brain syndrome begins relatively suddenly and its manifestations are those of a widespread, temporary disturbance of brain function. The syndrome usually lasts for several hours or days, and the patient's condition improves as the underlying disorder improves; however, in some patients the disorder may progress to a more prolonged subacute stage that leads to dementia or even to death.

The causes of acute organic brain syndrome may be (1) a trauma (e.g. concussion) (2) an infection (e.g. encephalitis, meningitis, or brain abscess) (3) a metabolic disorder (e.g. a hepatic disorder, anoxia, or uremia) (4) a neoplastic disorder (5) endogenous toxins (6) a cerebrovascular disorder or (7) deficiency disorders.

The patient usually shows a greater or lesser degree of delirium. He often exhibits a wide disorganization of mental functioning, especially disorders of cognition. He is conscious, but his consciousness is more or less clouded and the degree of clouding may fluctuate rapidly. He may retain some contact with his environment, and at times he may even appear fully alert and rational. However, this contact may be tenuous, and he often has misperceptions and illusions. Some patients have marked ideas of reference and even delusions of persecution and they are sullen, suspicious, and perhaps aggressive. The patient

may have hallucinations, which may involve any of the senses, but visual, auditory and tactile hallucinations are the most common. The patient's reality testing is defective, and thus his insight into his disorder is faulty and his reactions are inappropriate. His memory is affected so that his registration of events is poor, and he has a patchy disturbance of recent and past memory. At times he may have almost total amnesia. He cannot concentrate, his perceptions are blunted, and his thinking is woolly or frankly incoherent. He is often garrulous, but his conversation is vague and he tends to confabulate to cover gaps in his knowledge and memory. When he talks, he will cling to concrete topics because his capacity for abstract thought is impaired. His mood is often inappropriate and labile, and he may swing suddenly from euphoria to depression, then back to euphoria. Often he has a sustained underlying state of anxiety that can suddenly escalate into panic, sometimes in response to delusions, misperceptions, or hallucinations. Some delirious patients lash out at imagined enemies or monsters, and they may be difficult to restrain. Motor and autonomic symptoms are prominent, aimless overactivity alternates with inertia and, despite his reduced level of consciousness, the patient often appears tense, restless, and overalert.

Differential Diagnosis

In the differential diagnosis of acute organic disorders, the following should be considered: acute neurotic reactions, either undifferentiated or in the form of an anxiety state or hysteria; affective disorders; schizophrenia; paranoid states; personality disorders (in acute organic mental syndromes, less desirable personality traits may be temporarily exaggerated).

The features of delirium that differentiate it from the conditions just listed are clouding of consciousness and widespread cognitive dysfunction. Acute onset, lack of predisposing psychological factors, and absence of a personal or a family history may be significant. The association with a demonstrable physical disorder, and, in some patients, with abnormal electroencephalographic findings should make the diagnosis of acute organic brain syndrome certain.

Treatment

An acute organic brain syndrome is managed by treating the underlying disorder. Therapy includes the use of general measures, such as adequate hydration, correction of any electrolyte imbalance, and reduction of elevated temperature. It is also necessary to treat any incidental infection, to insure normal bowel and bladder function, to relieve pain, and to provide for adequate sleep. When behavior disturbance is prominent, the patient may require sedation. Barbiturates should be avoided because their depressant action may accentuate the patient's confusion, and because, in hepatic disease and in some other disorders, barbiturates may be inadequately metabolized. Phenothiazines should be given cautiously because they reduce the epileptic seizure threshold and may precipitate a grand mal attack.

For minor degrees of restlessness, a benzodiazepine (such as diazepam or chlordiazepoxide) given orally is effective, but for more severe restlessness, haloperidol given orally or parenterally may be necessary. None of those drugs causes significant respiratory depression or hypotension when given in therapeutic dosages. Haloperidol has a slightly lesser effect on the seizure threshold than have the phenothiazines; diazepam, on the other hand, is an effective anticonvulsant. Other medications such as paraldehyde, may be effective. In all cases of delirium it is wise to give concentrated vitamin supplements, especially of the B groups. Formal anticonvulsant therapy is sometimes indicated.

Good nursing care and observation are essential. The patient should be cared for in a calm environment, and sensory deprivation should be avoided. Equally, glare should be avoided (because the patient may have photophobia) as should harsh shadows (because the patient may suffer from illusional misinterpretations). The patient should not be allowed to wander because he might get lost or accidentally harm himself. If he is kept under sedation, he seldom needs to be physically restrained.

SUBACUTE ORGANIC BRAIN SYNDROME

Korsakoff's syndrome (Korsakoff's psychosis) is the most commonly seen subacute organic disorder in psychiatric practice. Essentially an amnestic disorder, it is characterized by a disturbance of recent memory, disorientation in regard to time and place, and confabulation. The patient usually displays a bland euphoria and a lack of concern about his disability. Korsakoff's syndrome is mainly the result of a nutritional deficiency, especially of thiamine and niacin, and it is often the end result of chronic alcoholism, although it can also follow other toxic and degenerative brain conditions. Polyneuropathy frequently accompanies it, and in very severe cases, Korsakoff's syndrome may be part of the presentation of Wernicke's encephalopathy, in which there is also clouding of consciousness, ophthalmoplegia, and ataxia.

In a number of uncomplicated cases of Korsakoff's syndrome, an adequate diet, vitamin supplements, and abstinence from alcohol produce good results in six to eight weeks. Unfortunately, many other patients recover only partially or not at all, and they often need to be hospitalized permanently.

CHRONIC ORGANIC BRAIN SYNDROME

Chronic organic brain syndrome is usually brought about by damage to nerve cells. The damage may be diffuse, or it may involve (primarily or exclusively) localized cortical and subcortical areas. Nevertheless, in addition to the crucial nerve cell damage, which may be focal or diffuse, the patient usually has a secondary dysfunction that is caused by pressure, edema, or circulatory alterations, depending on the pathological nature of the primary lesion. The psychological abnormality that is caused by chronic diffuse nerve cell damage is usually dementia (i.e., a lasting, global, deterioration of mental abilities). The psychological abnormality that is caused by predominantly localized chronic brain damage is either a disorder of specific functions, as in dysphasia, or a disorder that affects mainly certain aspects of the personality, as in frontal or temporal lobe damage.

The most common forms of the chronic organic brain syndrome are the diffuse disorders that are brought about by aging or by degenerative diseases. The elderly brain invariably shows signs of atrophy, but in most old people, the rate of mental decline is in synchrony with the rate of decline of their other constitutional processes. In some people, however, the brain deteriorates prematurely, and they have a pathological disturbance of memory and of other intellectual and social functions to a degree that constitutes dementia.

The disease process may affect much of the brain rather diffusely and directly, as in senile dementia, or it may be predominantly the result of multiple focal damage caused by the narrowing and occlusion of cerebral blood vessels, as in cerebrovascular dementia. Dementia may be due to an identifiable specific disease process, such as syphilitic infection, other chronic forms of intracranial infection, or chronic vitamin deficiency: or it may be idiopathic, in which case heredity is often suspected to play a part. Dementia most commonly occurs in old people. When it occurs before the age of 60, it is known as presenile dementia.

Clinical Forms of Dementia

Senile Dementia. The clinical findings, particularly the increased rate of deterioration, suggest that senile dementia is a pathological form of aging rather than a normal one. However, there are no distinct morphological findings in the brain to support that clinical dichotomy. When the senile dementing process is gradually progressive, the person's consciousness is clear for a considerable time. The symptoms the patient develops are exaggerations of his premorbid personality traits, as well as exaggerations of the mental changes shown by old people who are aging normally. The dementing person's social activities diminish, he becomes fixed in a routine, and he may be stubborn, cantankerous, and childishly demanding. His memory, especially for recent events, becomes progressively poorer, and he increasingly dwells in the past. His attention span, perception, and problem-solving capacity decline. Some patients become avolitional and apathetic, while others become restless and wander. When they become disoriented in regard to time and place, the wandering may lead to their being lost. As their other faculties decline, potentially dangerous incidents may occur; for example, gas or water taps are left open or meals are burnt. They may lose their ability to recognize relatives and friends, mistaking them for people from their distant past.

The person's social skills decline. He becomes untidy, forgets to fasten his clothes, or wanders outside inappropriately dressed. His eating habits deteriorate. He neglects cleanliness, and sooner or later he becomes incontinent. Eventually, it becomes obvious that he is unable to look after himself. If his family cannot care for him, he must be admitted to an institution for long-term care. As his dementia progresses, his speech becomes less coherent, and it may degenerate into incomprehensible jargon (word salad). His physical condition becomes increasingly frail and he may have to be confined to a chair or to bed. Eventually the patient dies from an intercurrent illness.

The cause of senile dementia is not known, although there have been suggestions that it, and Alzheimer's pre-senile dementia, may be due to the abnormal accumulation of aluminum in the brain (perhaps the result of an enzyme defect), or to the effects of a slow virus. Characteristically, the whole brain atrophies, the typical neuropathological findings in the cerebrum are widespread neurofibrillary tangles and argentophil plaques.

Many people who have senile dementa exhibit a loss of insight at quite an early stage of the disease, and so they seem relatively unconcerned as their disorder becomes more serious. However, some patients are aware of their progressive decline, at least at the start, and they may have severe neurotic depressive, or paranoid, reactions to it. Many dementing old people react to stress with severe anxiety, and they may suddenly develop what has been termed by Goldstein, a "catastrophic reaction." This reaction ranges from embarrassment to acute and total behavioral disorganization engendered by panic and triggered by anticipated or actual failure. The reaction gradually resolves when the stress is removed.

Cerebrovascular Dementia. In cases of multiple focal brain damage, especially in cerebrovascular dementia, the disturbances of the person's intellectual functions are often much patchier than they are in senile dementia and there is often a neurological deficit. The patient may suffer repeated subclinical episodes of brain damage due to the blockage of small cerebral arteries; he may have minor strokes caused by larger occlusions; or he may have a massive cerebral thrombosis or hemorrhage. The clinical course of the dementia insult may be accompanied by an episode of confusion or even delirium.

Depending on what area of the brain is most affected, predominating psychologi-

cal defects may be seen. Frontal lobe damage particularly affects judgement, volition, and ethical sense; temporal lobe damage may cause severe memory disturbance; damage to the paleocerebrum and midbrain may cause profound emotional instability; parietal lobe damage may cause dyspraxia and visuo-spatial disorientation. Any of these may thus complicate the patient's psychological condition. Damage to certain cortical and subsortical areas can cause various forms of dysphasia and other selective high-level defects.

In cerebrovascular dementia, it is not uncommon for the patient to retain at least partial insight into his disorder for a considerable time. He often exhibits emotional lability and sudden episodes of dejection. Because he realizes that he is mentally and physically disabled and because he readily becomes depressed, it is not surprising that he often becomes suicidal. The patient's general feelings of unhappiness and frustration are likely to be even more acute when he has trouble communicating, as when he has dysphasia. Although the incidence of senile dementia increases with age and occurs most often in women 70 years of age and older, cerebrovascular dementia is more common in men than in women, and not infrequently begins before age 60. Cerebrovascular dementia is often preceded by hypertensive disease or with diseases associated with atherosclerosis, such as diabetes mellitus.

Differential Diagnosis of Dementia in Old Age

In the early stage of any type of dementia, diagnosis may be difficult. Psychological testing is often of no help in old people, since even normal old people may perform poorly in certain aspects of the tests. However, some specially designed tests can help demonstrate neuropsychological deficits that may be related to coexisting abnormal physical findings.

Senile depressive illness is the most important condition to differentiate from senile dementia. A common disorder, senile depressive illness may mimic dementia, and it can even be associated with the early stages of a dementing illness. It is a condition that can be cured or at least improved and it should never be overlooked.

Other conditions that must be considered in the differential diagnosis are: involutional paraphrenia; delirium due to an underlying physical disorder; a neurotic reaction. Neurotic reactions, often thought to be restricted to younger people, are not uncommon in old people; intoxication due to the abuse of alcohol or drugs, the latter usually medically prescribed; intracranial tumor.

Treatment

Specific therapy is given when a treatable cause of the dementing illness is identified. Some patients who have been treated seem to recover almost completely, but the amount of their reserve cerebral function is usually significantly and permanently reduced. The reduction may show subtly, for example, in the person's reduced competence at work, impaired judgement, deterioration in his relationships with others, or an exaggerated response to stress. Of course, he may also have a permanent neurological dysfunction.

When the patient who has a progressive dementia becomes delirious, the treatment for delirium is instituted. In cerebrovascular dementia, the person who has episodes of confusion often has severe emotional lability. Such a person may be suicidal, and he should be put under special observation.

The only treatment for dementia is palliative care, making sure that the patient's physical health is maintained at its best possible level and that injuries are avoided. Unfortunately, there is a tendency to regard the dementing patient as a product of unavoidable deterioration and to ignore his remaining human needs. Kindness, attention, and a gently stimulating environment may encourage him to use what is left of his diminishing faculties and to retain some measure of dignity.

Specific Presenile Dementias

Alzheimer's disease. This is a progressive, diffuse cerebral degeneration that is identical clinically and pathologically to senile dementia except that it begins in middle life. Its cause is not known; heredity, abnormal aluminum accumulation, or the effects of a slow virus, may be factors. The disorder progresses to helplessness and death; its course may be from one to ten years. There is only palliative treatment.

Pick's disease. Much rarer than Alzheimer's disease, Pick's disease is sometimes familial. The cerebral atrophy shows a marked tendency to affect the frontal and temporal lobes, and in the early stages, personality and memory changes are prominent, and moral and social deterioration may be particularly conspicuous. As the atrophy spreads, the course becomes similar to that of Alzheimer's disease. There is no specific treatment.

Huntington's chorea. This disease usually appears when the person is in his 30's or 40's. The disease is characterized by involuntary choreic or athetoid movements and progressive dementia. It is transmitted by an autosomal dominant gene, and so, on the average, 50% of the person's children also develop the condition. Certain portions of the cortex and of the basal ganglia (especially the caudate nucleus), are severely involved, but the disease often progresses slowly. There is no treatment but genetic counseling may be necessary when a family is known to be affected. Research on the cause is being directed toward discovering a detectable genetic marker, but as yet with no success.

POST-TRAUMATIC DISORDER

When a person has had a severe accident, his general psychological reaction to it may be characterized by severe anxiety and its autonomic accompaniments, unpleasant dreams, and a phobic fear of situations that remind him of the accident. The reaction clears gradually, but sometimes the phobic fear must be dispelled by graded desensitization. At other times, the neurosis becomes chronic, and whether that happens seems to be determined by the patient's pre-accident personality. A chronic disorder seems more likely to appear if litigation or compensation is involved. So-called compensation neurosis often fails to improve until the litigation has finally come to an end, and often not even then. In many cases, the patient's dependency needs, aggressive drive, and other subconscious or conscious factors (rather than actual financial considerations) precipitate or reinforce the neurosis. The treatment should be tailored to the person but the outcome is often disappointing.

Sometimes the patient who has had serious brain damage as the result of an accident may have additional symptoms when he recovers. For example, his thought processes may be slowed, and he may be markedly obsessive in his thinking and behavior. His mood may be labile, but he often settles into a subacute depression, in which he is perpetually unhappy and dissatisfied. He tends to withdraw from society and to be irritable, sometimes even explosive, toward others. He may complain of persistent headaches, giddiness, and poor concentration. His insight may be relatively intact, and when he has some deterioration of intellect or a reduction in his psychic drive, his awareness of the difference between his former and his present self adds to his frustration and unhappiness. Epilepsy and the side-effects of anticonvulsant therapy may complicate his condition.

People with severe brain damage are often difficult to cope with; their constant complaining alienates others and their obsessive inflexibility defeats most attempts to help them reorganize their lives. However, they do need support and reassurance and some patients respond remarkably (if slowly) to prolonged encouragement. They should be helped to adjust their aspirations to their reduced capabilities. An actual depressive illness should not be overlooked; considerable improvement sometimes results from the administration of a tricyclic antidepressant. However, since the tricyclics tend to lower the epileptic seizure threshold, anticonsulsant therapy should also be provided.

CEREBRAL TUMORS

Most intracranial tumors have some psychological manifestations. However, most tumors affecting the brain manifest themselves at an early stage by producing symptoms arising from increased intracranial pressure, by triggering epileptic seizures, or by causing gross neurological signs and symptoms. Nevertheless, certain intracranial tumors have special psychiatric significance since they develop in areas that are relatively "silent" neurologically. Foremost in that category are frontal lobe and temporal lobe meningiomas and other pathological formations that compress or damage brain tissue locally rather than infiltrate it diffusely (e.g., scar tissue or cysts).

Localized frontal lobe lesions produce intellectual, affective, and vegetative disorders associated with changes in the personality as a whole. As in any early dementing process, the initial manifestations are exaggerations of the person's previous personality traits. Then the person's intellectual, affective, and social impairments become evident. He neglects his duties, and he loses his initiative, drive, and ability to organize his activities. His personal habits and his concern for others deteriorates. He becomes emotionally labile and irritable. Aimless overactivity, euphoria, talkativeness, and facetiousness may develop in some, whereas others may sink into a silent, neglectful, careless inactivity. The patient over-eats, loses his sexual inhibitions and sometimes becomes incontinent. Because the manifestations of frontal lobe lesions are predominantly psychological, the diagnosis may be difficult. The patient's intellectual and social deterioration, particularly if he is old, may be interpreted as a diffuse, degenerative dementing process. Thus a frontal lobe tumor may remain undetected in its early phase, when an operation could cure the patient.

On the psychological level, a temporal lobe disorder may lead primarily to poor control of affective functions and to aggressiveness. Thus a temporal lobe lesion may manifest itself by emotionally unstable, irritable, explosive behavior, with aggressive, destructive, or even violent attacks. The presence of olfactory and gustatory hallucinations and psychomotor-type epileptic seizures, however, is an important differential diagnostic clue. Nevertheless, it should be kept in mind that neurologically silent frontal lobe and temporal lobe lesions may remain undetected. Moreover, the findings on routine neurological, electroencephalographic, and radiological tests may be normal initially. Thus special tests, follow-up examinations, and retests may be necessary to detect those conditions, which are eminently curable.

FURTHER READINGS

Arie, T. (1973): Dementia in the elderly: diagnosis and management. *Brit. Med. J.* 4:540.
A good, brief account of the psychiatric aspects of dementia in old people and of its management.

Benson, D.F., and Blume, R.D. (1975): *Psychiatric Aspects of Neurologic Disease.* New York, Grune and Stratton.
A collection of monographs on a variety of organic brain syndromes and related problems.

Braceland, F.J. et al. (1977): Geriatrics. In *The Year Book of Psychiatry and Applied Mental Health.* Chicago, Year Book Medical Publishers.
This is an up-to-date, brief review of geriatric psychiatry from the U.S. viewpoint: easily readable.

Katzman, R., Terry, R.D., and Bick, K.L. (1978): *Alzheimer's Disease: Senile Dementia and Related Disorders.* New York, Raven Press.

Kolb, L.C. (1977): *Modern Clinical Psychiatry.* 9th ed. Philadelphia, W. B. Saunders.
A fairly massive account of the various organic brain syndromes, each described in a separate article.

Leading Article (1978): Dementia—The quiet epidemic. *Br. Med. J.* 1:1.
A very informative short article about the epidemiology of old-age dementia.

Lishman, W.A. (1978): *Organic Psychiatry: The Psychological Consequences of Cerebral Disorder.* Oxford, Blackwell.

Sim, M. (1974): Organic psychiatry. In *Guide to Psychiatry.* 3rd ed. Edinburgh, Churchill Livingstone.
Another massive account of the organic brain disorders, written from the British viewpoint by a man who has been involved in original research in this field.

Slater, E. and Roth, M. (1969): *Clinical Psychiatry.* London, Bailliere, Tindall and Cassell.
Known also as "Mayer-Gross' Clinical Psychiatry", the textbook contains fairly detailed chapters on various organic brain syndromes, integrating British and Continental approaches.

Wells, C.E. (1978): Chronic brain disease: an overview. *Am. J. Psychiatry.* 135:1–12.
An excellent review article on dementias, very readable.

28
Organic Disorders (Extracerebral)
Alistair Munro

A basically normal brain may be adversely affected by harmful influences arising elsewhere in the body. Interference with the brain's normal activity sooner or later causes psychological effects: at times these psychological symptoms may be only one aspect of a wide disorder of body and mind, but on other occasions the psychological disturbance may be the main, and virtually the only, presenting complaint. If cerebral function was already impaired to some degree prior to the onset of the harmful influence, psychological and behavioral ill-effects are all the more likely to manifest themselves. For example, the individual with established cerebral atherosclerosis is liable to develop the mental complications of severe metabolic disease at a much earlier stage than the patient with an intact blood-supply to the brain.

Depending on the nature of the harmful influence, its degree of severity, and the length of time it has been present, cerebral function may be differentially affected. The effects may be temporary and reversible, or may be permanent and irremediable. Symptoms can vary from mild slowing of thought processes to extreme intellectual malfunctioning, from slight confusion and minimal clouding of consciousness to stupor and coma. The pathological process can be gradual, as in many metabolic or endocrine disorders, or catastrophically rapid, as in severe carbon monoxide poisoning.

In general, the symptomatology in the earlier stages of such disease will resemble that of delirium (see Ch. 27), but if the condition is of longstanding, actual dementia may occur. In some of these cases of dementia, appropriate treatment of the underlying disorder can produce a surprising degree of intellectual recovery, although the brain may remain vulnerable to some extent. This type of recovery is strikingly seen in some patients with hypothyroidism who respond to thyroid treatment.

The brains of the very young and of the elderly are more readily affected by exogenous disease than those at other ages. Thus, a relatively minor systemic illness associated with fever, or a small shift in electrolyte balance, may precipitate confusion and disorientation in young and old individuals. In addition, the brains of children and adolescents are vulnerable to toxic or deficiency disorders produced by genetic abnormalities and in some cases this can lead to fatal dementia. For example, this may be seen in conditions like galactosemia, Tay-Sachs disease, and phenylketonuria.

A multitude of noxious, exogenous factors are capable of inducing malfunction in the adult brain. These are broadly categorized under the following headings: temperature change—pyrexia, or less commonly, hypothermia; anoxia; intoxications—endocrine overactivity, metabolic, drug-induced (including self-administered and prescribed drugs); deficiency disorders—vitamin deficiency, endocrine hypo-activity, mineral disturbances; sleep and sensory deprivation.

The aforementioned categories are not mutually exclusive. Anoxic effects may occur in an endocrine deficiency such as myxedema, or from an intoxication which produces respiratory depression, such as barbiturate poisoning. It can equally arise as a result of cardiac failure secondary to beri-beri.

Let us consider each category in more detail. Since the treatment of the abnormal mental status in every case is that of the underlying disorder, the emphasis is rather on the descriptive and diagnostic features of the various organic brain diseases.

TEMPERATURE CHANGE

As already noted, pyrexia is most likely to evoke mental complications in the very young and the very old, though no age group is totally immune. A high temperature may produce the classic symptoms of delirium, such as restlessness, confusion, clouding of consciousness, labile affect and, possibly, delusions and hallucinations. It may also induce convulsions, and this often adds to the patient's confusion but occasionally temporarily improves it, apparently in a way analogous to electroconvulsive therapy's effects. If the pyrexia is not relieved, fluid and electrolyte imbalance occur, with further deepening of the delirium. When the temperature returns to normal, the mental status usually follows suit, but in some cases a low-

grade, mild confusional state with disorientation and memory disturbance may persist for a time. This requires careful observation, treatment with a phenothiazine or haloperidol, and very occasionally, electroconvulsive therapy.

At the other extreme is hypothermia, seen in hypothyroidism, in elderly people who are too poor or too feeble to heat their houses adequately in winter, in the undernourished (including some patients with anorexia nervosa) and in chronic alcoholics whose peripheral vascular dilation encourages excessive heat loss. The hypothermic person's mentation is slow and there is often an element of confusion. Psychomotor activity is retarded and the overall picture may suggest a diagnosis of dementia. When the true diagnosis is made, the cause of the hypothermia must be treated, but especially in endocrine cases, one must be careful not to raise the temperature too rapidly; otherwise the sudden increase in cerebral metabolism may outstrip the brain's nutritional resources, leading to the danger of permanent damage.

ANOXIA

The brain is extraordinarily sensitive to changes in the supply of oxygen carried to it by the blood. Reduction of the supply can occur in various ways. For example, carbon monoxide competes with oxygen for hemoglobin transport; respiratory failure may reduce the absolute amount of oxygen absorbed through the lungs; blood supply may temporarily fail, as in acute syncope, or more permanently, as in cardiac failure or with occlusion of a cerebral blood vessel. In addition, if the brain cannot utilize oxygen adequately for a chemical reason, as in hypoglycemia, effective anoxia results.

Acute anoxia of sufficient degree causes faintness, then collapse and unconsciousness, leading rapidly to death if not remedied. Less severe oxygen-lack produces confusion, slowness of thinking and loss of judgement. Attention span and problem-solving capacity are seriously impaired, headache and nausea are common, and the individual feels restless and very apprehensive. Compensatory hyperventilation occurs in an attempt to increase the oxygen-intake. If this is not successful, symptoms of delirium are gradually overtaken by increasing drowsiness and, ultimately, coma. By this time, damage to brain cells is likely and the degree of recovery is always doubtful. If the underlying condition can be treated before death occurs, recovery may be only partial. Then the patient is often found to have both neurological and psychological deficits, the latter often resembling Korsakov's psychosis.

INTOXICATIONS

Endocrine Overactivity

A number of syndromes of endocrine hyperactivity are accompanied by psychological side-effects.

Hyperthyroidism. Many of the symptoms of thyrotoxicosis are very similar to those of anxiety neurosis. The patient is tense, restless, overactive and irritable, complains of fatigue, palpitations, and tremor, and often has insomnia (N.B. When asleep, a sleeping pulse rate may be diagnostically helpful: it tends to drop in anxious individuals but to remain high in thyrotoxicosis). Occasionally the patient's hyperactivity and emotional lability will escalate into manic-type behavior, often admixed with confusional elements. This can be highly dangerous as the patient may develop acute cardiac failure as a result of over-exertion and electrolyte disturbance acting on an irritable myocardium. Severe, untreated thyroid overactivity infrequently leads to a profound delirium in which collapse and death are an ever present danger.

Adrenal overactivity. Excessive glucocorticoids, either endogenous or as the result of medical administration, may cause restlessness and overactivity with insomnia. Euphoria is not uncommon, but this may give way to marked depression (possibly in predisposed individuals) and, on occasion, paranoid states which are often associated with confusion and some clouding of consciousness.

Pheochromocytoma. This tumor may produce symptoms which are mistaken for acute panic attacks. These are usually accompanied by paroxysmal headache, pallor and sweating and, of course, there is severe hypertension during the episodes.

Hyperparathyroidism. The hypercalcemia consequent on this disorder may be associated with lassitude, irritability, and anxiety. In a few patients there is marked depression and/or paranoia, and confusional states sometime occur.

Pituitary overactivity. When this occurs, the effects of stimulation of the thyroid, adrenals, etc., may be the most prominent manifestations. However, since the disorder is often the result of an anterior pituitary tumor, there may also be headache, irritability, depression, confusion or even apparent dementia. If there are pressure effects on the hypothalamus, additional phenomena can also appear, such as severe appetite disturbance, resulting in either cachexia or obesity, emotional outbursts of a bizarre nature, and various types of sleep disturbance.

Metabolic Disorders

Diabetic ketosis. An untreated diabetic experiences fatigue and lassitude for a time, but otherwise has no notable mental symptoms. However, as the ketosis worsens, he may develop confusional symptoms which can progress rapidly to stupor. These are due to a combination of the hyperglycemia and of electrolyte disturbance secondary to polyuria. Chronic diabetics are much more liable to dementia than normals (Bale, 1973).

Uremic encephalopathy. In severe renal failure, increasing confusion is seen, often associated with marked apathy, and memory and orientation are abnormal. Muscle-twitching and hiccoughs are common, and these cause much discomfort and a good deal of insomnia, both of which lead to additional confusion. Convulsions are not uncommon in the terminal stages, and further add to the symptoms of delirium. Incidentally, it should be noted that some patients on long-term renal dialysis show evidence of some degree of dementia (Sullivan et al., 1977).

Hepatic encephalopathy. A rise in the blood-level of nitrogenous substances as a result of hepatic failure leads to toxic disturbances in consciousness, with disorientation and restlessness. Gross EEG changes are frequently present and the patient shows a variety of behavioral and neurological abnormalities: the classical sign of flapping tremor may occur. The individual is agitated and may be aggressive. If he is a chronic alcoholic, there may already be potential brain dysfunction, accentuated by the liver-disease, and Korsakov's syndrome may be seen.

Acute intermittent porphyria. This condition can produce Raynaud's phenomenon, peripheral neuropathy and encephalopathy, the last-named being usually episodic. The disorder is the result of an autosomal recessive genetic defect and affects women more than men. Attacks may be precipitated by drugs, especially barbiturates, and during the active phase the urine turns a reddish-purple color if allowed to stand. Between attacks, excessive amounts of porphobilinogen G and delta-aminolevulinic acid may be present in the urine.

In the course of an attack, patients feel wretched and often have severe abdominal pain. In the early stages of their illness they are at risk of having an unnecessary appendectomy. Later they get a reputation for frequent whining and complaining and may be labelled as neurotic (and sometimes given barbiturates to "help" them!). During severe attacks, some patients evince delirious symptoms, and convulsions and unconsciousness can result.

Systemic lupus erythematosus (SLE). A wide spectrum of symptoms can occur with this serious disease. There may be direct effects of the disease process on the brain, or secondary effects due to pathology in other organs, such as the liver. In addition, in some cases, medications such as steroids may play a part in accentuating mental abnormalities. Some patients become markedly anxious and mood-labile. Some develop apparent depressive or schizophrenic-like syndromes, while others become delirious, often to a subacute degree. Occasionally, in severe and unremitting cases, dementia of a progressive type is seen (Bennet et al., 1972).

Drug Intoxications

Alcohol. This is the commonest intoxicant in our society and its unpleasant side-effects, if not too severe, are unfortunately hallowed to some extent by ancient custom. Alcoholism is discussed elsewhere (see Ch. 26) and only the toxic effects of ethyl alcohol are considered here. It is a central nervous system depressant, although in low blood-concentration its disinhibitory effect gives a spurious appearance of stimulation. As blood-levels increase, the individual shows loosening of thinking and impairment of concentration, insight and judgement. Thereafter, motor coordination becomes clumsy, emotional control is reduced, confusion appears and stupor and unconsciousness supervene.

In chronic alcoholics, a variety of accompanying physical disorders are likely, including peripheral neuropathy and a degree of brain-damage. These people are liable to develop delirium tremens, withdrawal seizures, Korsakov's psychosis and Wernicke's encephalopathy. As well as this, alcoholics develop cross-tolerance with certain drugs, especially barbiturates.

As a consequence, when sober, they can tolerate high dosages of these drugs, but when intoxicated with alcohol, the combined effects of the two substances may be highly dangerous, rapidly inducing coma.

In the late stages of chronic alcoholism, some individuals develop specific disorders such as alcoholic hallucinosis or pathological jealousy. At first these may depend on a degree of intoxication, but ultimately they can become independent of alcohol intake and occur in full consciousness. Their prognosis tends to be very poor.

Sedative drugs. These include hypnotics and minor tranquillizers. With all of these substances, central nervous system function is depressed to some degree. The barbiturates, which include sedatives and hypnotics, were at one time the most effective drugs available for treating insomnia and anxiety. They remain good anticonvulsants but most of their other therapeutic uses have been superseded by better and safer medications, and they have a bad record for habituation and abuse. Unfortunately, barbiturates are still prescribed far too often.

Acute intoxication causes drowsiness, coma, respiratory depression, and death, if untreated. Chronic overdosage leads to depressive symptoms, lethargy and inefficiency, and later to confusion and disorientation. Sometimes anxiety is a symptom and, not unnaturally, the patient tries to combat this with more barbiturates. Particularly in old people, paradoxical restlessness associated with confusion can occur, and this may result in abnormal, disinhibited behavior which is easily mistaken for dementia. At all ages, sudden withdrawal from barbiturates can cause severe physical symptoms, sometimes with convulsions, and delirium may appear a short time later.

Methaqualone is highly habituating, may produce severe confusion at times, and can cause convulsions. Overdoses are extremely dangerous because of respiratory depression. Despite its effectiveness as a hypnotic it should rarely, if ever, be prescribed. Glutethimide, too, has been described as causing seizures, but usually only following an overdose.

Of the minor tranquillizers, meprobamate is potentially addictive and several of the benzodiazepines have been reported to cause habituation. Although these drugs are remarkably safe to use in treating the symptoms of anxiety, toxic effects can certainly occur, particularly if patients are taking unwarrantedly high amounts. Especially in the elderly, benzodiazepines can precipitate depressive symptoms and confusion. Occasionally, restlessness and anger are manifested with normal dose levels, and, in some people, these medications accentuate insomnia.

Psychotropic drugs and antidepressants. Some patients receiving major tranquillizers become excessively drowsy and, occasionally, confusional states can occur. However, be aware that restlessness and confusion may be the result of concomitant administration of anti-parkinsonian drugs. Depressive symptoms are not uncommon, and may be dose-related. Phenothiazines are known to reduce the seizure threshold in a small proportion of patients.

Tricyclic antidepressants very occasionally cause convulsions, while some patients develop an unpleasant sensation of muscle-tension and subjective anxiety. Individuals in a depressive phase of bipolar affective disorder may be precipitated into mania, and some elderly patients have been reported to develop delirious states.

Opiates. These are invaluable for the treatment of severe pain but have a terrible record of addictiveness. A physically fit, nonhabituated person who takes morphine often reports that the mood-change it induces is somewhat unpleasant and that there is a subjective feeling of clouding of consciousness. On the other hand, the habituated individual usually experiences euphoria, the sensorium remains clear and there may be a good deal of temporary energy, although volition is reduced. A "fix," particularly intravenously, may cause orgasmic sensations but actual sexual activity is usually reduced. In many established addicts, somnolence and lack of directive activity become prominent. Sometimes, particularly if the sample of morphine happens to be pure and of high potency, the individual may receive a truly toxic dose and become confused, disoriented and stuporous. A potential combination thereafter of vomiting and respiratory depression is highly dangerous. In addition to direct effects of opiates on the brain, addicts are very liable to hepatic disease as the result of viral hepatitis and this, if severe, may have its own marked effect on mental functioning.

Stimulants. Amphetamines and related substances (including methylphenidate) nowadays have very narrow therapeutic indications (viz. hyperkinesis, narcolepsy) and probably have no real value in the treatment of obesity. They are apt to induce marked tolerance and are much abused on account of their euphoriant action. Taken for a short period and then stopped, they may cause a combination of depressive symptoms and lethargy. Taken in acute overdosage they can precipitate a confusional state with manic features. In some possibly predisposed individuals taking large amounts habitually, they evoke a psychotic disorder very similar to paranoid schizophrenia, associated with severe persecutory anxiety, excessive autonomic activity and, at times, an element of confusion. In the withdrawal state from this psychosis, the patient may become suicidal. Most patients recover when they stop taking the amphetamine but a proportion remains permanently psychotic.

Hallucinogens. These drugs profoundly alter sensory perceptions and produce hallucinations, with associated feelings ranging from euphoria to panic. On a "good trip" the individual feels capable of anything, including, tragically at times, the ability to fly. On a "bad trip," the experience is profoundly frightening and may result in persisting severe anxiety and, at times, paranoid symptoms. Frequent use may result in an amotivational state, and, in some cases, this may be associated with schizophrenia-like symptoms which can be permanent. Some individuals experience the "flashback" phenomenon in which, months after the ingestion of the hallucinogen and for no apparent reason, they spontaneously undergo a "trip" with all its attending sensations.

Cocaine. This drug experiences intermittent vogues, often in sections of high society. It produces euphoria and supreme self-confidence, but the effect is short-lived. Tolerance is built up, although some people seem relatively immune to addiction or ill-effects. It is a pernicious substance; acute overdosage can lead to confusional excitement and hyperpyrexia. Chronic abuse often causes physical debilitation and an accompanying low-grade psychosis with hallucinations in which "formication" (a sensation of ants crawling under the skin) is typical.

Cannabis (Marijuana). Cannabis can be smoked or eaten. Users claim that it induces relaxation, and detaches them pleasurably from their surroundings. Cannabis only occasionally causes hallucinations and rarely produces severe dependence. Some people get no pleasant response, and may even experience unpleasant anxiety to the point of acute panic. Most users find it sedative in effect, and heavy, chronic use seems capable of causing a lasting amotivational state. It has been claimed that it may precipitate severe neuroses or even schizophrenia; it is equally possible that individuals who already have these disorders become heavy users of the drug for its tranquillizing properties. There are many advocates for the legalized use of cannabis; however it is certainly not harmless and there have been reports that it can cause acute delirium or chronic toxic psychosis, sometimes with a paranoid coloring.

Bromide. This is an old-fashioned sedative which should no longer be used because of its liability to cause toxicity. It acts largely by displacing other halogen radicals from body fluids and it can insidiously build up a toxic state which, in its early stages, resembles a chronic neurotic disorder, with irritability, emotional lability, and lethargy. Later, it may mimic severe depressive illness and ultimately can produce a picture very similar to that of dementia. The possibility of bromism is often overlooked nowadays, and occasionally a serum bromide may prevent one from labelling a mysterious case of confusion or possible dementia as untreatable.

Other medications. Certain medical drugs have a marked tendency to produce untoward psychological effects. The following are a few of the most frequent offenders, with their principal mental side-effects:

L-Dihydroxyphenylalanine (L-Dopa) causes psychiatric side-effects in about one-third of Parkinsonian patients, including confusion, delirium, suicidal depression and, occasionally, mania.

Digitalis has been known to produce restlessness and apathy, which sometimes develops into full-blown delirium.

Antihypertensive agents, especially thiocyanates and reserpine, can cause confusion, depression, severe anergia and, occasionally, suicidal behavior.

Anticonvulsants may induce drowsiness and slowness in mentation. With prolonged usage, confusional or paranoid symptoms can develop: if relatively mild, these may be interpreted as evidence of chronic personality disorder.

Female hormones can produce depression and marked tension symptoms, mostly in women who already have neurotic personalities. Nowadays, all women with psychiatric symptomatology should routinely be asked if they are on an oral contraceptive.

Antipyretics (aspirin) in high dosage cause restlessness, excitement, confusion, tinnitus and even auditory hallucinations. Phenylbutazone has been reported as causing delirium and convulsions. Indomethazone frequently causes headache, less frequently depression, and, occasionally, delirium with hallucinations.

Some antibiotics, including occasionally penicillin, can precipitate toxic states, and sulphonamides not infrequently cause depressions. Isoniazid and cycloserine have been noted to reactivate mental symptoms in schizophrenics.

Lithium can cause an acute toxic state if given in too high dosage. This is often accompanied by agitation, altered consciousness and a variety of neurological signs and symptoms.

Gases. Carbon dioxide in excess produces headache, restlessness, giddiness, confusion and delirium. If inhaled chronically in small amount, it may cause a picture of mixed affective disorder, with both excitement and depression.

Carbon monoxide produces symptoms of anoxia. If intoxication has been severe, the patient may recover consciousness but demonstrate evidence of severe dementia and neurological damage. A Korsakov-like picture is not uncommon as a sequel.

Oxygen intoxication in the adult can result in irritability, depression, confusion and, eventually, loss of consciousness.

Hyperventilation is a common symptom in anxious individuals and habitually agitated people may hyperventilate chronically. Biochemically this results in a relative alkalosis and this may evoke tetany. The patient has the objective and subjective symptoms of anxiety, all of which are accentuated by the overbreathing. In particular, he experiences palpitations, lightheadedness, blurring of vision, paresthesias, bowel and bladder urgency and, possibily, syncope. The marked symptomatology often convinces the patient that he is seriously ill, physically or mentally, and a vicious circle of cause-and-effect is set up which may be very difficult to interrupt.

Heavy metals. Intoxication with these may result from occupational hazards or from environmental pollution. Lead intoxication may cause encephalopathy with irritability, headache, restlessness and insomnia, associated with a variety of neurological abnormalities. Confusion and delirium ensue and, if untreated, can lead to coma and death. Mercury intoxication causes widespread physical effects, and the most frequent mental symptoms are lethargy and/or excitement, with confusion. As a matter of interest, mercury was widely used in the hat-industry until the 19th century to produce the right type of "nap," or surface appearance. Poisoning was common among hat-workers, hence the phrase, "Mad as a Hatter" and "Mad-Hatter syndrome."

DEFICIENCY DISORDERS

Vitamin Deficiencies

Patients with scurvy due to vitamin C deficiency have severe pain due to hemarthroses, are irritable and often have marked depressive symptoms. In elderly people with nutritional scurvy, the physical inanition plus the distress and misery cause a degree of social withdrawal which may be mistaken for dementia.

Deficiencies of the vitamin B group are often multiple. Beri-beri, which is predominantly due to vitamin B1 deficiency, is associated with peripheral neuropathy and cardiac insufficiency. The patient is lethargic and apathetic, but also irritable and depressed. Anoxia due to cardiac failure may complicate the psychiatric picture and, if, in addition, there are brain changes due to, for example, chronic alcoholism, these may manifest in the ways described elsewhere.

Pellagra, largely due to lack of nicotinic acid, can cause headache, apathy, insomnia, confusion and, if untreated for a sufficiently long time, dementia. This dementia may prove resistant to treatment even when the other symptoms have improved.

Vitamin B12 deficiency produces a variety of neurological changes and, in addition, can cause unremitting anxiety and depression. It can also result in a confusional state with hallucinations and paranoid symptoms, and in the longstanding, untreated case, dementia can occur. Deficiency of folic acid may produce a similar mental picture: this condition may now and again arise with long-term anticonvulsant therapy and should be considered where epileptics appear to be undergoing a marked personality change.

Endocrine Hypoactivity

Hypothyroidism. This causes a slowing of mentation, with lethargy and memory disorder. Patients often appear depressed and may be confused. Occasionally they are deluded and restless, the condition sometimes known unkindly as "myxedema madness."

Hypoglycemia. Strictly speaking, hypoglycemia is often the result of endocrine *overactivity*, but the end-result is a deficiency state. The condition may be spontaneous or the outcome of excessive insulin-intake. Episodes often occur after exertion or in the early morning. In the early stages, mental symptoms include apprehension and muscular tension. Later, confusion and disorientation are common and the patient may appear to be in a drunken state. Hallucinations and delusions supervene with panic and severe restlessness. If not treated, stupor, coma, and convulsions can follow.

Adrenal insufficiency. Addison's disease is associated with lethargy and apathy. The patient is somewhat irritable and depressed, but emotional responses are muted. Sometimes, because of electrolyte or glucose abnormalities, intermittent confusion may occur, but this is rarely severe. An adrenal crisis may cause collapse and coma, and if not treated promptly and well, may result in brain damage and dementia.

Hypoparathyroidism. Characterized by reduced serum calcium, hypoparathyroidism causes an increase in neuromuscular excitability. Along with tetany, the patient may well be anxious and irritable, and, later, depression, confusion, and hallucinations may appear.

Pituitary insufficiency. Simmond's disease is characterized by mental apathy, lack of volition, and mild neurotic or depressive symptoms. The patient appears mentally passive, sexual libido is low, and there may be persistent hypochondriasis. As with pituitary overactivity, if an anterior pituitary tumor is present, it may add serious complicating psychiatric features.

Mineral and Electrolyte Disturbances

Serious disturbance of electrolyte or water concentrations in the tissues can induce profound mental symptoms, but the manifestations are not characteristic, and in many cases there are multiple electrolyte abnormalities. Sodium and water depletion cause apathy, weakness and confusion. Water intoxication will produce dizziness, headache, nausea and confusion, and ultimately convulsions. Both excess and diminished potassium levels are associated with apathy, weakness and confusion, and magnesium deficiency is manifested by depression, confusion, agitation, hallucinations and seizures.

Obviously none of these symptoms is pathognomonic and usually the biochemical disturbances are the result of underlying disease processes which in themselves may cause mental symptoms, such as diabetic keto-acidosis, uremia or severe diarrhea. It should also be noted that severe primary depressive illness may be accompanied by a raised serum sodium level.

Wilson's disease (hepatolenticular degeneration) is a familial disorder in which copper is deposited excessively in the tissues, notably liver and mid-brain. Along with the resulting neurological symptoms, the patient develops a progressive dementia, at times complicated by hepatic delirium.

A somewhat similar neurological and psychological outcome may be seen with excess iron deposition in untreated hemochromatosis.

OTHER

Sleep deprivation. There are, of course, other causes which lead to neurological and psychological symptoms. Individuals who are deprived of sleep for a prolonged period display a variety of physical and mental symptoms. Among the physical symptoms may be hypertension and muscular "fibrositis." The psychological symptoms include irritability, poor concentration, impaired judgment, and emotional lability. After a time the person begins to express feelings of persecution. He may experience disorientation, illusions, hallucinations, and delusions. The hallucinations are often visual and may be indistinguishable from vivid dreams. The full-blown sleep deprivation picture may resemble schizophrenia, but there are usually confusional elements and the symptoms rapidly clear when the subject regains his lost sleep.

An insomniac who regularly takes hypnotic drugs can suffer the effects of chronic sleep deprivation plus the side-effects of his medication.

Sensory deprivation. Prisoners in solitary confinement, castaways, and others who are forced to live for long periods in situations of environmental deprivation, are well-known to be subject to severe psychological disturbances.

Controlled investigations have been carried out on volunteers who are placed in stimulus-free environments for up to a week. Some individuals can only tolerate such situations for a very short time, and either become so anxious or else show such marked breakdown of ego-barriers that the experiment has to be immediately terminated. Those volunteers who continue throughout the whole course of the study tend to show a characteristic set of reactions. The experiment deprives the subject of the moment-to-moment interaction with his surroundings which is part of normal experience. Without this constant to-and-fro, the person is totally dependent on his inner self to regulate his mental set, his emotional state and his psychomotor activity. Under these conditions, reality testing is rapidly affected and the individual becomes highly suggestible. Alertness decreases, unconscious processes readily attain consciousness and, after a time, thought, affect and behavior become disorganized. During this period, the volunteer is usually aware of much amorphous anxiety. In addition, he has difficulty in concentrating on and in carrying out tasks. Sensory imagery becomes very vivid and illusions or hallucinations, usually visual, may be experienced. Delusions can occur and eventually the individual becomes quite dissociated from his situation and can act in an extremely bizarre fashion.

When returned to a normal environment, most people rapidly lose these symptoms. Occasionally, a subject will remain depersonalized and perhaps deluded for a considerable time. In such experiments it is obviously highly important to exclude subjects who may be predisposed to psychotic reactions. Information about environmental deprivation may be valuable in regard to selection procedures for personnel, or in altering work-patterns in particularly isolated occupations. Space-flight is the most dramatic present-day example.

Experimental sensory deprivation has been used as a model for psychotic illness (Pos, 1969).

POST-OPERATIVE PSYCHOSIS. A proportion of patients who undergo surgical operation show evidence of pathological anxiety and hypochondriasis postoperatively. This usually clears spontaneously, though sometimes rather slowly. A much smaller number develop psychotic symptoms, which may be functional or organic. The functional illnesses, depressive or schizophrenic, are usually regarded as expressions of a constitutional predisposition, with the operative stress acting as a trigger factor. However, in some cases the patient has actually had an unrecognized mental illness prior to the operation and this simply becomes more florid postoperatively.

Postoperative confusional states may arise from a variety of causes. The more prolonged the operation, the deeper the anesthetic, the longer a heart-lung bypass is in use, the more likely is delirium to occur. Some patients are particularly vulnerable and this may be indicated by a previous history of breakdown following operation, childbirth or abortion. A history of alcoholism or drug-abuse, the presence of a precarious cerebral circulation, or excessive preoperative anxiety, are all factors to be concerned about. The very young and the elderly are once more at higher risk than normal. Sleep-deprivation before and after the operation, though inadvertent, is common, and intensive care recovery areas are often noisy, highly mechanized and lacking in normal sensory cues, and together these circumstances may precipitate confusion. Febrile states and electrolyte disturbances are also important contributors. Elderly patients who have had bilateral cataracts removed may become very confused if their eyes are exposed too soon: they appear to need time to deal with the inrush of sensory data they had learned to do without.

Most postoperative confusional states make a rapid and complete recovery, but if significant brain-damage has occurred, the resolution of the delirium may reveal a permanent dementia.

Postpartum psychiatric disorder. For

psychiatric purposes, the postpartum phase is regarded as the six months following childbirth, since psychiatric illness is excessively likely to arise then. Psychiatric illness is relatively uncommon during pregnancy, but the rise in frequency after birth more than outweighs this. The causes are still not understood, but in the more severe forms of postpartum psychiatric illness, the woman often has a personal or family history of the disorder. Presumably, hormonal and stress factors around the time of birth are important, but to counterbalance the idea that the stress of the birth process itself is of great significance, postpartum psychosis can follow cesarean section.

About one in two women develop "postpartum blues" which can sometimes last up to six months. These cause feelings of dejection and weepiness but are usually fairly mild and do not interfere seriously with day-to-day life or mothering abilities. The blues are so common that they are probably physiological rather than pathological, and they usually clear spontaneously. Reassurance and support are adequate in most cases.

Roughly one in 100 women develop severe neurotic symptoms following childbirth, most commonly anxiety, but often with a depressive admixture. The mother is afraid that she is incompetent to care for the child and gets panicky if left on her own. Some women are phobic about dealing with their child and occasionally there are obsessional fears of causing harm. Whatever its form, the condition should be taken seriously and treated appropriately, on an outpatient basis whenever possible. The stability of the underlying personality is one of the best prognosticators.

About one woman in 1,000 develops a postpartum psychosis and nowadays this is almost always of a functional type, similar to those described elsewhere. Affective illnesses, both depressive and manic, are probably commoner than schizophrenic

ones, and a schizo-affective presentation is not infrequent. Since the onset is often acute, the picture may be atypical for a time and confusional symptoms can occur in the early stages. Treatment must be thorough and initially is best carried out in hospital, since some patients behave very irrationally and, on occasion, suicide and infanticide are real risks. Whenever possible, the infant should be admitted to hospital with the mother, who can gradually assume responsibility for its care as she improves. The prognosis is usually rather better than for corresponding non-postpartum illnesses. Favorable factors are a stable pre-morbid personality, lack of a previous or family history of psychosis, and acute onset (especially if associated with confusion or actual delirium) and obvious psychological or physical stress factors. Treatment is essentially the same as for other functional psychoses.

Prior to modern obstetric advances and to the introduction of antibiotics, postpartum psychosis was very much commoner and often took the form of an acute organic brain syndrome. This was related to underlying infection, electrolyte imbalance, severe blood-loss, and other physical factors. Nowadays, this should be rare, and if it occurs, can usually be remedied very readily. Very occasionally, following a severe postpartum hemorrhage resulting in pituitary necrosis, an acute delirium can clear up, to reveal chronic mental apathy due to the multiple hormonal deficits.

A woman who has had postpartum psychiatric illness of any kind, but especially one with functional psychosis, is more liable than normal to develop further attacks in subsequent pregnancies, following abortion, or after a surgical operation. The risk is not usually serious enough to warrant therapeutic abortion, but it should be appreciated by the physician and there should be careful observation in the postpartum or postoperative period. If there is a recurrent history, and especially if there is evidence of progressive psychological deterioration in the mother, further pregnancy is contraindicated.

CONCLUSIONS

Extracerebral causes of organic brain dysfunction are legion, and the mental symptoms range from the most minor to the profoundly psychotic. These symptoms are usually characteristic of organic disorder, but can mimic functional psychiatric illness. When the presence of a generalized physical condition which could cause secondary mental symptoms is known, then suspect that any concomitant psychiatric manifestations might be the result of that condition. If, in addition, a psychiatric disorder appears, which has no convincing psychogenic antecedents, which is out of character for the individual, which only tangentially resembles a functional illness, or which occurs at a time when an organic condition would not be surprising (e.g., postoperatively), then you must have extracerebral organic psychiatric disorder high on your list of differential diagnoses.

If potential psychiatric problems are foreseen in the course of a somatic illness or prior to surgical operation, prevention of a florid breakdown can often be effected by adequate psychological and psychopharmacological intervention.

REFERENCES

Bale, R.N. (1973): Brain damage in diabetes mellitus. *Br. J. Psychiatry.* 122:337.
Bennet, R. et al. (1972): Neuropsychiatric problems in systemic lupus erythematosus. *Br. Med. J.* 4:342.
Leading Article, (1974): Delirium after surgery. *Br. Med. J.* 3:702.
Pos. R. (1969): The biology of dreaming and the informational underload (sensory deprivation) theory of psychosis. *Can. Psychiat. Assoc. J.* 14:371.
Sullivan, P.A., et al. (1977): Dialysis dementia: recovery after transplantation. *Br. Med. J.* 4:740.
Willoughby, J.O. and Leach, B.G. (1974): Relation of neurological findings after cardiac arrest to outcome. *Br. Med. J.* 3:437.

FURTHER READINGS

Arieti, S. (1975): *American Handbook of Psychiatry.* 2d ed. Vol. 4. New York, Basic Books.
An overview of delirious disorders and extracerebral causative factors in organic brain disease.
Kolb, L.D. (1977): *Modern Clinical Psychiatry.* 9th ed. Philadelphia, W. B. Saunders.
A very good and readable account of the psychiatric aspects of brain disease produced extracerebrally.
Pitt, B. (1968): Psychiatric illness following childbirth. *Hospital Medicine* 3:815.
Slater, E. and Roth, M. (1969): *Clinical Psychiatry.* 3d ed. London, Bailliere, Tindall & Cassell.
A psychobiological review of the extracerebral brain disorders, with strong neurological bias.
Walton, J. (1977): *Brain's Diseases of the Nervous System.* 8th ed. Oxford, Oxford University Press.
An excellent account from the neurologist's viewpoint of cerebral dysfunction due to a multiplicity of external factors.

29
Childhood and Adolescent Disorders
Quentin Rae-Grant

This specialized area of psychiatry shares with general psychiatry the principles, precepts, and concepts with regard to etiology, interaction with the environment, intrapersonal and interpersonal psychic processes. The theoretical frameworks and constructions can be applied to both adults and to children. Differences in practice are substantially greater than are those in theoretical orientation. These differences are accounted for in large part by the simple fact that child psychiatrists must adapt what they do to the requirements of children.

and stage of the child. Thus temper tantrums at the age of three are rarely a matter of concern as they are so frequent as to be a normal phenomenon. Should they persist, however, till the age of ten, they carry by this time a major degree of social condemnation. At this age they need investigation and treatment. Children in their behavioral patterns also show much greater fluidity of presenting behavior. In mood they are more labile, and symptom presentation, which is relatively predictable in the adult, is confusingly and rapidly changing with the child.

DEVELOPMENTAL CONSIDERATIONS

In adult psychiatry the main decision that has generally to be made is whether the behavior that is being seen is within the normal range for that society, or whether it is deviant as judged by contemporary mores. If abnormal, into which category does it fall, and therefore which treatment is required? However with children and with adolescents one has to consider not only normality versus deviance in behavior but to consider a time axis as well. Whether the behavior is appropriate or inappropriate is only part of the question; the second part is whether this is so for the age

ACTION AS FEELINGS

Another factor which distinguishes child from adult psychiatry is the mode of communication. Children do not express their feelings in words as the majority of adults are able to do. They tend to communicate feelings of comfort, discomfort, dislike, opposition, or aggravation through their actions. This behavior has to be interpreted as having a meaning beyond being simply a matter of bad behavior or annoyance to others, although at times this may be the reason for its occurrence. The behavior has to be seen as an appeal for help, and an indication of where and why the hurt and pain is occurring. Conversely, it means that to communicate with children, particularly young children, one has to learn their language—the language of play. Much has been written about play therapy as if it were a separate, distinct, therapeutic technique. It is, in fact, no more than that method of understanding a child's expressive language, namely action, and of how to respond to it in a non-adult fashion. Play is the means of communicating with the child.

FAMILY AND ECOLOGICAL UNIT

The adult can be treated in relative isolation from his family. Children are more dependent organisms. Somebody has to care for them, be it the family, extended family, alternate family, or the state, through its various programs for children who are abandoned or need special care. The child spends a substantial proportion of time at school and is influenced by the events, positive and negative, that occur in that situation. The child depends for nurturance, indeed for life, on the presence of a supportive organization, family or alternative, and is influenced to a greater degree by the people-processing organizations to which he belongs involuntarily, particularly the school system. Thus it is impossible adequately to assess or to intervene, to change the situation of a disturbed or disturbing child without becoming involved in depth with the problems of the family and with the problems which are imposed upon him, as well as those presented by him to such organizations as school or group home. Concern for family of the patient may become similarly highlighted in adult psychiatry. To admit to a hospital a depressed, middle-aged mother and not take account of the impact of this on the children at home or the other members of the family may secure an excellent symptomatic result with modern day medication, but may create a continuing problem of concern, disruption, and dis-

equilibrium in the group to which she will have to return as she improves. So while the family, and dealing with the family and the extended organizations of society is necessary in child psychiatry, its importance is being increasingly recognized in general adult psychiatry. The bridging theoretical concept is systems theory which regards the breakdown of an individual as a result of a total system of forces, and the remedy as depending upon examination of and help to the system. The primary system is the family but may also include, in many cases, the place of work and the educational institution. Rather than confining intervention to dealing with the individual and making him "adapt" to the situation, more scrutiny is being given to the system of which he is a member and which may impose upon him, as if he were a lightning rod, the burdens of the unsolved problems of that system.

REASONS FOR REFERRAL

Children are brought for help for many and varied reasons which can be discussed along a developmental axis. Preschool children, in general, are brought to the attention of pediatricians, physicians, public health nurses, or mental health organizations because of delays in their development or problems of attachment and detachment from the parental figures. In school, in the first few years, the concentration is on behavior, socialization, and deviation from the expected norms. In older children the concern of the school and that which triggers referral is usually lack of achievement, "not working up to expected standards," and the frustration of having a child who is known to have good intelligence but seems unable to produce at the expected academic level.

During the shool years, the difficult, aggressive, pugnacious child, who can turn the classroom into a maelstrom in five minutes will certainly have a priority for identification and referral. Teachers are also becoming increasingly alert to the needs of the very quiet child; the one who disappears into the background, sits at the back of the class, and creates no problems whatsoever. Teachers are, in fact, among the best identifiers of deviant child behavior. They are accurate observers. They have experience of a large number of children from which to develop normal standards and expectations of behavior. They are, in many cases, basically optimists and have seen the value of not too quickly rushing in and identifying difficulties.

In adolescence the problems have become well known particularly through the work of Erikson (1968). They concern the question of identity—i.e. "who am I?" not "whom will I model and ape?" The sense of identity is developed slowly throughout adolescence. It is derived from the parents and other key individuals, from reading, and even from exposure to television. The various components should become synthesized into something which is comfortable and compatible, but unique to each individual.

In addition, adolescence is permeated by the problems of the emancipation from the family of origin, a process which can be mediated relatively smoothly, but can at times become a fiery battle in which the two generations are each convinced of the impossibility of the other. The generation gap may be more a myth than a reality; but if it appears anywhere, it is during this period when the child is no longer a child, not yet an adult. The adolescent has to move his attentions and interests outside the home. The parents are torn between a sense of gratification that their child is growing up, and one of regret that they will have little time to further enjoy his or her company as the peer group becomes important, and as the relative and absolute amount of time spent with them rapidly decreases. The other two tasks of the adolescent stage are the integration of the sexual drive, and whether or not this will be a successfully incorporated part of the functioning of the individual. Finally, the problem of career choice faces all adolescents, a problem which is most perplexing and difficult today. Education is no longer a guarantee of employment. The number of jobs available for unskilled labor is rapidly decreasing as machines take over; and if anything has sobered the dreams of the adolescents of the 60's, or brought a depressed and disillusioned atmosphere to the adolescents of the 70's, it is the present economic figures which indicate that it is exactly this age group for whom employment is least available.

TEMPERAMENTAL TRAITS

Thomas and Chess (1973) have demonstrated that children arrive in the world with very different temperamental characteristics; and that these early characteristics, which remain relatively stable throughout the child's life, interact with the personalities, the expectations, and the child-rearing styles of the parents. Thus the quiet, placid child who smiles, responds, eats, and thrives will give the anxious mother a sense of confidence and an ability to go forward and realize her capacities to bring up this child. But the same mother, given a fretful, difficult child who refuses to eat, who keeps her up all night to her annoyance, and to the annoyance of the neighbors, can wreck the mother's confidence very quickly and make her certain that she is doing the wrong thing. She becomes more anxious, and this is in turn communicated to the baby. Both are off to a totally different cycle, with potentially unpleasant consequences for both.

SEPARATIONS AND CONSEQUENCES

Certain events in children's lives are now known to have at least temporary and, in some cases, permanent effects. Of these, the most important are separations which include, for example, hospital admission.

The crucial age at which damage appears to occur from separation is from about one and one-half to four. Separations may occur suddenly, such as with the death of a parent or parents; or repeatedly, such as with several admissions to hospital; or when parents are separating and reuniting in the course of marital discord. Separations imperil the child's sense of security and interrupt a smooth historical flow of experience that allows the child to move from being dependent to being relatively independent by a process of, first, attachment, and then detachment from his parents. It should be emphasized, however, that separations, per se, may not be by any means the whole problem. Rutter (1972) in his classic work showed that what precedes and causes the separation, and that which follows the separation, may indeed be as important as the separation itself in terms of later problems; in particular that repeated short separations, rather than the single separation experienced with a good alternative, may be the more damaging.

Since divorce is becoming more frequent in our society many children are brought up by a single parent with the other parent visiting on a prescribed but sometimes erratic basis. No divorce can be accomplished without the children (and indeed all of the participants) being hurt emotionally in the process. But there is no reason to assume that recovery from this process is not possible in the majority of cases. Where the parents can continue to have the children's welfare in mind, the children can adapt to having father and mother live separately and even (with some difficulty) to the inclusion of a new father or mother figure in their lives. Divorce and separation are traumatic events known to produce short and long term adverse effects in children. Even more certain to make children unhappy and frustrated is an atmosphere of perpetual marital discord. The children become unwilling to be in the home as they derive little nurturance there and wait only for the day when they can escape. Parental discord has a most corrosive influence upon children.

PARENTAL EXPECTATIONS

Parental expectations, as they relate to a child's ability to respond, can create problems. The abusing parent becomes enraged when the child does not behave in a much more mature fashion than his age permits. Over-possessive and over-protective parents use a child's physical illness or fragility, real or imagined, as a reason for impeding natural growth, which would mean not only growing up, but growing away from the parents. The child becomes caught in a series of alliances with the family, the penalty for the breaking of which is intolerable guilt. Parental expectations can also be expressed in academic areas to the detriment of all concerned. The child who is in the lower range of IQ, and yet is expected to perform as a normal child, will indeed have problems in doing anything at all, let alone being able to function at his level of capacity. A similar situation occurs if a child of average intelligence is in a very bright family. He is almost as much of a thorn in the flesh to his parents as are many retarded children.

CHILD-PARENT INTERACTION

Children bring into the world temperamental characteristics that fashion the parents' response. But this is also influenced by other aspects of the child's functioning, e.g., chronic illness, intellectual potential, or congenital physical handicaps. In addition, the circumstances of the birth itself are important. Prematurity, for example, not only increases the risk of physical difficulties, but interferes with the mother-child bonding process. There are parallel factors that influence the ability of the parents to respond to the child's needs: their state of health, personal and marital happiness, and their needs as mirrored in the child; e.g. to help a failing marriage; to replace a child who died; or preferring male rather than female, the intellectual rather than the athletic type. Particularly important is the parents' own experience of childhood. Parents who were deprived as children have difficulty in turn in giving to the children. Parents who were beaten and abused when young are more prone to abuse their children, particularly if by temperament they are identifiable as "difficult."

The behavior that the child presents is the result of an interaction between him and his parents. The image of the child as the innocent and passive victim of the family environment clearly ignores the part he plays in fashioning the parental response. Further, both child and family are influenced by the larger society, its values, services, and institutions.

CLASSIFICATION

There have been many attempts to find a satisfactory classification scheme for childhood disorders. None has yet been devised that satisfied the requirements of precision, reliability, predictive value, or the link between diagnosis and specific etiology and treatment. But certain emphases have emerged in recent years. It has not led from factual observations to diagnosis, to treatment plans. It needs to be developed, and among the most promising attempts to derive such classification has been the multiaxial schema devised by Rutter et al. (1969). Three of these axes are: the normalcy or deviance of a child's behavior, the cognitive abilities of the child, and the psychosocial atmosphere in which the child is reared. Generally what one sees in child psychiatry are syndromes rather than identified diseases with clearly defined etiologies. There are exceptions in the areas of mental retardation, autism, and depression. One can talk of diseases, problems or deviations. In the remaining part of this chapter, except where otherwise indicated, the term deviation will be

chosen to indicate that behavior is outside the expected range of normality but still probably on a continuum with normality. These deviations will be discussed as descriptions of the major syndromes, epidemiological factors, possible etiology, and treatment approaches which have shown empirical value. The deviations which will be discussed are: deviations of development; deviations of cognition; deviations of attention; deviations of separation/attachment behavior; and deviations of socialization. The progression will be from the child's innate abilities to the ranges of feeling and attention required, particularly in school, to social behavior first, to the family, and second to the outside world. Finally, the major mental illnesses as occurring in childhood—psychoses and depression—will be discussed.

Deviations of Development

Motor development. The first of these areas is motor development, when progress is occasionally precocious but more usually a cause of concern because of delay. A child can be expected to be crawling by the age of six to eight months, to be able to stand without support and take his first steps by a year. While substantial individual variation occurs, the absence of walking by the age of 18 months is a matter clearly requiring investigation, including full neurological assessment, to investigate the possibility that there are organic components. However, when organic deficit is sufficiently severe as to cause this degree of developmental retardation, it is likely to be recognized in other ways. The most likely causes for this delay in motor development are: first, a generalized delay in all areas of function, which will be discussed under retardation; or, second, the possibility of degrees of cerebral palsy or other neurological conditions. Rarely seen today, but present at one time, was a picture of severely delayed development as the consequence of the lack of stimulation opportunity for children brought up in institutions. One still hears of the occasional case of children, unwanted, or for some reason unaccepted, who are locked away from the world and whose motor development is thus severely retarded because of lack of adequate stimulation.

Speech. As speech is the main way in which human beings communicate, its delayed or absent development rapidly becomes a cause of concern and brings the child to attention. Delayed onset may be caused by sensory impairment such as deafness, by organic CNS factors, or it may be part of the syndrome of the autistic child. Frequently the problem is not one of delay but of fluency or of use that the child makes of speech.

A frequent problem is stuttering. This decreases with age, but remains a problem into adulthood for about 1% of the population. It is four times more common in males, and more frequent in families when close family members also stutter. Essentially it is characterized by repetition or prolongations of sounds, syllables or words, or by unusual hesitations and pauses which disrupt the rhythmic flow of speech. Accompanying it, but as secondary features, are grimacing, tics, eye blinks, jerking of the head, very rapid or very slow pace of speech. These features have sometimes been acquired during the course of attempts at therapy, or have been found to speed up the process of vocalization by the patient. Stuttering often improves in reading aloud to oneself, talking over the phone, or singing. Fluency may be accomplished, for example, in singing when it appears to be impossible in general conversation. With children there is at first little awareness of the stuttering behavior, but society rapidly makes it clear that fluency is expected. Adding to the difficulty is the anticipation of the stuttering which in itself can promote a situation that verges on speechlessness. Many children have transient periods of stuttering at times of stress, particularly during adolescence. From these they recover without intervention. Stuttering embarrasses the stutterer and discomforts the listener. It impedes social relationships, unless the stutterer has come to very comfortable terms with this persistent problem.

Related to stuttering, but a quite different syndrome, is elective mutism. Here the child refuses to speak in certain situations although he has clearly demonstrated fluent speech in other situations. For example, the child may not talk in school but will talk at home, or vice versa. Reports of immigrant children (Bradley and Sloman, 1975), where one language is spoken at home and the other at school, indicate that elective mutism may be a prominent feature in the first year of their school life. Children who display this may also show other negativistic and oppositional behavior. A diagnosis of elective mutism should not be made unless clear evidence of normal intellectual functioning has been demonstrated, for example, by written work, communication by gestures, and by clear and verified reports of fluency and competent speech in situations other than the one in which there is elective mutism.

Among the developmental tasks, which are essential in the early years, is control over elimination so that it becomes voluntary rather than involuntary in terms of its time of occurrence. Two deviations are prominent in this area: (a) enuresis; (b) encopresis.

Enuresis. This is the persistent uncontrolled voiding of urine by day or night after the age at which most normal children have learned bladder control. Although some people have maintained that this control should be acquired by the age of four, it is probably premature to become greatly concerned with it until five. At that time it is estimated that 10% of children are enuretic; by the age of 10, 5%. About 1% retain the symptom into adult life.

Enuresis may be primary or secondary.

Primary enuresis involves the involuntary passage of urine after the age of five years, when there has never been a period in which this has either been under control or occurs infrequently. Secondary enuresis represents the reappearance of this symptom after a period of continence and dryness had been established, and when this has lasted for at least one year. In addition either of the two types can be classified as nocturnal or diurnal. Nocturnal enuresis is much more frequent; and diurnal enuresis, in general, should initially be regarded as perhaps indicating retardation, autistic behavior or some organic disorder when it occurs after the age of five. The reason for the division into primary and secondary is that primary enuresis probably represents a delay in development of the nervous system, or may be explained by an over-permissive family. Secondary enuresis, by contrast, is one way of expressing the unhappiness and inner turmoil associated with personal or familial disruption. Enuresis, despite what may be thought, is tolerantly accepted by many families. It has no known significant complications except that it can limit the child's activity and is an embarrassment. The treatment of primary enuresis consists of, in the first place, a relatively simple behavior modification program: keeping a chart of the dry nights (with rewards for these), encouragement to the child, no great emphasis on the enuresis, but involvement of the child in the change of sheets on the bed. If this is not successful, two main approaches can be recommended: the use of the imipramine hydrochloride in doses of 25 mgm in the evening for those aged six to nine, 50 mgm for ten and above, or the use of a simple operant conditioning device known as the bell and pad laid under the sheets. When the first drop of urine touches the pad, it rings an alarm which wakes the child who goes to the toilet. Over a period of time the child learns to become aware of sensations of the full bladder and to wake accordingly. Both

of these latter methods have success rates in the range of 80% to 90%. Innumerable other remedies have been tried for enuresis. Their results are no better than placebos. Finally, there are a number of devices which have direct electrical contact with the penis. These should be avoided as they are unnecessary and can lead to unpleasant physical and psychological complications with their misuse.

Encopresis. This condition has many features in common with enuresis. It is the persistent, voluntary or involuntary passage of feces in places and times inappropriate for that purpose. Like enuresis, it can be classified as primary or secondary, depending on whether continence has been established for a period of at least a year. It evokes in parents and caretakers the strongest feelings of opposition— disgust, anger, and hostility, even to the extent that children have been so severely beaten as to sustain fractures.

Childen who are encopretic are in general socially inept, silent, passively aggressive, difficult to deal with, and withholding. Although a number of these cases, particularly those in the primary category, may derive from developmental delays, there is good evidence that in this situation, as opposed to enuresis, the symptom is most often a reaction to severe familial conflict, with family disruption, and life stresses.

Both primary and secondary encopresis decrease, if untreated, with age, and by the adolescent period have disappeared. However, in a substantial proportion of these cases, antisocial and conduct disorders seem to be substituted for this more primitive developmental delay syndrome.

The differential diagnoses, in examining a case of encopresis, are those of structural abnormality such as anal fissure, and in particular the disorder of aganglionic megacolon known as Hirschsprung's Disease. Encopresis is treated, initially, by the evacuation of the bowel and the use of mild stool softeners, for frequently there is overflow incontinence from a grossly distended and impacted colon. But in most cases it will involve a somewhat prolonged course of psychotherapeutic intervention involving the family and the child. This will involve examination of the cause of the symptom, the role the child plays in the family, the reasons for the family hostility and antagonism to him, and the part he plays in perpetuating this situation. With the increased tolerance that some parents can acquire, the ability which the symptom has to annoy decreases and it tends to disappear. The less frequently that manipulations such as enemas or anal extraction are used in these children, the more likely it is that the syndrome will remit. Overzealous medical attention, when not justified by such a syndrome as Hirschsprung's disease, perpetuates the condition. There are as yet no effective drugs that can aid in the treatment of this developmental deviation.

Motor tic disorders. Tics are purposeless, involuntary movements—frequent, rapid, repetitive. Most commonly they affect the face and the eyes, but can extend to the whole head, torso or limbs. The symptoms are exacerbated by stress, disappear during sleep, and may become attenuated in distracting activities. The latest age of onset is in the middle latency period. Boys with tics outnumber girls, and the degree of disability relates more to the discomfort caused in the observer than to any particular impairment experienced by the individual. A particular specific disorder in this group is Gilles de la Tourette syndrome. This is characterized by motor tics accompanied by sudden vocalizations, grunts, sounds or phrases, frequently uttered in inappropriate places where their scatalogical nature is socially offensive. While psychological causes have been postulated for many of these cases, increasingly a possible organic etiology is being suggested. In both motor tics and Gilles de la Tourette syndrome substantial improvement can be obtained by the relief of tension, by a psychotherapeutic approach, or by the use of haloperidol or pimozide—two drugs which appear to have some specific effect on these conditions. Both these conditions have to be distinguished from schizophrenic disorders, various choreiform disorders, dyskinesias, and other neurological syndromes.

Deviations of Cognition

Mental retardation. Included under this term are a wide variety of conditions, the consequence of many different genetic and environmental factors. They share, however, one cardinal feature, a significantly lowered ability to acquire information and learn skills compared to the rest of the population. The population estimated to suffer such handicap is variously given as 3%.

Individuals suffering such conditions are found on testing by psychological means to fall at least two standard deviations below the mean and some may be untestable. Equally important for diagnosis and for management are the accompanying deficits in adaptive and self-help behavior.

In approximately one-fourth of the cases there are known somatic etiologic causes—chromosomal, metabolic or neurological. Down's syndrome is associated with autosomal trisomy. Phenylketonuria is a genetic disorder of phenylalanine metabolism which can be identified at birth, and if diet is suitably managed does not lead to retarded function. In such cases, the degree of impairment is likely to be more severe and capable of detection at an early age. The influence of socioeconomic factors is much less prominent although such factors as malnutrition or exposure to teratogens can enter as causal factors.

It is in the remaining three quarters that such factors play a major part. The degree of retardation is moderate, with an intellectual impairment in the range 50 to 70. No specific biological defect presently can be found to account for these disorders, although advances in genetics promise to reduce the proportion of this amorphous general retardation category. The diagnosis in these cases tends to be made at or near school entrance and, apart from the clear results on the intelligence tests, there are no positive physical or laboratory test results to guide us.

The incidence of mental retardation is disproportionately high among people in the lower socio-economic groups, perhaps because of hereditary factors, poor nutrition, poor prenatal care, sensory deprivation, lack of stimulation, and lack of status and opportunity.

Sub-categories of retardation have been developed—mild, moderate, severe, and profound. The principal purpose of this is for prediction as to the likely future and the likely value of remedial intervention. In mild retardation, which runs approximately from 50 to 70 on an IQ scale, we have the range of individuals who are educable. They can develop social and communicative skills. They are not in a major way retarded in sensory/motor areas and often are not distinguishable until later from normal children. They can learn up to approximately the sixth grade level by their late teens. They can learn social conformity and acceptability and can with guidance and assistance—when the economy is healthy—hold a job. In fact, they may be regarded as excellent workers because they tolerate repetitive work and perform it in a conscientious fashion. Those classified as moderately to severely retarded are more likely to require continuing supervision, and eventually perhaps, institutionalization.

Important in handling the situation of mental retardation are recognition of the following: (a) the findings of an I.Q. test are a guide to the present level of functioning, (b) the total functioning capacity has to be taken into consideration rather than simply the I.Q. level, (c) test results do vary significantly over a period of time (at best, one result can only give a guide), (d) the identification of mental retardation requires confirmation, specifically by a psychologist and by people in the educational stream, to determine that component and that series of educational services which would allow for the maximum learning at a pace geared to the intellectual capacities of the child, (e) the fact that learning that their child is retarded is a traumatic experience to parents. Parents listen but often do not hear, so the diagnosis may have to be repeated on a number of occasions. The parents go through the process of questioning, disbelief, anger, bargaining, hostility, depression, and eventual resolution—a process through which they can be very much helped by the support of their family practitioner. Having a retarded child places great burdens on both the parents and on siblings, particularly if the retardation is obvious to friends and neighbors. It may embarrass the older children, and it may skew the family attention towards or away from the retarded child. The parents usually worry about what will happen to the child when they are no longer around. This concern seems to intensify at particular times—at school entry, change from primary to junior high school, and the onset of adolescence and menarche, with the potentiality for sexual activity. A fuller discussion of the impact, the management and the implications of mental retardation can be found in Hawke (1977) as well as in Chapter 39.

Specific learning disabilities. To be distinguished from the general retardation problems discussed above are a number of specific disorders of cognitive development that are discrete in their focus, and particulary affect the areas of reading and arithmetic, the two basic components of learning. These children have adequate to above adequate general levels of intellectual functioning, but on psychological testing exhibit areas in which they have clear difficulties in particular modes of learning, either in the use and retention of visual material, or the use of auditory material. Frequently these children are referred because of failure to learn in school, and the delineation of the specific area of disorder is essential in terms of helping the school to design prescriptive and remedial teaching. Not infrequently these learning disabilities are accompanied by behavioral disorders. Because they are unable to learn they begin clowning, or getting themselves thrown out of class or school to avoid the embarrassment of being unmasked as the "dummy." Also in this group are children who show a marked drop off in intellectual capacity and functioning and inability to produce on standard test achievement as a result rather than a consequence of emotional problems and conflict.

This term—specific cognitive disorder—should not be used when it is part of another major picture; for example, infantile autism or mental retardation. The degree of incapacity of these children varies; the longer it goes without identification, the greater the problems in terms of achievement at school and in the behavioral concomitants of low self-esteem, truancy, dropping out, and anti-social behavior that occur. The diagnosis of these cases requires a skilled examination and discrete attention to various information processing procedures, utilizing school psychological services which are usually available, or the services of a psychologist and a mental health, or learning disorder clinic.

Deviations of Attention

A number of conditions under many different syndromes are grouped under this heading. The terms hyperkinesis, hyperkinetic syndrome, minimal brain damage, minimal brain dysfunction are used almost synonymously for what are increasingly being regarded as disorders of ability to attend. There are two main syndromes to be considered. The first is attention disorder with hyperactivity. The second disorder is characterized by the same features, but hyperactivity is not present.

Attention disorders with hyperactivity. Children so affected are excessively active from an early age. They are described at nursery school or elementary school as being impulsive, distractible, disorganized, inattentive, and with a short attention span. Fidgety, overactive, attention-demanding, and disruptive are other adjectives applied to their behavior. Similar complaints are applied to their behavior at home. The symptoms, however, fluctuate, and may vary from one situation to the other. Thus, they may be more prominent in the school or in the home.

On the first visit to a physician's office, the child may be subdued by the novelty of the atmosphere and fail to display the behavior which the parents described. On the second or third visit, however, the particularly hyperactive child may demonstrate in full measure his home and/or school behavior.

These children are difficult to control, and are difficult to discipline. Their temper outbursts are of greater duration than is normal and occur with less provocation.

Specific learning disabilities, previously mentioned, are frequent accompaniments of this particular syndrome. In a small proportion of cases there are clear neurological signs (hence the use of the term "minimal brain dysfunction" which argues by analogy that because some children with neurological disorders show hyperactivity, conversely, hyperactivity implies neurological damage). Many more children display soft neurological signs. EEG abnormalities may or may not be present. Typically this picture appears about the time when the child becomes independently mobile, approximately at age two or three or earlier. Mild cases of this syndrome are unlikely to be picked up until the child enters school.

The cause of this disorder is still in the process of being elaborated. While the hyperactivity and to some extent the aggressiveness decline with the onset of adolescence, it is clear that these children have a disproportionate number of brushes with the law because of antisocial behavior (Minde et al., 1972; Minde, 1975; Weiss et al., 1975). Worth noting is that this condition is most common in boys, in the ratio of ten to one. It occurs in as many as 3% of children of pre-school age, and seems to be associated with a family pattern of similar disorder in siblings and near relatives.

These children frequently benefit from a structured environment. Not infrequently, their homes lack that, and they do better in school, especially if small classes, personal attention, and a reduction of extraneous stimuli is provided.

Stimulant medication may be used as treatment, particularly methylphenidate in doses of up to 40 to 50 mg a day. This medication seems to be most useful after the age of five, although it sometimes produces dramatic effects before that age. When successful the response is immediate. This medication can be continued over a number of years. The side effects are loss of appetite or problems with sleeping, but frequently very hyperactive children on this medication show improvement in those areas. Medication should be given half an hour before food, with the last dose given not later than 4 p.m.

Opinions vary with regard to the advisability of drug holidays, namely during periods of less stress, for example on weekends. There are advantages to this. It allows one to assess the continuing need for the medication, and it diminishes the likelihood that over a period of time the impact of the drug will lessen.

Methylphenidate has disadvantages.

The drug has the potential to delay growth in the period of growth spurt. While the evidence for this claim is ambiguous, it is probably wiser to avoid the use of the medication during that period. A final adverse effect that occasionally occurs is an almost too successful response. A child who has been "destruction on wheels" suddenly becomes so slowed down that he is regarded by the parents as a zombie. Many parents would rather put up with the hyperactivity.

In addition to a more structured environment and the use of stimulant medication, behavior modification may be tried. The child is taught to curb his impulsivity and to say to himself, first aloud, and then within his mind, some phrase such as "stop, look, and listen." For this he is rewarded. Behavior modification may be an alternative to, or a supplement to the use of medication.

Attention disorders without hyperactivity. Closely allied to this syndrome of attention disorder with hyperactivity is that characterized by the same features but without the hyperactivity being present. These children are usually detected at entry into school and in the early school years because of their tendency to shift from one activity to the other, a lack of organization or care in the work that they produce, impulsive errors, and mistakes in material that they clearly know. Relatively unstructured situations accentuate this picture. These children, as do the hyperactive children, perform best in an organized and supervised environment. Unlike the hyperactive children, they are able to sit still and they do not cause the same degree of disturbance within the class or home. It is in their performance that the disorder is detected, by the inability to attend or concentrate, apply and complete assignments. As in the hyperactive group, this may be accompanied by soft neurological signs, specific learning disabilities, and EEG abnormalities, but the presence of these is not required to make the diagnosis. As with the previous group, the approach combines indivualized attention, a greater degree of supervision in class (for example, having the child sit close to the teacher), more structured rather than less structured situations and the use, under appropriate supervision and monitoring, of methylphenidate described above.

Deviations of Separation Behavior

The most prominent and indeed the most frequent syndrome occurring in this area is one known by various terms, namely school phobia, school refusal, or separation anxiety disorder. The basic feature of this picture is the inability of the child to tolerate separations from the parental home. Principally this is shown in a refusal to go to school. Further, these children do not stay overnight with their friends, or visit, or attend camp, and may even be unable to stay comfortably in a room by themselves. At the same time they display clinging behavior and shadowing of the parents. Typically, the picture begins with a number of somatic complaints on school mornings. These are vague, difficult to pinpoint, and are accompanied by considerable, obvious distress on the part of the child; but, if the decision is made that the child not go to school, the complaints clear up rapidly, only to recur the next day. The children who do go to school tend to stay a brief period, then leave and immediately return home. In their general behavior and functioning they show a combination of phobic features, shyness, or timidity. Occasionally, with siblings they show the opposite. Thus they have a vivid fantasy life with regard to what may happen to themselves, or more frequently to their parents, if they are not there magically to protect them, and this anticipatory anxiety brought on by the possibility of separation is a salient feature in the picture. There may be accompanying fears of animals, monsters, new situations, or intruders into the home. These children tend to come from intact, educationally concerned families, who appear on the surface to have a good and complementary relationship. However, the child can in an open or covert fashion manage effectively to gear the activities of the family round his or her particular interests. In the school situation they are frequently reported as over-compliant, creating no problems, over-achieving, and of above average intelligence, but somewhat distant and remote from close peer relationships. This picture of school refusal can be precipitated by any change in the child's pattern of life, for example, a move from one area to another, disruption within the family, separation or death of a parent, or the interruption caused by vacation periods. Thus the referral most frequently occurs soon after the summer or spring vacation when the pattern of going to school has been interrupted. Among the main etiological factors which have been suggested are: concern over the separation from the parents and the magical protection of being there to guard against danger (this phobic fear of separation is projected onto the school, but the basic fear is of leaving home); the perfectionistic nature of these children who set themselves extremely high standards and who, whenever they feel that these standards may be imperiled, (for example, by a period off school for illness) are reluctant to return in case this false image of themselves should be shattered; and a power struggle within the family in which, although the child may appear to be rather pathetic and in need of attention, has, when one looks at him more closely, effective control of the situation.

The first and non-negotiable component of treatment is the immediate return of the child to school. This is essential, as in its absence treatment is meaningless. The longer the child is out of school, the more difficult it is for him to return, particularly as he has lost ground and correspondingly is reluctant to take on the challenge of catching up. In addition there needs to be work with the child about his fears, and with the parents, one of whom at least not infrequently has experienced the same symptoms and the same feelings. Further, the parents should be encouraged to develop their own interests and live their own lives, moving away from the control that the child exercises on them.

The prognosis in these cases depends on the duration of the symptom—the longer the child is out of school, the greater the difficulty in returning; and upon the age of the child—the younger the age, the better the prognosis. The appearance of this picture in adolescence is of considerably more grave import than it is for the younger child. The essential component in the treatment is the return to school, the assurance and confidence of the position of the physician, counsellor, and parents that this will not adversely affect the child and, if necessary, the securing of help from the school to allow sufficient persuasion to be applied to get the child into the normal learning situation. The phase-in into the classroom may follow the sequence of sitting in the vice-principal's office, then sitting outside his own class, then becoming part of it; but generally the biggest first step—the essential first step—is simply unequivocal expression and implementation of the immediate return to school. Only occasionally, and in very persistent cases, is it necessary for a period of residential treatment to take place in a setting which combines psychotherapeutic and educational approaches.

This picture is to be distinguished from that of truancy which lies in the area of conduct or anti-social disorder. Truants come from, in general, deprived and disadvantaged families which do not value education. They often live in a subculture where truancy is an expected behavior. Frequently the parents do not know of the truancy until it is detected and brought to their attention by the authorities. The children's performance in school is below average, as in general is their intelligence. Their attitude, when confronted with the behavior, is one of bravado and denial, and the support that they receive at home has something of the same quality. They are not anxious and are frankly bored by the whole school procedure. In the situations of truancy, factors of the school probably deserve more attention, as frequently a change of class to what is more appropriate may be successful for the truant. A change of class for the school refusal child rarely, if ever, is indicated as the child simply transfers the problem from one class or one school to the other.

Deviations of Socialization

Among the categories of disorders which will be included here are general conduct disorders and anti-social behavior and a number of psychoses of childhood.

Conduct disorder. This term applies to persistent patterns of behavior which cause discomfort not to the individual carrying them out, but to the society and members of society which have to deal with them. These have to be distinguished from the normal degrees of exploration, mischief, and teasing which are characteristic of childhood and adolescence. The conduct disorder is characterized by a persistent and repetitive pattern of lack of concern for the feelings of others, an inability to be influenced by the hurt that others experience, aggressive and selfish antisocial behavior, difficulties in the school situation, and a persistent failure to develop close and age-appropriate relationships with friends. Thus this lack of concern can lead to uncontrolled bullying, aggression, teasing, and abusive behavior to adults and to other children alike. It is characterized by persistent episodes of temper, aggression, violence, truancy, and vandalism. In many of these cases the parents or community subtly condones or excuses this conduct.

Statistics of the incidence and frequency

of conduct disorders are difficult to obtain, as the diagnosis is made on social criteria which vary with the tolerance of the community, the degree of law enforcement, and other factors.

Continuous misconduct frequently leads to court appearances and correctional institutions. From this, the progression too often is to outright criminality; however, it should be remembered that of children who are sent to training schools, a substantial proportion do not reappear in court.

While moderate degrees of anti-social behavior can be taken care of by warning, parental guidance, or placing the child on probation, more serious degrees require removal from home, principally for the protection of society, and in such situations the eventual outcome is rather pessimistic. Predominantly the pessimistic prognosis relates not only to the behavior but to the fact that these children tend to be less successful in academic pursuits. They frequently come from homes characterized by poverty, large family size, single parent families, or neighborhoods where delinquency is sanctioned or condoned. Boys engaged in anti-social conduct substantially outnumber girls, although the ratio of this is changing.

These situations should be distinguished from a number of conditions that occur in adolescence and which relate to emancipation, the search for identity, and opposition to adult standards. These latter are noteworthy for their onset at adolescence, by the fact that the patient sees them as desirable and necessary rather than being indifferent to their consequence, and that they express the problems of facing independent decisions in breaking free from parental ties. They vary depending on the mood of the peer group with whom the individual is associated, and are fashioned along the lines that are current at that particular time. Individuals struggling with these problems are not in fact detached from parents or their peers. They

are very much dependent on them for their sense of well-being. They are in the process of moving their dependence on the adult world to that of their own age group. The frequency with which this occurs has led some students of the adolescent period to regard those who go through this without showing oppositional behavior as being retarded in development and likely to experience later difficulties. However the work of Offer (1973) makes it clear that at least one-third of adolescents are able to mediate this period without the actual sound and fury that has become by tradition associated with it. The solution is either a matter of time, parental tolerance, or the use of family therapy. In this, both sides have equal representation, and come to understand both the validity and invalidity of what each other is saying, and in the presence of a neutral observer are helped to re-define the contract of dependence, responsibility, and the relationships within the family situation.

Psychoses

Psychotic disorders, particularly in the form of early infantile autism and early childhood psychosis, can also be seen as disturbances in the relationship between the individual and the outside world. The clearest of these syndromes is that described by Leo Kanner to which the term infantile autism has become attached. This is characterized by: lack of responsiveness to other human beings; impairment, if not absence, of communicative skills; strange, unusual, and idiosyncratic responses to environmental stimuli; desire for sameness; fascination with inanimate objects; and use of parts of the human being as if they were a total human being. This picture appears within the first two years of life. Although, occasionally, it is reported that these children have a period of normality before "retiring into the psychosis," the more usual history is one of delayed development in a number of areas, including failure to cuddle, lack of eye contact, and indifference in affections, with delayed milestones and, particularly, delayed appearance of speech. Characteristic of these children, however, are islets of performance, both in tests and in behavior, in which they equal or surpass children of their own age. This may be in repetitive behavior, in ritualistic motor acts, or in their ability in music or in calculations of some particular rote area; for example, train time tables, historical dates, or arithmetical problems. Other features include a testable IQ, which is usually below normal. About 40% of autistic children test at an IQ of below 50; only 30% have an IQ of 70 or more, and with these standard tests, insofar as they can be applied, they show remarkable variability. They may do well with tasks which require manipulative skills and do poorly when verbal skill is involved.

The prognosis for these children is grave. For those who by the age of five have not established speech and do not have a testable IQ above 70, the likelihood is that they will never become self-supporting. However, a small proportion of cases are eventually able to lead independent lives with only minimal signs of the disorder, usually characterized by some social inappropriateness and by the selection of a career area that does not depend on skilled personal abilities. The prognosis is influenced by the availability of special educational techniques, and some of the more severe and bizarre components of the condition can be helped by the administration of antipsychotic drugs such as thioridazine or chlorpromazine. Despite the fact that much is written with regard to this syndrome, it is relatively infrequent (incidence of 0.4 per 1,000) in the field of child psychiatry, and more common in boys than in girls. Debate continues as to whether this particular syndrome of early infantile autism is related in any way to the onset and increased incidence of schizophrenia in adulthood. The increasing

opinion would regard the two as totally distinct conditions, with early infantile autism most probably now being viewed as an organically determined origin with some insult to the neural substrate. At times, arguments have been adduced that this syndrome appears as a consequence of remote, distant, highly intellectual parents; but the evidence for this is rather thin. Nevertheless, autistic children tend to appear in families with high socio-economic and educational levels more frequently than they do in families at the lower end of these scales.

Other psychoses of early childhood are characterized by a similar gross disturbance of emotional relationships, lack of appropriate direction, lack of ability to relate to their own age group, frequently accompanied by strange beliefs, ideas, and fantasies, without realizing that these are such, and preoccupation with morbid thoughts or interests. This leads to a restriction, diminution, and rigidity of areas of interest and makes special education essential. There is also disturbance in language, including delayed or echolalic speech and, in extreme cases, self-mutilation, including severe headbanging. Treatment includes the use of behavior modification, milieu therapy, residential treatment, antipsychotic drugs and special education programs.

Depression

This other major form of psychiatric illness has been, until recently, regarded as rare in children. However, over recent years the incidence of this and of its concomitants, successful and attempted suicide, has become increasingly frequent in adolescents. Suicide is the second most frequent cause of death in North America in 15 to 19 year olds. The fact that smaller numbers of children may be reported as committing suicide may be an artifact of the unwillingness to so label this in children. An excellent review of this is presented by Garfinkel and Golombek (1977). Suicide incidents in children occur most frequently in the late evening hours and at home. The incidence varies from country to country, and is influenced by such factors as predominant religious belief. Drugs are the most frequently used method, including diazepam, barbiturates, antidepressants, and aspirin. Violent methods are less often used by children than by adults. The motives behind suicidal behavior are many and include: the desire to punish parents, blackmail of the parents or others to change their attitudes or behavior, and incomplete comprehension of the meaning of death.

The management of attempted or threatened suicide should derive from findings in three major areas of investigation:

1. A complete history, including family, social, medical and peer relationships, and any recent changes.
2. A mental status examination that is comprehensive and emphasizes particularly factors related to elements of depression.
3. Consideration of and attention to the child's expression of feelings, both verbally and nonverbally.

Each attempted or threatened suicide should be taken seriously and should raise the question of admitting the child to an appropriate facility. The need for this can be determined with some degree of certainty by using the following criteria:

1. The more serious the method, the more likely this was a genuine attempt to commit suicide, and not an attempt to frighten the family.
2. When detailed plans have been made and indicated over a period of time, e.g., the giving away of treasured objects, leaving of suicidal notes, the intent, again, is serious.
3. The degree of present acute stress and whether or not this has been cumulative on pre-existing stress; namely, a long standing disorder in the family relationships.
4. The presence or absence of a family history of suicide.
5. The history of a previous attempt by the patient.
6. Evidence, on mental status examination, of the continuing presence of depression, particularly marked guilt feelings, ideas of unworthiness, and feelings of hopelessness.
7. The degree and competence of support available from responsible individuals to ensure that a repeated attempt is unlikely to occur.

It is to be noted that all children may, at times, make suicidal threats and gestures when they are experiencing difficulty. Further, when children and adolescents are depressed the features tend to be more "depressive equivalents;" namely, boredom, restlessness, fatigue, difficulties in concentrating, drop in school performance, isolation from peers, and somatic complaints. These may be accompanied by expressing feelings by running away from home, bullying other children, delinquency, or being prone to rather obvious accidents. The classical manic-depressive picture usually does not appear until late adolescence, although manic episodes in younger children have been reported in the literature occasionally.

Treatment. The treatment of depression in adolescents, and of suicidal attempts deriving from this, focuses primarily on relieving the acute and chronic stresses that are usually uncovered in the course of taken the patient's history. These stresses can be within the individual, in the family, or in his relationships with the outside— his school, friends, and society. Treatment is chosen accordingly, and may be in the nature of individual therapy or family therapy, with the objective of helping the child to find successful ways of coping with stress, or of helping the family towards more compatible functioning as a unit. In direct work with the child or adolescent, primary attention is given to the self-depreciation, lack of self-esteem and sense of rejection that are major characteristics of depression. The aim is to help the adolescent to deal with such situations as the recent experience of loss, a chronic sense of being under-valued, and patterns of coping that have been ineffective and against his best interests. At times placement in a neutral or therapeutic setting may be indicated, particularly to separate adolescent and family and to allow them to work out their difficulties without the constant aggravation of each other's presence. Thus brief hospitalization may be an effective form of crisis intervention and of initiating longer term treatment if this is required (Lucas, 1977).

When the depressive disorder continues to impair functioning, a trial of antidepressants is warranted. Several clinical studies, unfortunately not adequately controlled, suggest the value of this as part of the treatment program. Clinically, the tricyclics are to be preferred because of their greater safety, fewer side effects, and because they do not require dietary limitation during administration as do MAO inhibitors (Hersov, 1977). Because adolescents vary in their response to drugs, the physician should start with small doses, increasing to the adult level if there are no adverse effects. Currently, imipramine would appear to be the drug of first choice. If the patient does not respond in four to six weeks the drug should be discontinued. There is no place in the treatment of depression in adolescents for the use of chlordiazepoxide (Librium), diazepam (Valium) or hypnotics, and the place and value of lithium salts has not yet been established. All who advocate using drugs in the treatment of depression in adolescents, whether they do this with North American caution or European enthusiasm, agree that the drug treatment by itself is only one part of the treatment of the whole family and living situation required to handle the problems presented.

SUMMARY

It has not been possible to touch on more than the most frequently occurring syndromes in child and adolescent psychiatry in this chapter. Those noted are those likely to be encountered in practice. Psychosomatic conditions, covered elsewhere, were not included, although clearly the question of psychological factors in asthma, diabetes, cystic fibrosis, abdominal pain and particularly anorexia nervosa are very relevant to the area of adolescence. The emphasis, as was mentioned at the beginning, has to be not only on the child but on the child within the context of his family or family substitute, as well as within the context of the social environment. Disequilibrium in any of these components can be reflected in and through the child. The child may have the problem or he may be the expression of a problem within the system, particularly within the family system. Treatment of children is rarely possible without the involvement of the family or the family substitute caretakers. For most adolescents involvement of parents in the negotiating process towards emancipation, freedom, and the development of a sense of identity is an essential part of the treatment. Drugs are less used in child psychiatry but have an important part to play. Basically, however, the reliance has to be on common sense support, guidance and help to the parents as they deal with the child, basic psychotherapeutic principles and, where deemed important, manipulation of the environment. Children rarely need residential treatment or hospital care for psychiatric conditions. However, when needed it should be in the child's community. It should include an educational component; it should involve the parents in visiting and keeping contact with the child; and it should have available an array of individual, family, group, and psychopharmacological treatments which may be used as appropriate to the condition that requires admission.

Children are more flexible and labile than adults. One may therefore feel more optimistic about the occurrence of change in the process of growth as well as of treatment. Yet they have greater difficulties in determining their own choices for change. They are dependent economically, legally, and morally on the adults in their life. (In strict legal terms the only rights they have are the right not to be abused or neglected, and the right to education.) All other rights inhere in the parents, including the right to initiate treatment, to refuse treatment, or to withdraw from treatment. Indeed the child can only change when the family or caring unit permits and requires it.

REFERENCES

Bradley, S. and Sloman, L. (1975): The elective mutism in immigrant families. *J. Amer. Acad. Child Psychiatry.* 14:510.

Erickson, E.H. (1968): *Identity: Youth and Crisis.* New York, W. W. Norton.

Garfinkel, B. and Golombek, H. (1977): Suicide and depression in children and adolescents. In *Psychological Problems of the Child and His Family.* Edited by P. D. Steinhauer and Q. Rae-Grant. Toronto, Macmillan of Canada.

Hawke, W.A. (1977): Psychiatric aspects of mental retardation. In *Psychological Problems of the Child and His Family.* Edited by P. D. Steinhauer and Q. Rae-Grant. Toronto, Macmillan of Canada.

Hersov, L. (1977): Emotional disorders. In *Child Psychiatry: Modern Approaches.* Edited by M. Rutter and L. Hersov. Oxford, Blackwell.

Lucas, A.R. (1977): Treatment of depressive states. In *Psychopharmacology in Childhood and Adolescence.* Edited by J. M. Weiner. New York, Basic Books.

Minde, K.K., Weiss, G. and Mandelson, N. (1972): A five-year follow-up study of ninety-one hyperactive school children. *J. Amer. Acad. Child Psychiatry.* 11:595.

Minde, K.K. (1975): The hyperactive child. *Can Med. Assoc. J.* 112:13.

Offer, D. (1973): *The Psychological World of the Teenager.* New York, Basic Books.

Rutter, M. (1972): Maternal deprivation reconsidered. *J. Psychosomat. Res.* 16:241

Rutter, M., Lebovici, S., Eisenberg, L., et al. (1969): A tri-axial classification of mental disorders in childhood. *J. Child Psychol. Psychiatry.* 10:41.

Thomas, A. and Chess, S. (1973): Development in middle childhood. In *Annual Progess in Child Psychiatry and Child Development.* New York, Brunner/Mazel.

Weiss, G., Kruger, E., Danielson, E., et al. (1975): Effect of long-term treatment of hyperactive children with methylphenidate. *Can. Med. Assoc. J.* 112:159.

FURTHER READINGS

Anthony, E.H. (1974): Child therapy techniques. *American Handbook of Psychiatry.* 2d ed. Vol. 2 Edited by S. Arieti. New York, Basic Books.
An excellent review of the principles of psychotherapy with children, the role of the therapist and evaluation of effects.

Anthony, E. (1974): Psychotherapy of adolescence. In *American Handbook of Psychiatry.* 2d ed. Vol. 2. Edited by S. Arieti. New York, Basic Books.
A similar review for the treatment of adolescents.

Barker, P. (1976): *Basic Child Psychiatry.* 2d ed. Baltimore, University Park Press.
An introductory text particularly useful for phenomenology and syndrome description, written from a British psychiatric viewpoint.

Freedman, A.M., Kaplan, H.I., Sadock, B. (1975): *Comprehensive Textbook of Psychiatry.* 2d ed. Vol. 2. Baltimore, Williams & Wilkins.
Appropriate and detailed section within a most comprehensive and referenced text in the field of psychiatry.

Ginott, H.G. (1965): *Between Parent and Child.* Toronto, Macmillan of Canada.
A popular and useful guide for parents that answers a number of the questions they may ask about the management of their children and minor day to day problems of training and discipline. An up-to-date alternative to Dr. Spock's classic work.

Halpern, H.M. (1963): *A Parent's Guide to Child Psychotherapy.* New York, A. S. Barnes.
An excellent and useful guide to supplement the above reading. This again emphasizes the basic principles and particularly de-mystifies the process of working therapeutically with children.

Rutter, M., Hersov, L. (1977): *Child Psychiatry: Modern Approaches.* Oxford, Blackwell.
A most comprehensive, detailed and critical review of the literature and practice in child and adolescent psychiatry. An excellent reference for detailed in-depth examination of such issues as adoption and different theoretical approaches to etiology and treatment.

Steinhauer, P.D., Rae-Grant, Q. (1977): *Psychological Problems of the Child and His Family.* Toronto, Macmillan of Canada.
A comprehensive introductory text dealing with the child and his family, methods of clinical assessment, common syndromes, psychological crises and principles of intervention. Contributors from the Faculty of the University of Toronto, Department of Psychiatry. This gives more detail and clinical examples relating to issues summarized in this chapter.

30
Psychiatric Emergencies
George Voineskos and Frederick H. Lowy

Psychiatric emergencies are as important as medical or surgical emergencies, and often they are as dramatic. Primary care physicians and psychiatrists are most often called upon to deal with psychiatric emergencies, but specialists of all types may be involved.

Regrettably, many physicians are intimidated by psychiatric emergencies and attempt to deal with them rather superficially before making a rapid referral to a psychiatric facility. This is unfortunate, not only because in the end a superficial approach will often lead to greater time demands on the physician but also because the emergency situation often offers an opportunity for useful therapeutic and preventive intervention.

DEFINITION AND INCIDENCE

The psychiatric emergency patient has been defined as "any individual who develops a sudden or rapid disorganization in his capacity to control his behavior or to carry out his usual personal, vocational and social activities." Such disorganization, however, may have been taking place over a period of time but the behavior is recognized as that of a psychiatric emergency only when the patient comes or is brought for treatment. Therefore a practical definition of a psychiatric emergency is "any situation which compels a person to seek immediate psychiatric treatment, or which impels his family, friends, or an official agency to seek such treatment for him."

As many as 50% of patients attending general hospital emergency clinics have been found to suffer from some form of psychiatric condition, either relating to a presenting somatic complaint or independent of it. Primary psychiatric cases seen in the emergency department constitute on the average 5% to 10% of the total, although figures as high as 30% have been reported.

The incidence of psychiatric emergencies in family practice is not known but it must be high since a substantial proportion of patients seen in family practice suffer primarily from a psychiatric disorder.

CHANNELS AND HOURS OF REFERRAL

Studies of referral patterns in North America show that well over 50% of the patients are self and/or family referred; police referrals account for 10% to 20% of the total; patients referred by family physicians amount to approximately 20%. This last source of referral is in marked contrast to Great Britain where referrals from general practitioners account for two-thirds of the total, a fact that reflects the different organization of health services.

While late night psychiatric emergencies will be easily remembered by the staff, it should be noted that about 50% of emergency psychiatric patients come to the emergency department during the regular working hours of the week, and about 80% come between 8 a.m. and 10 p.m.

DEMOGRAPHIC CHARACTERISTICS OF PSYCHIATRIC EMERGENCIES

Emergency departments usually serve a younger population than the remainder of the hospital. Fifty percent of psychiatric emergency consultations are provided for patients 20 to 39 years of age; patients between 20 and 29 years of age make up the largest single group. There are variations in the reported ratio of males to females, some studies reporting a preponderance of males. The most frequent finding, however, is that females outnumber males in a ratio of 3:2. The divorced, separated, widowed and single are overrepresented, as are unemployed people.

PREVALENCE OF DIAGNOSTIC CATEGORIES AND PREVIOUS TREATMENT

Psychiatric emergencies are not confined to particular diagnostic categories; they can develop in those with psychoses, organic brain syndromes, neuroses, personality disorders and psychosomatic disturbances, and also in people without psychiatric illness during periods of crisis. Whiteley and Denison (1963) in London, England, found approximately one quarter of their patients to be suffering from psychosis, just under half from neurosis, and one quarter from personality disorders, including alcohol and drug addiction. Lowy et al. (1971) reported similar figures from Montreal.

TABLE 8:   TEN COMMON PSYCHIATRIC EMERGENCIES

1. The suicidal patient
2. Marital or family crises
3. The depressed patient
4. The intoxicated or delirious patient
5. The acutely psychotic patient
6. The anxious or panic-stricken patient
7. Medical emergencies presenting as psychiatric emergencies
8. The confused patient
9. The aggressive, assaultive patient
10. The homicidal patient

At least two-thirds of patients presenting with psychiatric emergencies have had previous psychiatric contact. Miller (1968) reported that 52% of patients had an ongoing significant treatment relationship at the time of presentation; 37% were involved in current psychiatric treatment and 15% in non-psychiatric medical treatment.

PRESENTING BEHAVIOR AND CRISIS SITUATIONS

Contrary to popular belief or fear that the mentally ill are dangerous to others, aggressive and assaultive behavior in psychiatric emergencies is uncommon. The patient who is dangerous to himself is much more common than the patient who is dangerous to others. Glasscote et al. (1966) concluded, with respect to the behavior of emergency patients, that: there is high frequency of depression; the combined number of emergencies presenting as depressed or anxious is three and one-half times as great as the number who are assaultive, aggressive, or destructive; and there is high frequency of intoxication. Miller (1968) reported suicidal behavior in 30% of emergency patients, those who had actually made a suicidal attempt accounting for 13%. Only 1% were considered homicidal.

When there is a threat of suicide or assault to persons or property, almost everyone in the patient's environment becomes alarmed and this leads to public intervention, even if the affected individual does not himself seek help. Other less dramatic situations may also call for attention, for example, severe depression, panic states and dramatic or incomprehensible changes in a person's behavior, but whether these are perceived as emergencies in a given situation depends upon the stress or threat experienced by the individual, or the concern created to those around him.

Jim, a 24 year old immigrant from southern Europe, was brought to the emergency department by his brother. During the previous week the mother had found out that Jim kept a knife under his pillow at night. His mother asked him the reason for keeping the knife but Jim was vague. When his brother insisted, Jim explained that he wanted to protect himself from his father. He was afraid that his father would kill him while he slept. His brother tried to reassure him that his fears were unfounded and asked him to give up the knife. Jim refused, became angry and punched his brother. Three years earlier, while Jim was doing his military service in his country of origin, he spent four months in a psychiatric hospital for a "nervous breakdown."

Glasscote et al. (1966) and Morrice (1968) concluded that most psychiatric emergencies are also social emergencies, although, of course, the converse is not necessarily true.

In most emergencies it is possible to identify crucial events or experiences which appear to have triggered the emergent behavior. Social factors are considered to be primary in almost two-thirds of psychiatric emergencies; family conflicts such as marital disharmony, impending separation or divorce, desertion and conflicts with parents account for 50% of the referrals. Crises relating to job, income and other financial difficulties also occupy a prominent position.

Mary, a 38 year old widow, had a few friends in for supper, including her current boyfriend, on a Saturday night. Around 11 p.m., when everyone was in good spirits her 14 year old son returned home. Holding a glass of wine, she invited him to greet the guests. Her son took a look and said to her that he was fed up with her drunk friends. Her boyfriend then criticized him for speaking to his mother in that manner. Her son shouted back that he was indeed fed up and he was going to pack and leave at once. He then went to his room. Mary screamed and rushed to the bathroom upstairs. Her boyfriend followed her a few seconds later, saw her swallowing a handful of pills and prevented her from taking any more. She continued screaming. He then drove her to the downtown hospital where she had been treated for a depressive illness. They arrived at the emergency department at 1:30 a.m. At the time of presentation her chart read that her depressive illness was in remission, she was on maintenance Amitriptyline 100 mg at night, and was seen by her psychiatrist every two weeks. At interview she was tearful, desperate and suicidal. She was admitted to hospital.

It is important to consider the patient and the social environment as playing a joint role in producing the psychiatric emergency. A useful concept is that of "the ecological group" which refers to the patient and those people in the social environment with whom he has major dynamic relationships. The family, close friends, the work environment and, in many instances, the medical environment often constitute the most important systems, and interact with the identified patient. The emergency or crisis arises in the ecological group, the breakdown more often being that of an unstable social system than merely that of an unstable person.

Mary's entire family situation was unstable and precarious. Nine months following her admission to hospital her son was brought to the emergency department after he threatened to kill himself during another domestic argument.

CRISIS THEORY

In dealing with psychiatric emergencies the emphasis has shifted from the mere disposition of patients, to case finding, to brief but definitive treatment, and to preventive work. Crisis theory and crisis intervention provide a useful framework for the assessment and management of psychiatric emergencies.

Crisis theory, as originated by Lindemann (1944) and developed by Caplan (1964), recognized that most people and their ecological groups usually deal adequately with problem situations and maintain equilibrium by using their habitual coping mechanisms. Crisis occurs when there is an imbalance between the magnitude and importance of the problem (the hazardous event) and the resources and coping mechanisms available to deal with it. The term "crisis" generally indicates a disruption of adaptation, in which the customary problem solving techniques do not work. The crisis emerges as an acute, unexpected upheaval in a previously stable equilibrium and, in proportion to the intensity of the upset, it poses a threat to the individual and/or social system. For the individuals in the social system a state of psychological helplessness, coupled with anxiety, fear and panic may be the result. The individual in the crisis situation is vulnerable because of the magnitude of the hazardous event, reduced capacity to adapt to the particular stress, or sociodynamic factors in the ecological group and is fortunately accessible to helpers during this phase of intense disequilibrium. The patient's vulnerability makes the help of outside persons practically always necessary. Such help is termed "crisis intervention."

Crisis intervention, therefore, can be defined as systematic professional (and non-professional) aid to the individual and/or social system in acute psychological disequilibrium. If such help is successful, there is not only a reduction of distress but also often a growth process resulting in a high level of functioning. The problem-solving capacity of the individual and the social system has been increased. If the crisis is not mastered, the result can be regression in the individual, with the onset or exacerbation of psychiatric illness, and disintegration in the social system.

From this perspective, crises must be regarded not as nuisances but as situations full of potential for growth. The crisis, mobilizing emotions and energies, can provide leverage for change, and act as a catalyst which disturbs old habits, evokes new responses and becomes a major force in charting new developments. The motivational force of the crisis and the dynamics for change, which exist in the open state of the organism in crisis—in sharp contrast to the non-crisis state—can facilitate the accomplishment of maximum change with minimum effort. The readiness of the individual to reach out to others for help, and the helping responses his distress evokes in others are positive forces for change.

The usual process of response to a crisis is short, lasting approximately six weeks. In crisis intervention and therapy, therefore, brevity is essential and professional steps including assessment, intervention and termination must take place rapidly within a limited time.

ASSESSMENT

The fundamental objective of the emergency assessment is to gather information as a basis for defining the problem or problems, identifying the desired outcomes and suggesting means of achieving them. In defining the problem the key questions are: "Why now?"; "Why does this person present with this problem, at this setting, at this time?"; "Whose emergency is it—the patient who is disturbed, or the environment which finds him disturbing?".

The information relevant to the patient's present psychological, social, and biological functioning must be obtained by interviewing the patient, family members, and others who accompany him. Ideally, this is done in calm surroundings which afford privacy though often the examination takes place in crowded and busy cubicles of emergency departments. The date of commencement or exacerbation of the symptoms should be ascertained as accurately as possible. A thorough mental status examination is important. This will include evaluation of the anxiety level, ego functioning, alterations in emotional state and tone, suicidal or homicidal potential, and presenting symptoms.

In order to consider the patient within his ecological group, the current life situation must be well explored and understood. This includes living and work arrangements, and interpersonal relationships with emphasis on recent changes in these areas. Of particular significance are actual or threatened losses to which the patient may be reacting. Detailed inquiry is made of the previous coping mechanisms and responses of both the individual and the ecological group to problems of similar nature, and why these coping mechanisms have failed in the present instance.

> Harvey, a 32 year old writer working for a broadcasting department, came to the emergency department on his own on a Monday afternoon. He was tearful and explained that he had had hardly any sleep in the previous three nights. He had a deadline for a screenplay but he had done no work during the weekend as he was unable to concentrate. He emphasized that he was homosexual, that he had come to terms with it and did not want that changed. For the past four years he lived with his lover in a house they had bought, and he described the relationship with him as satisfactory from the social, financial, and sexual point of view. However, on Friday, 3 days before Harvey came to the emergency department, his lover told him that he had a relationship with another man, that he preferred to be free to relate to others, and that he was planning to move out in two weeks. They had a lengthy discussion and were able to reach agreement on the financial aspects regarding the house and the furniture. That night Harvey felt upset and drank four bottles of beer and half a bottle of whiskey. He slept three hours. The following day he felt depressed and at times tearful. He tried to work at home, but he could not concentrate, his mind wandering on events of his past life. He felt rejected by his friend and could not come to terms with the proposed separation. Around lunch time he began drinking. He

> slept for two to three hours at night and when Sunday came he was feeling more depressed and tearful. He made an attempt to persuade his lover not to leave but the latter was insistent. He drank again, though less, and slept restlessly for three hours. On Monday morning he went to work, but he could not concentrate, and was tearful. He spoke to a fellow writer who took him out for lunch and suggested to him that he should see a psychiatrist. Harvey had been a heavy drinker for a period of six years during his twenties. However, in the past four years he had remained abstinent, and he attributed this to the relationship described above.

> Harvey was an only child. His mother was 40 years old and his father 45 when Harvey was born. When Harvey was 8 years old his father died from a heart attack. Harvey was raised by his mother and grandmother, and he was close to both of them. He had no previous psychiatric contact. During the interview in the emergency department he was tearful and distressed. He spoke at some length about his relationship and stressed that he could not cope with the thought that it was ending. He feared he might start drinking heavily again. He was concerned about the lack of sleep and asked for sleeping pills. He had no suicidal ideation. Harvey agreed to engage in individual psychotherapy twice a week as an outpatient for a period of two months.

The evaluation of the medical status of the patient is crucial. For example, many physical conditions (hypoglycemia, bronchopneumonia), brain syndromes (epilepsy, encephalitis), prescribed medications (phenothiazines, barbiturates) and drugs which have not been prescribed (amphetamines, L.S.D.) can often cause psychiatric emergencies. A careful review of systems and a physical examination are, therefore, essential parts of the assessment of psychiatric emergencies.

> Domenico, a 27 year old overweight schizophrenic man, was brought to the emergency department by his mother at about 8 p.m. His mother explained that Domenico could not eat at supper time because he had difficulty in swallowing, and his head had turned to the right. While coming to the hospital, he told her that he had some difficulty in breathing and that his tongue was going into his mouth. On examination, he could not pro-

trude his tongue, his neck was stiff and his head was turned 45 degrees to the right. On physical examination there was cogwheel rigidity in both arms. The patient said he was fine until 6 p.m. At about 10 a.m. he had been given fluphenazine decanoate 50 mg intramuscularly. This injection was his third and he had not required antiparkinsonian medication before. The diagnosis was made of an acute extrapyramidal syndrome due to fluphenazine. He was given benztropine mesylate 2 mg I.V. and within 15 minutes he was able to move his tongue and swallow well; the experienced difficulty in breathing disappeared, and he was able to move his head. However, a degree of cogwheel rigidity remained. He was given benztropine mesylate 2 mg tablets and was asked to take one twice a day.

MANAGEMENT

In the management of psychiatric emergencies the following crisis intervention techniques are stressed.

Definition of the problem. Defining the problem and clarifying it to the patient and his family in concise and understandable language are essential steps in intervention, and often reduce anxiety.

Focus on the current problems. The focus is on the current life situation with a view to providing help in coping with current problems. The emphasis is on improvement of the present emergent situation, rather than on cure of longstanding antecedent problems. These, if required, can be tackled once the crisis is resolved.

> The focus in brief psychotherapy with Harvey was the separation and what it meant to him. Loss, abandonment and rejection were key themes in therapy. These themes had roots in Harvey's childhood experiences. These were explored, however, only inasmuch as they were related to his present problem. The focus was on resolving the present problem and coping with the crisis rather than the childhood traumata.

Task mastery should be encouraged and fostered. The patient, in most crises, should be assisted to overcome his problem by confronting it, despite the unpleasant affect that this might arouse. Meaningless activities are discouraged. The patient is encouraged to explore actively alternative ways of viewing and solving the problem.

A systems or ecological group approach to therapy. Identification of the members of the ecological group is required. The intervention should be family focused, with involvement of key members as soon as possible. In face to face conjoint meetings of the patient, the family and therapist, open communication about problems and expression of pertinent feelings is encouraged.

> During Mary's brief admission, following individual interviews with her son and her boyfriend, the three of them were seen in joint family meetings. The purpose of these meetings was to explore the way in which they related to one another and resolve some of their difficulties which were partly at a feeling level and partly at a practical level. The meetings continued after Mary was discharged, and her 16 year old daughter, who played an important role in the family dynamics, joined in.

Family supports are preserved whenever possible. Mobilization of outside supports, such as the help of friends, clergy, etc., and linkages with appropriate community agencies are instituted.

Goals of treatment are time-limited. This is important for the patient and his family and, not infrequently, for the staff. The patient is encouraged in the idea that there is a limited time in which to come to grips with difficulties which must not be allowed to become chronic. Nor must the patient's family and friends begin to regard him as a hopeless psychiatric casualty.

Timing of therapy. Therapeutic contacts should be frequent, and, if necessary, short rather than infrequent and lengthy. Often it is appropriate for patient and therapist to collaborate in deciding this, as well as the form of treatment, and even the need for, or continuation of hospitalization. At other times these must remain professional decisions.

Harvey's therapy was time-limited, with well defined goals. The therapy sessions were frequent; they occurred twice a week.

Medication. With some patients, psychotropic agents are employed early for symptomatic relief. Medication is used for alleviating ego-alien symptoms and facilitating rapid return to premorbid levels of functioning. Being able to maintain role performance, and to obtain the needed sleep and anxiety reduction to effect this, are integral parts of crisis intervention.

Techniques of rapid neuroleptization have been developed recently (Ayd, 1977), permitting rapid control of acute psychotic symptoms, such as delusions, hallucinations, agitation, destructiveness, etc. The neuroleptics used are the short acting ones, specifically haloperidol, or the piperazine phenothiazines such as trifluoperazine or fluphenazine. These are administered intramuscularly hourly, until the target symptoms are controlled. Rarely is it necessary to continue the intramuscular neuroleptics beyond six to twelve hours. The following day treatment is continued with oral doses. The oral daily dosage should be 1.5 times the amount that was given the first day by injection. This dosage is continued for two to three days and then gradual reduction begins until the optimum amount is reached. With many patients medication will not be required and psychotherapeutic techniques will be both preferable and sufficient.

Crisis intervention and crisis therapy techniques are employed from the time of assessment and are continued in outpatient follow-up, or if necessary, on an inpatient basis. Some hospitals have developed small (6 to 12 beds) brief-stay inpatient units for the crisis management of psychiatric emergencies. These units operate on crisis intervention techniques, including time-limited stay which varies from 3—14 days.

Between 15 and 45% of psychiatric emergencies require immediate admission, and up to 60% are referred for outpatient psychiatric treatment. It is interesting to note that the number of those referred for immediate psychiatric admission is usually in inverse proportion to those referred for outpatient care. This possibly reflects the organization of the psychiatric services and the alternatives which are available to the emergency department staff.

The reader who wishes a detailed description of the manifestations and management of specific psychiatric emergencies should consult Bridges (1971) and Glick et al. (1976).

REFERENCES

Ayd, F. (1977): Guidelines for using short-acting intramuscular neuroleptics for rapid neuroleptization. *Int. Drug Ther. Newsletter.* 12:5.

Bartolucci, G., and Drayer, C.S. (1973): An overview of crisis intervention in the emergency rooms of general hospitals. *Am. J. Psychiatry.* 130:953.

Bridges, P.K. (1971): *Psychiatric Emergencies: Diagnosis and Management.* Springfield, Ill., C. C Thomas.

Caplan, G. (1964): *Principles of Preventive Psychiatry.* New York, Basic Books.

Caplan, G. and Grunebaum, H. (1967): Perspectives on primary prevention: a review. *Arch. Gen. Psychiatry.* 17:331.

Glasscote, R.M., Cumming, E., Hammersley, D.W., et al. (1966): *The Psychiatric Emergency: A Study of Patterns of Service.* Washington, D.C., The Joint Information Service, A.P.A. and N.A.M.H.

Glick, R.A., Meyerson, A.T., Tobins, E. et al. (1976): *Psychiatric Emergencies.* New York, Grune & Stratton.

Lindemann, E. (1944): Symptomatology and management of acute grief. *Am. J. Psychiatry.* 101:141.

Lowy, F.H., Wintrob, P.M., Borwick, B., et al. (1971): A follow-up study of emergency psychiatric patients and their families. *Compr. Psychiatry.* 12:36.

Miller, W.B. (1968): A psychiatric service and some treatment concepts. *Am. J. Psychiatry.* 129:924.

Morrice, J.K.W. (1968): Emergency psychiatry. *Br. J. Psychiatry.* 114:485.

Voineskos, G. (1974): Psychiatric emergencies: the crisis intervention approach. *Univ. Tor. Med. J.* 51:85.

Whitely, J.S., and Denison, D.M. (1963): The psychiatric casualty. *Br. J. Psychiatry.* 109:488.

31

Suicide and Attempted Suicide

George Voineskos and Frederick H. Lowy

The evaluation of the potential for suicide is one of the major responsibilities of a physician. It is a common problem. In the United States between 25,000 and 30,000 people die each year from suicide. In Canada 2,773 people took their own lives in 1973, giving a crude death rate from suicide of 12.7 per 100,000 population. Allowing for underreporting in official statistics, it is not unreasonable to assume that the true figure was around 3,500, a death rate from suicide of the same order as the combined rates from bronchitis, emphysema, and asthma, and exceeding the separate death rates from hypertensive disease, carcinoma of the breast, leukemia, rheumatic heart disease, and cirrhosis of the liver.

During the past few decades suicide rates have continued to increase, the rise being more pronounced among the young. Death from suicide in those between 15 and 30 years old ranks second among all causes, being exceeded only by motor vehicle accidents. In Ontario 30% of the officially classified suicide deaths in 1975 were people under the age of 30.

SOCIOLOGICAL AND PSYCHOLOGICAL THEORIES

Besides medicine, suicide has attracted the attention of theology, philosophy, an-thropology, psychology, sociology and so on. The French sociologist Emil Durkheim's monumental work on suicide is just as important today as it was in 1897 when it was first published. Durkheim suggested that suicide was explicable etiologically with reference to "the social structure, and its ramifying functions." Of the types of suicide that he described the most commonly recognized are the egoistic and the anomic. The *egoistic* type results from lack of social integration. Individuals are either not integrated into or become divorced from society and from their social groups such as family, religious, and political groups, thereby losing their sense of belongingness and social involvement. *Altruistic* suicide, the antithesis of the egoistic, represents instances where the individual is overly integrated in the society. The *anomic* type refers to loss of societal regulation; societal values and customary norms of behavior lose their force, thereby leaving the individuals with no standards to guide them in times of stress. The *fatalistic*, the antithesis of the anomic type, refers to overregulation of the individual by the social group.

Freud viewed suicide as a failure to externalize aggressive feelings which are turned inward. The individual turned back on himself the repressed anger toward a love object. Zilboorg (1935) suggested that suicide was an attempt to thwart frustrating external forces, to gain immortality and to maintain the ego rather than to destroy it. Other psychodynamic conceptions of suicide speak of an attempt to punish specific external forces or objects, or view it as retroflexed anger and self-punishment with atonement or expiation as goals.

SOME CHARACTERISTICS OF SUICIDE AND ATTEMPTED SUICIDE

Suicide is more common among men than women (a ratio of 3:2). For men there is almost a linear increase with age, while for women the suicide rate begins to drop after 65. Upper class males have higher rates than lower class males at all ages up to about 65, at which point the pattern is reversed. The divorced constitute the group with the highest rate, followed by the single and the widowed. Suicide is more common among those suffering from social isolation or from physical handicaps limiting daily activities. Suicide is higher among the unemployed, particularly those without a personal or social network of supportive relationships.

Among the psychiatric illnesses, affective disorders contribute the highest toll to suicide. It is estimated that those suffering from major affective disorders carry a risk of dying by suicide 30 times higher than the general population, and have a 15% eventual mortality rate by suicide. Alcoholism, with an estimated 5 to 10% eventual mortality by suicide, and psychopathy are the other two major contributors. Suicide in schizophrenia is less frequent but when it does occur it is often a very determined act.

Attempted suicide is much more frequent than suicide, a conservative ratio being 10:1. Higher rates have been reported. A study from London, Ontario gave a crude annual attempt rate of 730 per 100,000 population.

In contrast to completed suicide, attempted suicide is more common in women than in men (a ratio of 2:1). Suicide attempters tend to be young, about 50% being under 30 years. Stengel's classic work based on data from the late 1950's and early 1960's put the peak age for attempted suicide between 24 and 44. Recent studies have shown that the peak has moved downward to between 20 and 25. The divorced and the separated are most at risk for attempted suicide. Attempted suicide is also more common among unemployed males, and it is higher in the lower social classes.

An acute situational reaction involving interpersonal stress is the most common precipitant of suicide attempts. Depression is the most frequently recorded diagnosis among attempters, accounting for 35 to 79%. Alcoholism becomes a major factor among early middle age men. Persons suffering from adolescent crises, young women with hysterical personality disorders, and delinquent young men are well represented.

Suicide attempts are frequently preceded by excessive alcohol intake (Weissman, 1974. Holding et al., 1977). Most attempts are unplanned and impulsive, with little opportunity to clarify objectives. Motivations are multiple, confused, and often contradictory. A strong ambivalence between the wish to live and the wish to die has often been noted. Stengel called attention to the underlying wish to resolve an unbearable, intrapsychic or interpersonal situation and get help, rather than to die. The suicide attempt is often a "cry for help" as pointed out by Stengel and Cook (Stengel, 1967) and by Shneidman (Farberow and Shneidman, 1961).

Since the time of Durkheim, at the turn of the century, it has been known that there is a seasonal variation in the incidence of suicide, the cause of which is still not clear. In Europe, Canada, and the northern United States suicide rates peak in the spring; the same is also the case with hospital admissions for depressive illness.

METHOD OF SUICIDE AND ATTEMPTED SUICIDE

The most common method in the United States, Canada, Britain, and Australia is poisoning by the ingestion of drugs, which accounts for a least one-third of suicides and well over two-thirds of suicide attempts. The drugs used in each country are those most widely prescribed or available there. Not surprisingly barbiturates are well ahead on the list, followed by analgesics, including aspirin, and by newer psychotropic drugs, including minor tranquillizers. Firearms are the second leading cause of death from suicide, and, for males, of the same order of frequency as poisoning.

ASSESSMENT AND MANAGEMENT

No attempt or threat at suicide should ever be dismissed as trivial. Kreitman (1973) suggests that more effective attention should be paid to suicidal hints or threats in view of the fact that a considerable number of people who commit suicide have communicated their suicidal ideas or plans beforehand to a physician, relative or close friend (Kreitman, 1973, Robins et al., 1959, Rudestam, 1971). It is essential to remember that the "medical seriousness" of a suicide attempt, while it impresses clinicians and the public alike, is no predictor of the likelihood of further attempts or of death from one of these. Nor is there any association between the toxicity or amount of injury sustained by the patient during an attempt and the severity of the psychiatric illness.

A complete psychiatric evaluation should be made including mental status and the social circumstances of the individual. Interviewing members of the family or significant others is essential, since shame and social disapproval frequently lead to denial and minimization of the suicidal act by the individual patient.

In assessing suicidal risk we are now past the stage of subjective clinical intui-

TABLE 9 ASSESSING SUICIDE POTENTIAL

Take all attempts or threats seriously.
Perform complete psychiatric evaluation.
Ask about suicidal intent and plans.
Interview "significant others" (family, friends).
Ask about consequences of suicide (to family, friends, business, etc.)
Ask about alternative solutions.
Know high risk factors.

tion, which must be complemented by knowledge of factors known to be associated with high suicidal risk. The more closely a patient who attempts suicide approximates the demographic and clinical characteristics of those who commit suicide, as described earlier, the higher the suicide risk. Particularly vulnerable among patients with an affective disorder are those who had childhood or recent bereavements, and those with marked guilt feelings, ideas of unworthiness and feelings of hopelessness. Previous suicide attempts, a history of previous psychiatric treatment, depression and the heavy use of alcohol are highly associated with suicidal acts (Johnson et al., 1973). Bagley and Greer (1971) were able to predict 80% of repeaters by identifying the presence of five variables: antisocial personality, organic brain syndrome, previous attempts, marital status of widowed, separated or divorced, and membership in higher social class. Of those attempting suicide, between 20 and 30% make further attempts within 12 months (WHO, 1968). Persons who make an attempt are at a much higher risk of death by suicide in the future than those who do not. The death rate from suicide among attempters who had initially been hospitalized following an attempt has been estimated at about 1 per cent per year (Weissman, 1974). It has been estimated that the eventual mortality rate for those who have attempted suicide is 20% (Dorpat and Ripley, 1967). The suicide risk appears to be higher during the first two years after the attempt, espe-

TABLE 10   MANAGEMENT OF SUICIDAL ATTEMPT

General Principles
1. Preserve life—medical and surgical measures.
2. Establish therapeutic alliance with patient and relatives.
3. Hospitalize when necessary—involuntary admission may be required—treat psychiatric, social and medical problems vigorously.
4. When hospitalization is not necessary
   —plan for crisis resolution.
   —provide or arrange for psychological and environmental support.
   —arrange for "lifeline" if emergency recurs.
   —arrange for follow-up or referral.

cially the first three months, and it plateaus thereafter.

In management, preservation of life is the immediate goal, using appropriate immediate medical measures and subsequent admission to a psychiatric facility, if required. At times admission may have to be arranged on an involuntary basis under mental health regulations. Since "suicide attempt" is not a diagnosis, ascertaining the nature of the psychiatric disorder, if there is one, and/or the situational crisis that led to the act, will permit intervention aimed at treating the psychiatric disorder or altering the environmental situation. Such intervention is the next goal in management. A most important point in the management of the patient is the diagnosis and vigorous treatment of psychiatric illness, particularly affective disorders. Barraclough (1972) has estimated that if the recurrent depressives among a group of suicides had been treated prophylactically with lithium, one-fifth of the deaths might have been prevented.

For the physician providing emergency psychological support Littman (1957) has the following useful suggestions: establishing communication with the patient, reminding the patient of his identity, involving family and friends, and stimulating toward constructive action. He further suggests that psychological support is

transmitted by a firm and hopeful attitude. Hope is a powerful medicine which should never be withheld.

The physician should remember that what often hampers management is that attempters show an excess of generalized hostility and generate considerable hostility among those around them. However, those who accept psychiatric treatment following the act do better than patients who do not, and those who eventually commit suicide tend to be people who have not become involved in treatment.

The non-psychiatric physician who is aware of these characteristics of suicide attempters and recognizes the overt signal, has the best opportunity for early case finding, since many potential suicidal persons are frequent attenders of medical outpatient clinics and have frequent hospitalizations. Motto and Green (1958) found that 17% of those who committed suicide and 40% of the attempters had seen a physician within a month of their act, and that almost 50% of the former and 60% of the latter had seen a physician within the previous six months. Robins et al. (1959) reported similar findings. Here, then, is an unusually challenging public health problem for the physician and other health workers.

Kreitman (1973) suggests that one of the main priorities in suicide prevention must be to increase the capacity of medical students and general practitioners to recog-

TABLE 11   PREVENTION OF SUICIDE

1. Never forget to inquire about suicidal ideation and previous suicide attempts.
2. Know high risk factors.
3. Do not be talked out of hospitalizing high risk patients.
4. Do not prescribe lethal amounts of drugs, particularly antidepressants, when risk is high.
5. Do not prescribe barbiturates as hypnotics.
6. Do not stop anti-depressant drugs abruptly or prematurely.
7. Beware of sudden well being in depressed patients.
8. Work to reduce availability of firearms.

nize high risk cases. The same is true for social workers, lawyers, clergymen and others, who often are the people to whom the future suicide first turns.

Physicians can take two steps in their prescribing practices which will contribute to primary prevention. First, they must cease prescribing barbiturates as hypnotics; not only are barbiturates no longer the drugs of choice as hypnotics but also such a step could help remove a very lethal drug which is still the most popular suicidal poison. Second, psychotropic medication, particularly antidepressants during the early phase of outpatient treatment, should not be prescribed in lethal quantities. It is far safer to prescribe for a week at a time rather than four weeks. While skeptics might argue that removal of a lethal agent will result in its replacement by another, it should be remembered that impulsivity is a frequent feature in many suicidal acts, and that the suicide rate in Britain was reduced by almost 50% when the domestic coal gas was replaced by a mixture that contained no carbon monoxide.

Restriction of the availability of firearms should be seen as an important objective of primary prevention for every citizen; the 25% increase of suicide by firearms in Metropolitan Toronto from 1974 to 1975 is just one supportive illustration for such an objective.

REFERENCES

Bagley, C. and Greer, S. (1971): Clinical and social predictors of repeated attempted suicide: a multivariate analysis. Br. J. Psychiatry. 119:515.

Barraclough, B. (1972): Suicide prevention, recurrent affective disorders and lithium. Br. J. Psychiatry. 121:391.

Dorpat, T.L., Ripley, H.S. (1967): The relationship between attempted suicide and committed suicide. Comprehensive Psychiatry. 8:74.

Durkheim, E. (1951): Suicide: A Study in Sociology. Glencoe, Ill., Free Press.

Farberow, N.L. and Shneidman, E.S. (1961): The Cry for Help. New York. McGraw-Hill.

Freud, S. (1951): Mourning and melancholia. In The Standard Edition of the Complete Psychological Works of Sigmund Freud. Vol. 4. London, Hogarth Press.

Greer, S., and Bagley, C. (1971): Effect of psychiatric intervention in attempted suicide: a controlled study. Br. Med. J. 1:310.

Holding, T.A., Buglass, D., Duffy, J.C., et al. (1977): Parasuicide in Edinburgh—a seven year review 1968–1974. Brit. J. Psychiatr. 130:534.

Johnson, F.G., Ferrence, R., and Whitehead, P.C. (1973): Self-injury: identification and intervention. Can. Psychiatr. Assoc. J. 18:101.

Kreitman, N. (1973): Social and clinical aspects of suicide and attempted suicide. In Companion to Psychiatric Studies. Vol. 1. Edited by A. Forrest. Edinburgh, Churchill Livingstone.

Littman, R.E. (1966): Acutely suicidal patients: management in general practice. Calif. Med. 104:168.

Motto, J.A., and Green, C. (1958): Suicide and the medical community. Arch. Neur. Psychiatry. 80:776.

Robins, E., Gassner, S., Kayes, J., et al. (1959): Communication of suicidal intent: a study of 134 cases of successful (completed) suicide. Am. J. Psychiatr. 115:724.

Robins, E., Murphy, G.E., Wilkinson, R.H., et al. (1959): Some clinical considerations in the prevention of suicide based on a study of 134 successful suicides. Amer. J. Public Health. 49:888.

Rudestram, K.E. (1971): Stockholm and Los Angeles: a cross cultural study of the communication of suicidal intent. Journal of Cons. and Clinic Psychology. 36:82.

Stengel, E. (1967): Suicide and Attempted Suicide. Harmondsworth, Penguin.

Weissman, M. (1974): The epidemiology of suicide attempts 1960 to 1971. Arch. Gen. Psychiatry. 30:737.

World Health Organizaiton (1968): Prevention of Suicide: Public Health Paper #35. Geneva, WHO.

Zilboorg, G. (1935): Suicide among civilized and primitive races. Am. J. Psychiatry. 92:1347.

CHAPTER 32

Treatment: General

Frederick H. Lowy

Since treatment in psychiatry is based on the same principles as is medical treatment in general, it seems best to review those principles before discussing the problems and techniques that are specific to psychiatric treatment.

1. Treatment is most likely to succeed when it follows a sound diagnosis. That observation implies not only that the clinical problem has been labelled as accurately as the current state of knowledge permits but also that other diagnostic possibilities have been considered and ruled out, particularly those that are life threatening and treatable.

2. Treatment is based on an understanding of etiological factors to the extent that those factors are known and discernible. Although the precise causes of most psychiatric disorders are not known, current concepts of psychobiology and psychodynamics usually permit the identification of important predisposing, precipitating or contributing factors in a given patient's illness. When those factors are delineated and a formulation is made of why and how the patient became ill at the time that he did, it is easier to decide when to intervene. Almost all psychiatric disorders result from multiple causes and they usually require a multiple-treatment approach that is directed at those contributing biological, psychological, familial and sociocultural factors that can be changed.

3. Treatment must be individualized. The advantage of having an accurate diagnosis is that the physician can categorize the patient's illness and behavior with other illnesses he has treated or learned about and whose responses to various treatments are known. That permits a routinization that makes for efficient as well as effective treatment. (Not all hernias call for the same operative procedure and the same drug dosage can have quite different effects in different patients). Yet the best treatment is one that is tailored to the individual. That is particularly the case in psychiatry (and especially in psychotherapy), where the object of the clinician's concern is not an isolated area of tissue damage or even a diseased organ system but a malfunctioning, complex person.

4. The results of treatment depend on the mobilization of the patient's defenses and strengths, which must be as carefully assessed as the pathogenic stressors. "Host factors" are as important in psychiatry as they are in immunology; host factors determine the selection of a program

of psychotherapy just as they determine whether a kidney transplant should be done.

5. Treatment in psychiatry, as in all of medicine, more often leads to the patient's adaptation to his disability than to his complete cure. It is a truism that physicians cure sometimes, relieve often, and comfort always. When confronted with a psychiatric disorder, the physician rarely has the satisfaction of a job completed such as he would get from having removed a diseased appendix or having successfully treated a bacterial pneumonia. A more accurate analogy is to the treatment of diabetes mellitus and its complications or of congestive heart failure due to non operable disease. In those conditions and in most psychiatric disorders, the challenge is to restore the patient's physical and mental homeostasis to the best level possible.

6. Treatment by specific scientifically proven measures, when they are available, is superior to supportive therapy alone. Examples of such measures that are pertinent to the treatment of psychiatric disorders are: the replacement of metabolites, such as vitamin B12 and folic acid in delirium due to pernicious anemia; the use of drugs such as lithium carbonate in bipolar affective disorders; the use of behavior modification techniques, such as desensitization, in simple phobias; and the use of intensive psychotherapy, in some neuroses and personality disorders.

7. Treatment by non-specific supportive techniques is sometimes all the physician can offer. But even specific treatment is enhanced by the use of the non-specific, time honored healing arts. The sick patient suffers from the symptoms of his illness but also fears disability and death. He faces the shame of being dependent or the stigma of having mental illness and suffers from the consequences of his, at times maladaptive, attempts to cope with the disorder, and from irrational fantasies, and so on. Thus he is impelled to seek help from a professional, whom he endows with healing potential. The patient usually brings to the physician not only his symptoms but also the wish and the expectancy that he will be helped. That attitude favors the development of a positive therapeutic alliance that is helpful in all kinds of medical practice and indispensible in most kinds of psychotherapy.

8. Treatment should involve the patient's family unless the patient does not wish it or it is not in his interest. The patient's illness must be seen in the context of his social system to be fully understood and treated. Usually that means interviewing his family and enlisting their help in making the diagnosis and in treating and rehabilitating the patient. Sometimes psychotherapeutic treatment of the family, or part of the family, in a group is more effective than treating only the patient. Members of the patient's family are almost always concerned about him, and they deserve an explanation of and reassurance about the patient's illness that is consistent with the physician's obligation to protect the patient's privacy. The patient's family often feels frightened, guilty, ashamed or hopeless about the illness. The physician must see that they receive appropriate support and that any reactive illnesses they may have are prevented or diagnosed early.

THE THERAPEUTIC ALLIANCE

The therapeutic alliance is formed by two parties—the patient (or the family) that is being treated and the physician who is treating him. The physician has the advantage of having attributed to him the prestige, authority, and benevolence that all societies grant those who are designated as healers. But the physician does not keep that for long unless he reinforces it by his personality, attitude, and performance. Most good physicians intuitively build therapeutic alliances, but some otherwise capable physicians do not. Moreover, many psychiatric patients sorely test the alliance, often unwittingly, by acting toward the physician in hostile, suspicious, clinging, or seductive ways.

The therapeutic physician has the following attributes:

He is competent and knowledgeable.

He is able to inspire confidence.

He is able to emphathize accurately.

He genuinely wishes to help.

He is compassionate and warm but not possessive or smothering.

He is able to use himself as a therapeutic tool.

He is able to kindle hope.

He treats the patient as a person, not as an object.

The therapeutic alliance has the following attributes:

The patient and the therapist are committed to the alliance.

The patient and the therapist agree about the goals of treatment.

The patient and the therapist agree about the conditions of the treatment, such as schedules, place, procedures, and payment.

The patient and the therapist agree about confidentiality (including any limits to it).

The patient and the therapist trust each other.

The bedrock of the therapeutic alliance is the competence of the physician which is based on sound training and continuing upgrading of knowledge. But the practitioner must not only *be* competent; he must *be seen* as competent, and he must be able to inspire the patient's trust and confidence by maintaining a respectful, nonjudgmental attitude, by refraining from premature conclusions and, perhaps most important, by not amplifying or even participating in the patient's anxiety, shame, or despair. Every crisis, no matter how grave, can be contained if it cannot be resolved; and doing so calls for a calm, reassuring, and hopeful attitude on the part of the physician.

THERAPEUTIC TECHNIQUES

The techniques that are most useful in the managment of psychological symptoms and disturbed behavior are listed in Table 12. The techniques are divided into those used by all physicians, psychiatrists, and nonpsychiatrists alike (Table 12) and those ordinarily used by specialists— psychiatrists, other mental health professionals, and physicians with special interest and training in the field (Table 13).

Since a detailed consideration of techniques for specialists is beyond the scope of this book, they are discussed only briefly. The nonpsychiatric physician should be able to determine when a patient should be referred to a specialist for treatment and when the patient would be best cared for by his family physician or internist.

TECHNIQUES FOR ALL PHYSICIANS

All physicians can use supportive techniques, which are intended to strengthen the patient's coping capacity so as to permit him to master or at least adapt to the stresses that have disturbed his equilibrium. Their use is based on the assumption that in most psychiatric disorders the patient's characteristic defenses, although not adequate to deal with the stress at hand, continue to function to some extent. With support, the patient can mobilize his defenses and strengths so that he can carry on despite his difficulties. That is particularly true of patients with a reactive psychiatric illness, including acute situational stress reactions and many neurotic and psychophysiological disorders.

The physician too often does not give enough attention to the general supportive techniques and to supportive psychotherapy (Table 12) and relies too heavily on hypnotics and minor tranquilizers. Although prescribing drugs for troubled people is simpler for the physician, it is not recommended. Many patients become drug dependent, substituting pharmacological well being for real health.

The general supportive techniques listed in Table 12 can be remarkably helpful when they are prescribed wisely. However, like drugs, they must not be used indiscriminately. The techniques are most useful when they are employed either to reduce specific internal or external stresses that have been identified, or to strengthen specific defenses that are potentially available to the patient although he is not at present using them effectively. Like most medical prescriptions, the supportive techniques should be individualized.

A successful but harried 35 year-old businessman came for treatment with nonspecific somatic complaints and evidence of anxiety, tension, and depression. He had become short tempered and irritable. He complained of headaches, indigestion, and occasional diarrhea, and he had not slept well for several weeks. He had trouble concentrating and he found it harder and harder to keep up with the heavy work load at the office, where he both resented the additional demands that were made on his time and worried about his inability to satisfy them. He was preoccupied with morose thoughts, and unrealistically, he considered himself a failure.

His history showed no previous physical or psychiatric disorder. He had always been an intense, hard-working person who was eager to please others in order to gain their approval. He had always been exceedingly conscientious, and he became critical of himself when he was not sure that he was doing well in his work or as a husband, father, and son.

During the previous six months, he had been trying to master a new job, to which he had been promoted. The new job had coincided with greatly increased responsibilities in his personal life; his fourth child, unplanned, had been born four months before and his wife felt overburdened. In addition his father was convalescing from an almost fatal myocardial infarction.

Characteristically, the patient had attempted to deal with those challenges single-handedly by working hard at the office and being supportive to his wife and his parents, but his strategy did not work. He felt that he had not met his responsibilities and that he was letting everyone down. He had not had a vacation in three years, and in recent months he had felt guilty even about taking an evening or a weekend off. He pushed himself harder and harder until he felt he was on the point of collapse.

Working with those facts, which he gathered during two office visits in which he ruled out any physical illnesses and major affective disorders, the physician had to make a diagnosis and a plan of treatment. The patient obviously had a neurotic disorder in which depressive features predominated. The patient's habitual style of coping with his problems—attempting to master them by hard work—failed him when too many problems came at once. Knowing that he had not mastered his problems, especially those connected with his family, led him into a vicious cycle. Self-doubt and depression impaired his performance and led to self-criticism and more severe depression.

As discussed in the following paragraphs, the physician might use some or all of the methods listed in Table 12 to treat the patient.

GENERAL SUPPORTIVE MEASURES

The patient might be able to accept the physician's firm prescription to go on a vacation—even though the patient might feel "unable to go away at a time like this." Similarly, the physician might "order" the patient to incorporate periods of exercise or relaxation into his daily schedule.

The patient might be able to accept the physician's advice about his job, his father's illness or his wife's situation even though he had rejected similar suggestions when others made them. The physician might also interview the wife to determine whether she needs supportive treatment. Any of the steps just described might decrease the pressure on the patient and reduce the stress to a level he can handle.

MEDICAL SUPPORTIVE MEASURES

The physician might prescribe the use of minor tranquilizers (e.g. diazepam, chlordiazepoxide) for a specific period of time

TABLE 12   THERAPEUTIC TECHNIQUES IN PSYCHIATRY: METHODS FOR ALL PHYSICIANS

1. *General Supportive Measures*
   a. Prescribing activity
      (1) rest, vacations, exercise, daily routine, recreation and diversions, work, etc.
   b. Giving advice and guidance
      (1) specific suggestions to remove external stresses; change of job, living arrangements, family contacts
      (2) fostering socialization
   c. Modifying the environment
      (1) help in changing attitudes of other people in the patient's environment
      (2) referral of the patient to other professionals and institutions (social service agencies, unemployment insurance agency, etc.) or intercession with them on the patient's behalf
   d. Eliminating sources of inferiority and shame
      (1) by cosmetic surgery, retraining and rehabilitation, dermatological treatment, obesity control, etc.
2. *Medical Supportive Measures*
   a. Improving the patient's nutrition: advice about diet and judicious use of vitamins
   b. Improving sleep; use of hypnotics, sparingly
   c. Controlling the patient's pain and other symptoms of chronic illness: using analgesics and narcotics appropriately
   d. Controlling the patient's tension and anxiety: careful use of minor tranquilizers
3. *Supportive Psychotherapy*
   a. Creating a therapeutic alliance
   b. Listening to the patient and helping him to ventilate his feelings
   c. Reassuring and supporting the patient and giving him any explanation he needs
   d. Suggesting and persuading
   e. Improving communication with the patient's spouse or other family members by conjoint and family interviews
   f. Reinforcing the patient's adaptive defenses and eliminating his maladaptive defenses

to reduce the stress level, in conjunction with other measures. The short-term use of a hypnotic drug (e.g., flurazepam) may help to restore the patient's normal sleep patterns.

SUPPORTIVE PSYCHOTHERAPY

Supportive techniques can be used to strengthen the patient's coping capacity to the point where he achieves not only relief from his symptoms but even growth in his personality. The opportunity to talk about and face his situation with a sympathetic listener can bring the patient great relief. In the presence of an authority figure who is not critical or judgmental, the patient may be able to look at his problems and his performances more realistically and to admit and assess any feelings of shame, inadequacy, anger, and guilt. In a series of appointments that are at least 30 minutes long, the physician should create an atmosphere that encourages the patient to speak freely about himself. The physician should arrange not to be distracted by the telephone or other interruptions during the sessions. The physician should listen attentively to the patient and encourage him to express his feelings. The focus is usually on the patient's current problems, and attention is given both to what the patient thinks, feels, fears, and fantasizes about his problems and to what is happening in his relationships with people who are important to him. Consideration of the patient's current problems sometimes leads to discussions of his past problems. While those discussions can occasionally be helpful, it is usually best in supportive psychotherapy to center on those aspects of the past that are troublesome in the present, such as memories that still produce anxiety or shame or that illustrate coping patterns that are relevant to the patient's current problem. The therapist's techniques include listening empathically, encouraging ventilation, clarifying and explaining his symptoms, gently but firmly confronting the patient with the consequences of his actions and offering him suggestions, reassurance, and hope.

The patient's relationships with the people who are important to him should be examined. If those relationships are deteriorating, it is important to find out why. At times joint sessions with the patient's spouse and other members of his family are indicated. Such sessions might alleviate the patient's feeling of isolation and restore to him some of his sources of support and strength. The supports will be particularly important to the patient after he has completed the course of psychotherapy. As the patient gets better, he will tend to become more dependent on the physician. The dependency is inevitable and desirable during and immediately after the crisis. But the goal of psychotherapy is to help the patient to find gratification from "permanent" sources—his family, friends, job and so on. The physician who allows his patients to become unnecessarily dependent on him is doing a disservice to them and to himself.

In regard to the case example, the physician might have decided to refer the patient to a specialist for intensive psychotherapy if it became apparent that the patient's former level of functioning was less healthy than it seemed at first or if the patient did not respond satisfactorily to the measures described in the preceding paragraphs.

TECHNIQUES FOR SPECIALISTS

The techniques listed in Table 13 require more time and training than most non-psychiatric physicians have. Patients who require these techniques should be referred to a psychiatrist or another suitably trained psychotherapist, marital therapist, or behavior therapist.

TABLE 13   THERAPEUTIC TECHNIQUES IN PSYCHIATRY: METHODS FOR SPECIALISTS AND SPECIALLY TRAINED PRIMARY CARE PHYSICIANS

1. *Intensive Individual Psychotherapy*
   a.   Relationship therapies and re-educative therapies
   b.   Reconstructive therapies (including psychoanalysis)
   c.   Hypnotherapy and narcotherapy
   d.   Abreactive therapies
2. *Intensive Group Psychotherapy*
   a.   Abreactive therapies
   b.   Transactional analysis therapies
   c.   Psychoanalytically oriented group therapy
   d.   Intensive marital therapy and family therapy
3. *Advanced Behavior Therapy*
   a.   Desensitization techniques
   b.   Flooding
   c.   Advanced operant conditioning techniques
   d.   Aversive techniques
   e.   Biofeedback techniques
4. *The Use of Pharmacological Agents in Acute Psychosis*
   a.   Major neuroleptics, e.g. phenothiazines, thioxanthenes, butyrophenones
   b.   Antidepressants (tricyclic compounds and monoamine oxidase inhibitors)
   c.   Lithium carbonate
5. *Electroconvulsive Therapy*
6. *Psychosurgery*

FURTHER READINGS

Berne, E. (1964): *Games People Play.* New York, Grove Press.

Bruch, H. (1974): *Learning Psychotherapy.* Cambridge, Harvard Univ. Press.

Frank, J.D. (1961): *Persuasion and Healing.* Baltimore, Johns Hopkins Press.

Fromm-Reichmann, F. (1950): *Principles of Intensive Psychotherapy.* Chicago, Univ. of Chicago Press.

Jackson, D.D. and Weakland, J.H. (1961): Conjoint family therapy. *Psychiatry:* 24:30.

Lazarus, A. (1971): *Behavior Therapy and Beyond.* New York, McGraw-Hill.

Luborsky, L. et al. (1975): Comparative studies of psychotherapy—Is it true that "everyone has won and all must have prizes?" *Arch. Gen. Psychiat.* 32:995.

Marmor, J. (1975): The nature of the therapeutic process revisited. *Canad. Psychiatric Assoc. J.* 20:557.

Rogers, C.R. (1951): *Client-Centered Therapy. Its Current Practice, Implications and Theory.* Boston, Houghton-Mifflin Co.

Wolberg, L. (1971): *The Technique of Psychotherapy.* 3rd ed. New York, Grune & Stratton.

Wolpe, J. (1969): *The Practice of Behavior Therapy.* New York, Pergamon.

33

Treatment: Psychotherapy and Behavior Therapy

Frederick H. Lowy and Robert Pos

The therapeutic procedures most widely used in psychiatry are the psychotherapies and the behavior therapies. Both are attempts on the part of a trained professional (the therapist) to influence favorably the thinking, feeling and behavior of a patient by specific psychological techniques. Although some of these techniques involve aspects of ordinary human communication (listening, encouraging, clarifying, advising, and so on) formal psychotherapy and behavior therapy are specific procedures that have indications and contraindications, involve techniques that require formal training, and produce measurable results and side-effects.

These techniques have evolved historically from the comfort-giving activities of socially sanctioned healers found in all societies, such as priests, shamans, physicians, etc. To this heritage has now been added almost a century of recorded clinical experience and the research findings of social psychology and sociology, psychoanalysis, learning theory and cognitive psychology.

Unlike other medical and surgical procedures that affect the activity of specific biochemical systems, organs or organ systems, the psychotherapies and behavior therapies attempt to influence the functioning of an entire human being or family. Because of the incredible complexity of the interactions among the therapist, the patient and the environment, the scientific measurement of the process and outcome of these procedures has been extremely difficult. However, the advent of videotape recording, computers and modern statistical techniques has led to considerable progress in psychotherapy research in recent years. For the future there is the promise of much better delineation of the patient, therapist and technique variables that correlate with good outcome.

More than other therapeutic procedures in medicine, the psychotherapies are influenced by the personality and attitudes of the therapist as well as by socio-cultural factors. It is not surprising that some therapists are more successful than others, especially when treating certain problems and certain types of patients. It is tempting for these therapists to give undue credit to their particular theoretical perspectives and techniques and this has facilitated the development of a wide range of psychotherapies. But despite the existence of several large schools of psychotherapy and a larger number of variations, the approaches have more in common than they have differences. At present only broad guidelines are available for prescribing the type, frequency and duration of psychotherapy that is best for specific clinical problems but this is an area where progress can be anticipated as research techniques improve.

The major psychotherapeutic approaches used in America and Europe are classified in Table 14.

The dynamic therapies and behavior therapies are the most widely used of these groups, and they will be discussed briefly in this chapter. The discussion is introductory and for orientation and is mainly intended to facilitate the referral process (see Chap. 38). Additional information about these and the other psychotherapies may be obtained from the publications listed under Further Readings.

Psychotherapy is most often conducted in a professional office between a therapist and a single patient (*individual therapy*) but a therapist or two co-therapists may meet with 6 to 10 patients (*group therapy*) or with a marital couple or family (*conjoint or family therapy*). As might be expected, there are important modifications of technique specific to each of these modalities. However some goals, procedures and therapeutic stances are basic to all types of intensive psychotherapy.

INTENSIVE PSYCHOTHERAPY

The term "intensive psychotherapy" is used here in contrast to "supportive psychotherapy," as discussed in Chapter 32. It will be recalled that the goal of supportive psychotherapy is to strengthen the patient's coping capacities to permit a return to the premorbid level of functioning or to prevent further decompensation. In intensive psychotherapy the goal is more ambitious: to help the patient acquire better ways of functioning, including the capacity to deal effectively with those con-

TABLE 14   MAJOR PSYCHOTHERAPIES

A. Psychodynamic
   1. Psychoanalysis   ⎫ (Freudian and
   2. Psychoanalytic psychotherapy ⎭ Neo-Freudian)
   3. Analytical psychology—(Jungian)
B. Behavioral
   1. Systematic desensitization (Wolpe)
   2. Cognitive restructuring (Meichenbaum, etc.)
   3. Operant conditioning (Skinner)
   4. Modeling (Bandura)
   5. Biofeedback techniques
C. Existential-Humanistic
   1. Existential therapy (Binswanger, May)
   2. Logotherapy (Frankl)
   3. Client-centered therapy (Rogers)
D. Group and transactional
   1. Group psychotherapy
   2. Marital and family therapy
   3. Transactional analysis (Berne, Harris, Steiner)
   4. Psychodrama (Moreno)
E. Others—Some newer therapies
   1. Primal therapy (Janov)
   2. Gestalt therapy (Perls)
   3. Reality therapy (Glasser)
   4. Rational-emotive therapy (Ellis)

flicts that he was previously unable to master and that gave rise to symptoms. In the course of achieving this goal, patients usually experience personality growth, improved self esteem and better interpersonal relations. Thus the intensive psychotherapies are reconstructive therapies.

The difference between supportive and intensive psychotherapy might be clarified by a cardiovascular analogy. If a patient is subject to bouts of congestive heart failure, a search for the cause is undertaken. If the major cause is a correctable cardiac valvular defect then reconstructive surgery is indicated—provided that the patient is well enough to undergo the procedure, and that a trained surgeon and appropriate operating facilities are available. If the major causes of the cardiac decompensation cannot be reversed then long term medical management is undertaken, using digitalis, diuretics, and a variety of supportive measures. Similarly, when there is personality decompensation manifested by neurotic symptoms or a behavior disorder, intensive reconstructive psychotherapy is attempted if this is feasible. If not, supportive psychotherapy is offered as part of a rehabilitative regime.

Intensive reconstructive psychotherapy can require frequent (2 to 4) weekly sessions for up to several years when there are serious and pervasive character disturbances that have been present since childhood. But in recent years it has been demonstrated that some ambitious reconstructive goals can be met in brief intensive psychotherapy (12 to 20 sessions) that is focused narrowly on a single important area of malfunction.

PSYCHOANALYSIS AND PSYCHOANALYTIC PSYCHOTHERAPY

In North America for decades the most influential forms of intensive psychotherapy have been psychoanalysis and its derivates, the psychoanalytically oriented (dynamic) psychotherapies. Psycho-analysis is not only a particular type of intensive psychotherapy but also a comprehensive theory of human motivation and behavior, created primarily by the Viennese neurologist, Sigmund Freud. His work generated both enthusiastic followers and critics and has had a powerful impact beyond psychiatry, for example on education, child rearing practices, philosophy and literature. Of course its influence on the understanding of personality development and psychopathology and on the practice of psychotherapy has been immense.

The psychoanalytic psychotherapies are derived from psychoanalysis and they largely share its theoretical assumptions. Although there are many varieties of psychoanalytic psychotherapy, reflecting modifications to theory or practice proposed by Freud's colleagues and followers, they all share with psychoanalysis several basic assumptions. These include the following:

1. Human behavior is purposeful and motivated, but the person in question is not aware of all his motives, and indeed these are usually more evident to others than to himself.

2. Although some behavior is conflict free, adaptive and oriented to personal aspirations, other behavior is defensive and self-defeating. In addition to having to cope with external threats and painful life events, people feel threatened by some of their own desires and impulses which they have come to regard as unacceptable. When these impulses arise, they mobilize anxiety which acts as a signal that activates psychological defenses. These tend to be largely adaptive in healthy people and frequently maladaptive in those with serious psychiatric disorders.

3. Psychogenic symptoms result from attempts to cope with the anxiety arising from unresolved intrapsychic conflicts. Acute symptoms reflect the conflicting demands of the patient's wishes and drives on the one hand, and conscience-dictated

or reality-imposed prohibitions against them on the other. Chronic symptoms in addition are complicated by other factors, such as reinforcement by social rewards associated with the sick role.

4. Vulnerability to neuroses and personality disorders stems from constitutional factors interacting with traumatic childhood relationships. These factors distort the emotional, cognitive and social development of the child leading to reduced ability to master the developmental challenges of life, e.g. separation from parents, establishing personal identity, the changes of puberty and adolescence, marriage and so on.

5. There is a strong tendency to repeat again and again in challenging new situations the old maladaptive attempts to cope with unresolved problems. This leads to restricted stereotyped behavior and limits the degree of choice available to the person in many situations.

Technique. Psychoanalysis as a treatment has a highly structured format. There are three to five sessions per week, usually at a fixed time, and analyses often take a number of years to complete. Sessions last 45 or 50 minutes, the psychoanalyst sitting to the side or behind a couch on which the patient reclines. The only instruction to the patient is to try to say whatever comes to mind. This involves both free association of random thoughts and the relating of present and past life events, dreams and fantasies. The regular, structured and intense contact generates a climate in which the patient gradually comes in touch with feelings, impulses, memories and fantasies that were previously beyond awareness. The analyst facilitates this process and helps the patient understand how his symptoms, and indeed his personality traits, arose from attempts to cope with both external stresses and internal conflicts.

A number of nonspecific curative factors present in all psychotherapies are also at work in psychoanalysis, including ventilation and abreaction, learning, reassurance, suggestion and the support inherent in a prolonged relationship with a helping person. However, the major therapeutic activity of the psychoanalyst involves three additional processes: *confrontation*—bringing the patient face-to-face with aspects of himself that are revealed during the analysis but that he had hidden from himself; *interpretation*—explaining the feelings or behavior in question in relation to the patient's motives, both overt and covert; and *reconstruction*—linking all these with the patient's previous experiences and relationships, thereby filling gaps in his memory and in the continuity of experience produced by repression and other defense mechanisms.

In psychoanalysis (and indeed in all intensive psychotherapies) establishing a therapeutic alliance is of the utmost importance (see Chaps. 7, 32). In an atmosphere of trust and confidentiality, highly personal feelings and impulses are confided, often for the first time, and a relationship of considerable intensity develops. This facilitates the emergence of a process called "transference"—the tendency of the patient to behave towards the psychoanalyst or psychotherapist as he has behaved in previous relationships (e.g. with mother, brother, uncle, etc.) when there is nothing in the present treatment relationship that calls for this behavior. It is as though the patient has transferred to the analyst or therapist feelings that were held towards the person in the previous relationship. These misplaced feelings give rise to behavior that is inappropriate in the present treatment situation, though the feelings might well have been appropriate responses in the original relationship. The identification and analysis of these transference phenomena bring to light important fantasies, memories, attitudes and assumptions that determine aspects of the patient's behavior even though he has been unaware of them.

The technique in psychoanalytic

psychotherapy differs from psycho-analysis in several important respects. There are one to three sessions per week, the patient and therapist sit facing each other and the therapist tends to be more active. Instead of waiting for the unfolding of unconscious processes, the therapist confronts the patient more directly and generally focuses the flow of the session on specific problems. There is greater attention to problem solving than to reconstruction of gaps in the memory of past experience. Transference phenomena are noted by the therapist but he may or may not bring them to the patient's attention depending upon the therapeutic goals.

Indications. Psychoanalysis and intensive psychoanalytic psychotherapy are the treatments of choice for most severe neuroses and crippling personality disorders, provided the personality distortion is not extreme. That is, these treatments are probably not required for very mild neurotic disability and they are rarely curative (though they may help) where there is extreme personality distortion. In recent years there have been major efforts to modify the treatments to make them effective with a broader range of personality disorders. Psychotic patients are not generally considered good candidates for intensive psychotherapy, though there are exceptions. The patients who seem to benefit most from psychoanalysis and psychoanalytic psychotherapy are those who have had at least some healthy interpersonal relationships, who have some introspective capacity and curiosity about themselves. Since these treatments, especially classic psychoanalysis, require considerable tolerance for frustration and the need to work hard in therapy for quite some time before results are apparent, patients who demand quick solutions and immediate gratification have difficulty.

When intensive psychotherapy is successful, not only symptom relief but far reaching favorable life changes result. These can be quite dramatic. For example, a long standing hypochondriacal patient with a history of multiple physician contacts, many hospitalizations and psychogenic complaints that led to exploratory surgical procedures abandons a life of chronic patienthood; a persistent underachiever in school, work and interpersonal relationships becomes freed to realize his potential and begins to succeed; a bitter, chronically depressed, overweight and unpopular person with very low esteem and crippling neurotic symptoms is able to reverse these and achieves a normal life.

As with all powerful treatments, there are also side effects and treatment failures. The most common undesirable side effect is excessive dependency upon the therapy and the therapist, leading to therapeutic stalemate and interminable treatment. Further treatment does not produce further gains but when treatment is halted there is a return to crippling symptoms and a neurotic lifestyle. A variant of this is the situation where the patient focuses his attention inward to the point of totally ignoring important concrete problems in his life outside the therapy. The therapy here becomes an end in itself rather than the means to a more successful life.

As has been mentioned above, there are other forms of intensive therapy which do not derive primarily from Freudian psychoanalysis. Discussion of these treatments is beyond the scope of this chapter. The same is true of the use of adjuncts in psychotherapy such as hypnosis and narcotherapy (drug facilitated psychological exploration and treatment). Interested readers are referred to the bibliography at the end of this chapter.

BEHAVIOR THERAPY

Behavior therapy includes a group of procedures designed to directly alter undesired and maladaptive behavior, including both overt actions and "internal behavior" (thought, affects).

The focus is on behavior change *per se* rather than on searching for or providing insight into underlying motivation or intrapsychic conflicts.

The roots of this therapeutic approach lie in the experimental physiology and psychology laboratories of Pavlov, Thorndyke, Watson and Miller where the principles of behavior acquisition and change were delineated. These principles were then applied systematically to altering human maladaptive behavior by Eysenck in Britain, Wolpe in South Africa, Skinner in the United States, and their followers.

The behavioral approach is based on the premise that much of human behavior is the result of simple social learning, being dependent on such factors as conditioning through association, reinforcement, stimulus generalization, and modeling (imitation). Behavior which is learned can also be unlearned, or extinguished, by applying known principles of learning theory. Most behavior theorists today acknowledge that these principles, discovered experimentally with laboratory animals and healthy human volunteers, are not sufficient to understand and treat those psychiatric disorders which involve complex interactions of symbolic psychological factors, neurophysiological mechanisms, and social modifiers. Yet it is certainly true that neurotic symptoms, which originally resulted from such complex interactions—arising from attempts to defend against and cope with perceived threats (psychodynamic mechanisms)—can be perpetuated by internal and external reinforcement long after the original factors have ceased to be operative. Behavioral techniques are especially useful in such situations whereas attempts to gain insight into the psychodynamic roots of the problem can be lengthy, arduous and unproductive.

Technique. Once the decision has been made to use behavior modification techniques, the therapist proceeds in stages.

BEHAVIORAL ANALYSIS. The various psychological symptoms (fears, obsessional thoughts, etc.) or actions (excessive timidity, aggressive behavior, sexual dysfunction, etc.) to be altered are specifically identified together with the factors which precipitate, perpetuate and suppress them. Complex symptoms are broken down to components which themselves are studied with respect to precipitants. Usually the patient himself is enlisted as an ally, as self-observer in the process of behavioral analysis.

THERAPEUTIC CONTRACT. Once this analysis is complete, the therapist is in a position to propose specific attainable behavioral objectives that he and the patient agree to try to achieve. Such a "contract" ensures congruence regarding goals, an important feature of virtually all therapist-patient interactions, and also enlists the patient's active collaboration in the treatment.

CHOICE OF PROCEDURE. This will of course depend upon the types of behavior to be changed, the nature of the underlying disorder and the personality motivation and expectation of the patient. These techniques usually fall into four categories:

1. Response decrement procedures. These reduce the frequency of maladaptive behaviors occurring in the patient's current repertoire.

2. Response increment procedures. In this group of techniques desired behaviors which are occurring too seldom are caused to occur more frequently.

3. Response acquisition procedures. At times, patients do not have necessary behavioral skills in their repertoire and treatment is aimed at teaching them.

4. Cognitive restructuring. Phobic and other patients commonly have characteristic ways of thinking about their abilities and experiences which help to maintain their avoidance behaviors. Cognitive restructuring involves changing these ways of thinking.

A growing number of procedures of each type are becoming available as modern behavior therapists add methods derived from other psychotherapies and social therapies to those which originated in learning laboratories. Three of the most important techniques will be described briefly and the reader is referred to Lazarus and Wolpe for further details.

Systematic desensitization attempts to reduce the patient's sensitivity to stimuli that produce unwanted reactions, such as fears. Wolpe, who largely developed this method, stated, "If a response incompatible with anxiety can be made to occur in the presence of anxiety-evoking stimuli so that it is accompanied by a complete or partial suppression of the anxiety responses, the bond between these stimuli and the anxiety responses will be weakened." For example, fear of heights in a patient is analyzed into its components, and a hierarchy is constructed of situations which increasingly produce anxiety. With or without the aid of medication, the patient is then taught how to achieve deep muscle relaxation, a state incompatible with anxiety. While deeply relaxed, the patient is asked to imagine the least anxiety-provoking scene in the hierarchy, say climbing several flights of stairs in an office building. When he can do this without anxiety, the therapist asks him to vividly imagine the next scene, which might be to stand near a closed window on an upper story of the tall building. This is continued until it is possible for the patient to meet the objective, which might be to ply his trade as carpenter on a construction project. While the hierarchy is pursued in fantasy with the therapist, the patient has the tasks of continuing to rehearse the relaxation techniques he has learned and to carry out in his life situation the things he has mastered in the therapy. Desensitization can also be carried out in vivo with the therapist accompanying the patient in a "real life" progression toward the goals.

Flooding (or implosion therapy) involves immediately exposing the patient, in fantasy or in vivo, to the most anxiety producing situation in the hierarchy. For example, the carpenter is repeatedly asked to imagine, or taken to, a work situation on an exposed high building until he is progressively able to master the accompanying anxiety.

Operant conditioning techniques depend on the principle that behavior is determined by its consequences. Actions on the part of the patient that are positively reinforced in selective fashion are likely to be learned and will be repeated. For example, an institutionalized, regressed, chronic psychotic patient who is incontinent can be motivated to change by reinforcing attempts at continence, whether by praise and attention on the part of staff or by a tangible reward, e.g. a token which can be cashed in for candy. Or a patient with anorexia nervosa whose weight has fallen to dangerous levels can be motivated to eat by enforcing bed rest and making activity (in those patients who very much wish to be active) contingent upon weight gain.

Indications. Behavior modification techniques are now widely used, having been found effective in removing many troublesome neurotic symptoms (e.g. phobias). They have also been employed successfully, in combination with other measures, in the management of certain personality disorders (e.g. in passive, dependent, timid persons), sexual function disorders (e.g. in premature ejaculation, frigidity), somatoform and psychophysiological disorders (e.g. anorexia nervosa), chronic psychoses and conduct disorders of children.

When they are appropriately prescribed, behavior therapy techniques are highly effective. For example, the results in the treatment of uncomplicated phobias are probably the most impressive in psychiatry, with stable cure rates approaching 90%. Similarly, when combined with other approaches in more complex problems, behavioral methods can make a most valuable contribution. An example is the

Masters and Johnson technique for the treatment of sexual dysfunction which makes use of behavioral and physiological approaches together with marital psychotherapy.

FURTHER READINGS

A. *Psychodynamic Therapies*

Freud, S. (1933): *New Introductory Lectures on Psycho-Analysis*. Standard Edition of the Complete Psychological Works of Sigmund Freud, Vol. 22, 1964, London, Hogarth Press.

Greenson, R.R. (1967): *The Technique and Practice of Psychoanalysis. Vol. 1*. New York, International Universities Press.

Jung, C.G. (1968): *Analytical Psychology: Its Theory and Practice*. New York, Aronson.

Small, L. (1979): *The Briefer Psychotherapies*. New York, Brunner-Mazel.

B. *Behavioral*

Lazarus, A. (1971): *Behavior Therapy and Beyond*. New York, McGraw-Hill.

Masters, W.H. and Johnson, V.H. (1970): *Human Sexual Inadequacy*. Boston, Little, Brown.

Meichenbaum, D. (1977): *Cognitive Behavior Modification*. New York, Plenum Press.

Wolpe, J. (1974): *The Practice of Behavior Therapy*, 2nd Ed. New York, Pergamon.

C. *Existential-Humanistic*

Frankl, V. (1965): *The Doctor and the Soul*. New York, Knopf.

May, R., Angel, E., Ellenberger, H.F. (Eds.) (1958): *Existence*. New York, Basic Books.

Rogers, C.R. (1951): *Client-centered Therapy: Its Current Practice, Implications and Theory*. Boston, Houghton-Mifflin.

D. *Group and Transactional*

Minuchin. S. (1974): *Families and Family Therapy*. Cambridge, Harvard University Press.

Moreno, J.L., in *Comprehensive Textbook of Psychiatry/II. vol. 2*. Baltimore, Williams & Wilkins.

Steiner, C. (1973): *TA Made Simple*. Berkeley, Ca., Claude Steiner.

Yalom, I. (1970): *The Theory and Practice of Group Psychotherapy*. New York, Basic Books.

E. *Other Therapies*

Ellis, A., Harper, R.A. (1971): *A Guide to Rational Living in an Irrational World*. Englewood Cliffs, N.J., Prentice-Hall.

Glasser, W. (1965): *Reality Therapy*. New York, Harper and Row.

Perls, F.S. (1973): *The Gestalt Approach and Eye Witness to Therapy*. Ben Lomond, Ca., Science and Behavior Books, Inc.

Wolberg, L.R. (1975): Hypnotherapy in S. Arieti (Ed), *American Handbook of Psychiatry*, 2nd Ed. Vol. V. pp. 235–253. New York, Basic Books.

34

Treatment: Somatic

Edward Kingstone

ELECTROCONVULSIVE THERAPY

ECT is the use of electrical current to produce a grand mal seizure. In properly selected cases it can be shown that ECT is more effective than placebo in ameliorating the symptoms of depression. Furthermore, investigations have shown that the therapeutic effect of ECT is due to the convulsion, and not to fear of the use of electricity, or the anesthetic agent. Few if any treatments in the fields of psychiatry have stood the test of time better than ECT. Furthermore, no treatment has been subjected to such continuing outbursts of criticism and still has continued to remain available for the treatment of certain well delineated and indicated conditions. Until the advent of tricyclic antidepressant medication, no other effective therapy of severe and serious depression was available. Despite its safe and life-saving effectiveness and the progressive refinement of technique, there still exists an air of opprobrium about convulsive therapy in the minds of both professional and lay people. Much of the continued criticism stems from the perpetuation of erroneous beliefs about the application of this treatment, which bears no relationship to what actually transpires in modern psychiatric settings. One such be-

lief is that ECT is used to control and punish patients who do not conform to hospital rules and regulations. In actuality, ECT is known to be ineffective in dealing with personality disorders. Another misconception is that numerous attendants are needed to restrain a patient during the process of a violent seizure. This belief continues despite the use of muscle relaxants for over 20 years. A recent film, "One Flew Over the Cuckoo's Nest," perpetuates this false view: it also depicted convulsive therapy as capable of producing permanent, irreversible, massive brain damage akin to frontal lobotomy. Partly because of this widespread and widely held sentiment, convulsive therapy tends to be a treatment of last resort.

Of course, no pill or physical treatment can resolve psychological conflicts, or remove the inevitable sadness and distress that is bound to be encountered in everyday life.

ECT is frequently referred to as an empirical therapy; that is to say, one which works but whose method of action is still under debate. Until the advent of the major tranquilizers and tricyclic antidepressants, ECT was widely used in the treatment of all psychoses. Its use is limited now to certain resistant forms of depression and to other psychoses where drugs are temporarily inadequate.

ECT may, occasionally, have some side-effects. Initially, there may be a transient organic state involving confusion, headache, and some amnesia. The majority of such individuals develop a mild transient anterograde and retrograde amnesia, the latter particularly for very recent events, and, sometimes, for proper names. It must be emphasized that the ability to remember some things and the ability to learn new material is not affected by the use of ECT in recommended amounts.

Indications

Affective disorder. This therapy is used essentially in depression, in particular that depression called primary or unipolar. Nowadays, the term autonomous is frequently used instead of endogenous. This latter differentiation is used to indicate relative absence of reactive factors. As a rule, these depressions also represent the major indication for the use of tricyclic antidepressants, and hence is the category of depression which gives the best results with either tricyclics or ECT.

Mania and hypomania. ECT is mainly indicated in these conditions when drugs are ineffective, or are being relatively ineffective and measures are needed to prevent dehydration, malnutrition and paradoxical effects from drugs, or toxicity.

Schizophrenia. Catatonic states, particularly the stuporous variety, respond extremely well to the use of ECT. However, most of these conditions respond equally well to pharmacotherapy and there must, therefore, be additional reasons for the use of ECT in such conditions. In other forms of schizophrenia, generally, the use of ECT is not indicated, since the evidence shows that this treatment offers very little and pharmacotherapy and psychotherapy are the treatments of choice.

Other. From time to time it is necessary, usually life-saving, to use ECT in other conditions. Such an example may be anorexia nervosa.

Convulsive therapy is rarely the primary treatment and is usually used only if other methods of treatment are either not indicated, or not effective:

1. In cases of depression, almost always ECT will be recommended after a suitable trial of antidepressants has been attempted. This may in practice amount to the use of one or more tricyclics in effective doses and may actually include a trial of MAO inhibitors alone, or in combination with tricyclics.

2. In patients in whom it has been demonstrated during a previous attack that there has been good response to ECT, the decision to use this form of treatment will be made after a shorter, but still adequate trial of tricyclics.

3. Patients suffering from chronic myocardial conditions, where the risk of cardiotoxicity from tricyclic antidepressants is sufficient, the cardiologist may rule against a trial of tricyclics, but approve, instead, the use of ECT as a safer modality. As this phenomenon becomes understood and widespread, there may indeed be an increase in the use of ECT in the older age groups.

4. Generally speaking, the other indications for the use of ECT stem from the presence of behavioral manifestations not responding to adequate pharmacotherapy, for example, in mania and hypomania, uncontrolled despite the use of adequate doses of neuroleptics and lithium.

5. In some severely suicidal patients, ECT is administered earlier, since it is "fast acting," and the suicidal risk is thereby more rapidly diminished.

Most patients treated with ECT are followed up by maintenance doses of tricyclic antidepressant, lithium or major tranquilizers. Some patients, usually individuals with a depression of later life, may not respond to the prophylactic effect of medication and may require further ECT when relapse occurs. Any patient who has frequent relapses not preventable by pharmacotherapy, should be considered for maintenance treatment with ECT. These cases, however, are not frequently found.

Technique and Procedures

When the patient has been selected for ECT treatment, if it has not already been done, then a thorough physical examination is required. Further examination involves x-ray examination of the skull, chest and spine, the latter to be certain that there are no major deformities and to provide a baseline for comparison in the future. An ECG should be done. In addition, adequate laboratory examination of the blood is done in accordance with hospital requirements. This usually involves an examination of the hemoglobin, white cell count and differential. In addition, a BUN and urinalysis is performed. The vast majority of patients selected for ECT treatment may have it performed upon them quite safely. The absolute contraindication is the presence of increased intracranial pressure. Relative contraindications are myocardial infarction and active pulmonary inflammation. Since barbiturate anesthesia is most widely used, the presence of allergy to barbiturates, or history of porphyria should be sought.

The patient is prepared for general anesthetic. The procedure is performed in a special room with an anesthetist present and adequate resuscitation equipment on hand. A sufficient dose of short acting barbiturate, either Pentothal, or Methohexital, is injected intravenously. Usually, atropine sulphate 0.4 mg is given subcutaneously or intramuscularly about an hour before the treatment, though it may also be given intravenously at the time of treatment. Atropine is given because of its

effect in inhibiting the secretion of saliva, and also to prevent excessive cardiac slowing due to vagal stimulation during the seizure. Following the administration of the barbiturate anesthesia, a dose of succinylcholine hydrochloride is given to produce muscle relaxation. It is this relaxant which allows the convulsion to take place with minimal risk of fracture or later muscular discomfort to the patient. A sufficient amount of electricity, which varies from machine to machine, is administered to produce a grand mal convulsion. This is noted by the presence of an initial tonic contraction, usually best seen in the toes, lasting about 15 seconds, followed by clonic movements lasting up to a minute. The first seizure is generally the longest and succeeding treatments may require more electric current to produce grand mal convulsions.

Placement of electrodes. Two forms of ECT are generally spoken of, bilateral and unilateral. Bilaterally, ECT involves the placement of the electrodes in the bitemporal position, each electrode being midway between the external canthus of the eye and the external meatus of the ear. In order to minimize post-convulsive confusion and amnesia, unilateral ECT has been devised, in which the electrodes are placed so as to spare the dominant temporal lobe: one electrode is placed as for bilateral ECT (in right-handed patients on the right side in the temporal area) and the second electrode is placed on the mid-forehead. In both methods, sufficient electricity has to be passed to produce a grand mal seizure. Achieving a grand mal seizure of both sides of the body requires care and skill when the electrical stimulation is unilateral. Therefore, in properly administered treatments, bilateral and unilateral ECT are equally effective with the latter much to be preferred.

Number of treatments. Ordinarily, a minimum of four treatments is necessary in order to have any effect. Between eight and twelve treatments is usually the necessary number. Following adequate symptomatic improvement, two treatments are generally given to "seal in" the effect. The rate of treatment is two to three times weekly. Treatments given more frequently tend to produce a greater degree of confusion and no acceleration of therapeutic effect.

DRUG THERAPY

The discovery of drugs to deal specifically with heretofore intractable and chronic psychiatric conditions has revolutionized modern psychiatry in much the way in which the introduction of psychoanalysis did fifty years earlier. A new discipline, that of psychopharmacology was born, giving rise to the study of brain chemistry; action of drugs on neurotransmitter systems—a term that was only vaguely postulated at the time when these drugs were introduced; and therapeutics with psychoactive agents.

There has always been a belief that, sooner or later, such drugs would be discovered. Fifty to sixty years ago, pharmacological advances of great importance were made but these have since been made obsolescent, or have been superseded by further advances. The first was the discovery that artificially induced malarial fever could be effective in the treatment of tertiary syphilis. The second was the use of insulin coma in the treatment of schizophrenia. The former treatment has been replaced by antibiotics and the latter by specific drugs. First on the scene was chlorpromazine, followed closely by imipramine, shortly thereafter by chlordiazepoxide. Although lithium carbonate had actually been introduced prior to any of these other compounds, it did not become available for widespread use until the early 1960's. Disulfiram, in the treatment of alcoholism, was introduced into medicine about the same time.

The ensuing two decades since the introduction of these drugs has seen activity in elucidating the mechanisms of their ac-

tion, along with the knowledge of the effects of the parent compounds and their analogues; this, in turn, has provided a deeper understanding of the illnesses which the drugs help to treat.

A specific and effective therapy always galvanizes a field and discipline when it becomes available. Nowhere is this more true than in the field of psychiatry, where the treatment of hospitalized patients has changed dramatically. Locked doors, the symbol of the mental hospital, began to be a relic. The use of these drugs reduced considerably the suffering of the afflicted patients and increased enormously the range and efficacy of the psychiatrist's ability to intervene. Research has also been stimulated.

The drugs used in psychiatry are only slowly being named by their generic term. "Tranquilizer" has a descriptively pleasant sound, but it is, at once, too broad and too narrow. Probably the best general term is that of "psychoactive" or "psychotropic" agents. The following categorization of drugs is often utilized:

CATEGORIES	INDICATIONS
(1) Major tranquillizer Neuroleptics Antipsychotics	Major psychoses Schizophrenia Mania and agitated depression
(2) Antidepressants	Depression Major, retarded Manic depressive illness
(3) Antianxiety drugs Minor tranquillizers Muscle relaxants	Anxiety states Insomnia "Neurotic states"
(4) Psychoactive cations (lithium)	Mania and hypomania Manic depressive illness
(5) Hypnotics & sedatives	Insomnia Epilepsy
(6) Enzyme inhibitors Disulfiram (Antabuse); Calcium Carbimide (Temposil)	Alcoholism

All classifications in this still changing field are somewhat controversial. The simplest classification is using the concept of target symptoms. In effect, this means describing the class of a drug in terms of the target symptom of patients' illnesses that is most descriptive and understood. The categories may then be simplified as follows: (1) Antipsychotic (2) Antidepressant (3) Antimanic (4) Antianxiety (5) Hypnotic and (6) Anti-alcoholism.

It follows, therefore, that the choice of a drug will depend, in large measure, upon accurate history taking and examination of the patient for particular signs of mental dysfunction. It is only with such clear cut ideas concerning diagnosis and differential diagnosis that a correct approach to pharmacotherapy can occur. Proper physical examination is important, in order to estimate the ability of a patient to tolerate given drugs, and in what dose. While these drugs have a specific effect on both target symptoms and certain syndromes, they also have the potential for a considerable variety of side effects, involving nearly all organ systems. An understanding of the essential pharmacology of these agents becomes important, particularly in the earlier phases of therapy, when dosages are often changed to provide a therapeutic effect before accommodation has taken place. In the long term use of these drugs, vigilance is extremely important, in order to detect the development of late appearing side effects; therefore, monitoring of the patient, from both the point of view of mental functioning and physical functioning, at reasonable intervals, is mandatory.

Antipsychotic Drugs

The main indication for the use of these drugs is in the treatment of schizophrenia, acute and chronic. They are often used, as well, for the acute short term treatment of mania and hypomania, particularly their behavioral aspects, and for the severe restlessness of agitated depressions.

The advent of the antipsychotic, neuroleptic drugs marked a turning point in psychiatry. The significance of the introduction of these drugs can, perhaps, be best understood by comparing their impact on psychiatry with the impact of anti-biotics on general medicine in the treatment of infections. Although many humanistic movements in psychiatry had already begun, such as opening locked wards, individual and group therapy, there is no question that these movements were significantly helped by the availability of the antipsychotic agents. The area of the treatment most dramatically changed was that of psychotics and, particularly schizophrenia, which, while having an incidence of only 1 to 3%, nevertheless, because of its chronicity, accounted for 50% of all mental hospital beds and 25% of all hospital beds in North America. Efforts could now properly go forward with studies on prevention and rehabilitation. The expectation of psychiatry went from custodial to treatment-oriented, with early discharge the rule rather than the exception.

Historically, the introduction of phenothiazines into psychiatry came by way of anesthesia. These drugs were introduced as an improvement or change in the "lytic cocktail" being administered to patients for surgery, to reduce the amount of anesthetic agents. The relative tranquilization of these patients without accompanying sedation or hypnotic effect was noticed and then applied in the treatment of disturbed psychiatric patients. It is this characteristic of being able to interfere with motor and sensory components of the brain without producing profound cortical depression, which characterizes these neuroleptics.

Pharmacology. There are currently six major classes of antipsychotic compounds available for clinical use. These classes differ one from the other by virtue of relatively small changes in the cyclic core of the molecule resulting, however, in significant changes in the frequency and intensity of side effects. Interestingly some small changes in structure may change significantly the basic action of a drug; for example from antipsychotic via dopamine blocking to antidepressant via catechol-

TABLE 15   COMPARISON OF SOME COMMONLY USED ANTIPSYCHOTIC AGENTS

Generic Name	Trade Name	Relative Antipsychotic Potency	Range of Total Daily Dose Mg/Day
Phenothiazines:			
Aliphatic:			
Chlorpromazine	Largactil	100	50–1600
Methotrimeprazine	Nozinan	100	50–1000
Piperidine:			
Mesoridazine	Serentil	50	25–400
Piperacetazine	Quide	12	10–160
Thioridazine	Mellaril	100	50–800
Piperazine:			
Fluphenazine	Moditen	2	1–60
Perphenazine	Trilafon	10	8–64
Trifluoperazine	Stelazine	5	4–60
Thioxanthines:			
Aliphatic:			
Chlorprothixene	Tarasan	65	25–400
Piperazine:			
Thiothixene	Navane	5	6–120
Dibenzazepines:			
Loxapine	Loxapac	15	15–160
Butyrophenones:			
Haloperidol	Haldol	2	2–100
Diphenylbutylpiperidines:			
Pimozide	Orap	0.3–0.5	2–12

Dosage: 1. Lower values apply to maintenance.
2. Upper values apply to acute cases.
3. Starting doses are 20–25% of upper values.

"LONG ACTING" PREPARATIONS			*DOSAGE*
Fluphenazine Enanthate	Moditen	25–100 mg.	im every 1–4 weeks
Fluphenazine Decanoate	Modecate		
Pipothiazine Palmitate		25 mg.	im every 3–6 weeks
Fluspirilene			im weekly

amine blocking. These are shown in Table 15.

The neuroleptic effects may, in the long run, become equated with the mechanism of action of these drugs although the mechanisms are not yet completely understood. The action at the following anatomical sites correlates reasonably well with the behavioral and clinical effects as well as the side effects of the antipyschotic drugs.

(a) at the reticular activating system of the midbrain, where sensory input is monitored;

(b) at the amygdala and hippocampus, structures in the limbic system which provides the emotional coloring attached to incoming signals;

(c) at the hypothalamus, which governs the peripheral responses to meaningful sensory information through both the pituitary-endocrine system and the autonomic nervous system;

(d) at the globus pallidus and corpus striatum, where extrapyramidal syndromes are elicited.

At the synaptic level, all these drugs have the effect of blocking central neurotransmission which is mediated by dopamine. Recent work has shown that these localized sites of action, correlated to the action of the drug, are in the cell membranes. The sedative effect of the antipsychotic varies as indicated in Table 16. Unlike the sedative-hypnotic drugs, they increase muscle tone and lower the convulsive threshold but do not produce either anesthesia or drug dependence. Moreover, patients sedated by antipsychotic drugs are easily arousable.

Indications and use. The primary indication is for the treatment of schizophrenia. Secondary indications (in that drugs with a more specific effect exist) are mania, agitated depression, and, at times, severe anxiety.

Having decided that an antipsychotic drug is indicated, it is often a problem to the student and young physician to choose from what appear to be a bewildering variety and array of similar drugs. Table 15 notes the differing equivalences among the drugs. It should be noted that, despite many attempts at proving otherwise, all drugs currently in use have an equally beneficial effect on the treatment of schizophrenia when used in equivalent doses. Moreover, it has still not been possible to select drugs for any particular "subgroup" of schizophrenia. Some general principles have been arrived at on a pragmatic basis to enable the physician to understand how a drug may be chosen, and to come to some conclusion about selecting a drug for the initiation of therapy.

It may be important to keep in mind that a large number of acute schizophrenic cases seen are, in effect, relapses in patients who have stopped taking their medication, or whose maintenance medication has been inadequate or insufficient. The main problem may be to determine which medication was helpful to the patient in a previous attack and institute treatment on that basis. A useful approach is for the physician to become familiar with one member of each class or subgroup, when there is more than one, and in this way he will be able to switch to another class or type in the event that in-adequate results are obtained, or severe side effects occur. The following principles may, therefore, be helpful in the selection of an appropriate drug:

1. Response to previous therapy—this "Rule" has held up over the last 10 to 15 years as the best criterion for selecting a drug in the treatment of a patient in acute schizophrenic relapse.

2. Desirability of sedation—in patients who are agitated and present a behavioral problem, the use of medication which is highly sedative can be selected. While initially this can be seen as a desirable benefit, as time goes on this may be seen as a side effect. Before switching to another drug, it is *imperative* that an adequate dosage range has been reached.

DOSE AND DOSE RANGE. Because of the wide therapeutic margins which exist in this category of drugs, it is very difficult to be specific about dose ranges. These will, therefore, depend on current practice, patient need and careful observation. Some basic principles concerning dose and dose ranges are as follows:

1. Patients who are acutely ill can tolerate greater doses than patients whose illness is on the wane, or in remission.

2. Finding the correct dose, which will hold in abeyance the acute symptomatology, is a matter of titration over a period of some two or three days.

3. Initially, the drug should be given in divided doses to establish the tolerance of the patient for the medication. Once this has been established, it is then possible to prescribe the drug in one daily dose, usually at night, to minimize side effects. The biological half-life of the major metabolites is such that this form of dosage is possible.

4. If it is necessary to use a parenteral form of medication, then concern over autonomic effects (particularly cardiovascular ones) becomes paramount. If a compound such as chlorpromazine, which has sedative and cardiovascular effects, is chosen, then small doses to start with are mandatory; it is standard procedure to check blood pressure each time an injection of chlorpromazine is administered. This is not the case with a drug such as haloperidol which has recently been used increasingly in a technique known as rapid neuroleptization where 2.5 to 10 mg of the drug is administered intramuscularly every 30 to 60 minutes until symptoms are controlled. Usually one to four such injections are adequate. Patients are then switched to oral medication in a range of between half to twice the total injected dose. This treatment is indicated particularly where patients are excited and belligerent, a situation not uncommonly found in cases of acute functional psychosis brought into the emergency room.

These drugs find their greatest usefulness in the treatment of schizophrenia. Numerous studies have shown their effectiveness, especially as compared with any other form of treatment. This was shown particularly in the studies of May who compared drugs, individual psychotherapy, milieu therapy and ECT. Results unequivocally show that, in the treatment of acute schizophrenia, the use of antipsychotic medications is a key element in any treatment program, with other treatments being possibly helpful, definitely adjunctive and, therefore, not indispensable.

Even though there is a modest natural recovery rate, most observers now agree, since antipsychotic drugs have quantitatively produced a better result than use of placebo, that it is poor medical practice to withhold such medication in acute cases. The experience of a psychotic schizophrenic reaction is one of great and acute pain for the patient. Attempts at ameliorating this situation constitute sound practice. Following the remission of the acute phase, the question inevitably arises of whether to continue with medication or not. Experience has shown that there is a high relapse rate when medication is discontinued immediately upon discharge from hospital; and in general, the most common antecedent of relapse is discontinuation, or inadequate intake, of mainte-

TABLE 16   ACTIVITY PROFILES OF LOW vs HIGH POTENCY ANTIPSYCHOTIC AGENTS

Activity	Low (Chlorpromazine)	High (Butyrophenones Piperazines*)
Antipsychotic Effect	Equal	Equal
Sedation	High	Low
Extrapyramidal	Low Frequency and Severity	High Frequency
Tardive dyskinesia	Equal	Equal
Autonomic (Anticholinergic)	High	Low
Allergic (Rashes, Blood Dyscrasias)	High	Low
Cardiovascular (Hypotension)	High	Low
Weight Gain	High	Low
Endocrine	Equal	Equal
Photosensitivity	High	Low
High Oral Dosage	Risky	Relatively safe
IM Injections	Risky	Relatively safe

*Piperazines fall midway between low and high potency compounds.

nance medication. Either because of the relatively slow clearance rate, or because of other factors, there is usually a delay of some six weeks to two months following the cessation of medication before relapse occurs. It is, therefore, recommended that all patients who have acute illnesses which have remitted with medication be kept on medication for six months to a year, or longer. It is important as well to introduce as many factors as possible which might lead to adequate patient compliance. Once-a-day dosage of medication, cutting down the dose to the minimum (which must be fixed for each patient), maintaining a good therapeutic relationship—usually within a clinic setting—will all help.

In cases where numerous relapses have occurred and the situation is viewed to be chronic, greater efforts may have to be made to maintain a patient on medication, particularly if, as happens in some cases, the patient shows little appreciation of, or is actually negative to, the self-administration of medication. In these cases, the use of injectable, long acting antipsychotic compounds, such as fluphenazine enanthate, is extremely helpful.

One of the problems of maintenance treatment is the fact that the target symptoms in chronic cases are social withdrawal, anhedonia and apathy, none of which are particularly well treated at the moment with the antipsychotic medications available. Many of the more newly released medications are said to be particularly beneficial in the area of social withdrawal. This may be particularly true of the diphenylbutylpiperidines such as pimozide, and fluspirilene.

In general, the continuation of maintenance medication must be judged according to the following criteria: the risk of relapse; the risk of developing chronic, irreversible, neurological side effects (tardive dyskinesia); and any beneficial or therapeutic effect on current functioning.

It is in the cases where patients have been suffering from chronic illness for many years, have not been successfully rehabilitated into the mainstream of society, and where small amounts of medication are as effective as large amounts, that it becomes difficult to judge the necessity of the continuation of this kind of treatment.

Despite much effort, some patients remain resistant to the currently available antipsychotic drugs. The possible effectiveness of such drugs as the beta-blocking agent propranolol indicates that in some cases at least other transmitter systems may be involved in both the pathogenesis and the treatment of the illness.

Side effects. Though side effects are frequent with this category of drugs it must be emphasized that toxicity is extremely low. These drugs have been in widespread use for some twenty five years, and they are considered to be among the safest drugs in medicine today. Because of their psychic activity, there is almost always a slight sensation of being aware of taking these drugs, even in relatively small doses, and this accentuates the reluctance of patients to take these drugs regularly. Some of these side effects are a sense of heaviness and sluggishness, and are referable to the autonomic activity of these drugs, e.g., a variety of mild anticholinergic effects, including dry mouth and blurred vision. The most important side effects are the extrapyramidal syndromes. These can occur in a number of different ways.

1. *Parkinsonian-like syndrome*, which may include any, or all, of the following features: altered posture, "pill-rolling" tremor, muscular rigidity, shuffling gait, akinesia, immobile facies, fine tremor of the extremities, seborrhea.

2. *Akathisia*, usually manifested by a sense of not being able to sit still or stand still, a sense of extreme restlessness, constant pacing, almost involuntary movements of fingers, hands and legs. This syndrome is often mistaken for increased psychotic agitation, hysteria or anxiety; its recognition is vital.

3. *Acute dystonic reaction*, usually appearing in the first few days after the start of medication. This is seen more in younger patients and may include torticollis, opisthotonus, or oculogyric crisis.

The management of these side effects can be achieved generally by reduction in dosage and/or by the administration of antiparkinsonian agents. Some commonly used agents are: biperiden, 2-8 mg/day; procyclidine hydrochloride, 10-20 mg/day; benztropine mesylate, 4-6 mg/day; trihexyphenidyl, 2-10 mg/day. The latter two are also available as parenteral preparations for the treatment of acute dystonic reactions. If the reaction has been severe, the antiparkinsonian medication should be continued for some two or three months after which side effects tend to disappear. Therefore routine use of antiparkinsonian agents for greater than a 3 month period is not indicated. These drugs should be reinstituted only if there is a further emergence of side effects.

In milder cases, especially where reduction in dosage of drugs has been accomplished without interference with the antipsychotic treatment, it may be necessary to continue with antiparkinsonian agents. In almost all cases, it is unnecessary to continue the use of antiparkinsonian agents indefinitely. These agents, moreover, should be used in the minimum effective dosage, because of their tendency to exacerbate anticholinergic effects.

4. *Tardive Dyskinesia*. The term "tardive" means late, and this is, therefore, usually a late appearing dyskinetic form of extrapyramidal syndrome. Because it may occur with greater frequency than previously suspected, and because of the possible chronicity and irreversibility of the symptoms, and the unsatisfactory treatment currently available, it is imperative to evaluate and reevaluate the wisdom of prolonged, indefinite, high dose maintenance therapy. Use of drug holidays and drug-free intervals is of great importance.

The main feature of tardive dyskinesia is repetitive, involuntary movement of a choreoathetoid type, involving the mouth, lips, tongue, trunk, and extremities. There is no definite neuropathological explanation for the development of this syndrome. The most acceptable current hypothesis runs along the following lines: Initially, the antipsychotic drugs produce a block of dopamine receptors in the postsynaptic neurons in the areas where these drugs work. Initially, in the dopamine system, this block may produce the extrapyramidal side effects. After prolonged use, the dopamine lack becomes, through overcompensation, dopamine excess, and, when combined with dopamine sensitivity, leads to the development of tardive dyskinesia. The syndrome is often discovered on the reduction, or the withdrawal, of medication. Because of the irreversibility of the syndrome, some form of neuronal change must also take place.

Treatment of this condition is still in the experimental stage. It is possible to suppress these symptoms by maintaining or increasing the dose of the antipsychotic being used. However, eventually this requires a still further increase. This approach may have to be resorted to, particularly if the patient's psychotic symptoms recur and, therefore, require the continued use of antipsychotic medication. In the long run, the approach to treatment will be related to methods which will decrease dopaminergic activity. It, therefore, cannot be too strongly stated that a conservative approach to long term use of these drugs is of greatest benefit. While it may not be possible to reduce the incidence of this difficult side effect completely, careful attention to the possibility of tardive dyskinesia will make sure that the smallest number of cases develop this complication. Long term treatment, therefore, should be reserved for those patients who can really benefit from the use of the agent.

There are two other forms of dyskinesia which bear mention—withdrawal dyskinesia and overt dyskinesia. The former occurs immediately on withdrawal of medication while the latter occurs two weeks after stopping medication, and persists like tardive dyskinesia.

AUTONOMIC SIDE EFFECTS. Hypotension is occasionally seen, more commonly with phenothiazines given orally in high doses. The elderly and debilitated patients are particularly prone to develop this side effect. Anticholinergic side effects include blurred vision, dry mouth, tachycardia, and occasionally constipation.

METABOLIC AND ENDOCRINE EFFECTS. Patients taking antipsychotics often show a troublesome weight gain, even when the medication is reduced to maintenance levels. Molidone, an indole derivative, is the only antipsychotic which may produce weight loss in patients who are obese or who have difficulty losing weight following recovery from their psychosis. Galactorrhea may occasionally be seen in women, and is probably caused by the elevation of prolactin levels.

HEMATOLOGICAL EFFECTS. Any of the antipsychotic medications may produce agranulocytosis. This usually occurs within the first six weeks of treatment and is probably due to a direct toxic effect on the bone marrow. In many patients who are treated with antipsychotic medications, a decrease in white blood cell count occurs. Very few patients, however, develop agranulocytosis. Because of the fact that the leukocyte count is often normal just prior to the onset of agranulocytosis, the practice of following patients with regular leukocyte counts has been abandoned. Inasmuch as agranulocytosis is a potentially fatal condition, patients on antipsychotic medication, who develop fever and sore throat, should have their leukocyte count recorded. Treatment of this condition must be done in consultation with infectious disease specialists.

OTHER SIDE EFFECTS. Chlorpromazine frequently induces photosensitivity. Patients must be cautioned about this possibility and take suitable precautions. Using a sun screen preparation is often quite effective. For a small number of patients, who also develop an allergic skin reaction the offending agent should be stopped but then may be resumed when the rash is cleared.

Thioridazine in doses of over 800 mg a day may produce retinitis pigmentosa. This drug is also cardiotoxic and has been shown to cause sudden unexplained death which some claim to be cardiac standstill secondary to ventricular arrhythmias. It is therefore safer to avoid using high doses, i.e., exceeding 400 mg per day.

In summary, therefore, the antipsychotic compounds found their greatest source of usefulness in the treatment of schizophrenia. Not curative and hardly ideal, they have been responsible for the ameliorations of much pain and the prevention of relapses. Particularly because of the inevitable development of many, and potentially serious side effects, the search for new drugs of greater potency and specificity and few side effects must continue. In the process much is also learned about the neuropathology of the illness itself.

Lithium

Although it has been investigated for a variety of mental and emotional conditions, so far lithium's most important and vital place is in the treatment of acute manic and hypomanic conditions, and in their prophylaxis. Actually, lithium was first introduced as a specific pharmacological agent by Cade in Australia in 1949, but it remained in a shadow and under a cloud of suspicion because of a number of deaths associated with lithium when used as a salt substitute in the treatment of hypotension. Schou, in Denmark, persevered in the investigations and use of lithium, which has now received worldwide acceptance.

Pharmacology. Completely absorbed from the gastrointestinal tract, it is also somewhat irritating and may cause a transient nausea after ingestion. It is excreted almost entirely by the kidney, with a half-life of about twenty-four hours. The amount of lithium excreted by the kidneys varies directly with sodium intake. It is, therefore, a matter of importance to maintain adequate sodium intake.

Properties of lithium are extremely similar to those of sodium, save for the fact that it crosses cell membranes relatively slowly and, therefore, plasma steady states are built up only slowly. It is, therefore, not surprising that this ion has major effects on a number of body systems, including the endocrinological, cardiovascular, gastrointestinal, and central nervous systems. Lithium probably alters a number of bodily functions simultaneously. The mechanism of action of lithium is still unknown. Several hypotheses are under consideration. Lithium's specificity of action may go a long way to help in the investigations of some of the basic pathophysiological mechanisms of manic-depressive illness and other important psychiatric disorders.

Some of the hypotheses which may account for the action of lithium are as follows:

1. Increase in the concentration of norepinephrine or other neurotransmitters, in the presynaptic nerve terminals in areas where the major nerve transmitters are of a catecholamine variety.

2. Addition of hormone-activated adenyl cyclase in the CNS, resulting in decreased production of cyclic AMP.

   Both of these explanations would fit in with the notion that in mania there is functional overactivity of the catecholamines in the brain.

3. Alteration of electrolyte levels.

4. Alteration of physiological processes depending on ion transport or distribution in the CNS.

   Both (3) and (4) may account for lithium's anti-manic effect on the basis that these latter phenomena can alter membrane excitability.

5. Interference with neuronal carbohydrate metabolism. It is of interest to note that in the dog, lithium administration can produce a stability and immunity to amphetamine-induced changes.

Indications and use. Studies have shown that lithium and antipsychotic drugs are equally effective in the treatment of acute episodes of hypomania. However, antipsychotic drugs and lithium have significant differences.

1. Antipsychotics—produce an effect by tranquillization. The illness is initially contained within a chemical straightjacket. The onset of action is speedy. These factors apply to patients regardless of diagnosis.

2. Lithium is nonsedative. It has a normalizing effect on the patient so that thought processes become slowed, and there is no outward appearance of being drugged. It is slow acting. It is ineffective in patients not suffering from manic or manic-like disorders.

In practice, however, the two agents are almost always combined. The behavioral manifestations of a hypomanic attack are initially controlled by an antipsychotic drug, while lithium levels are building up to therapeutic levels.

The initial medical evaluation includes laboratory tests of renal, electrolyte, and thyroid function, complete blood count and electrocardiogram.

Initiation of treatment. Lithium in the form of lithium carbonate, in tablets or capsules of 300 mg, is usually given in amounts of 600 to 900 mg, three times daily. Serum levels should be checked during the initial period three times weekly. Blood for lithium should be drawn 8 to 12 hours following the last dose. After 7 to 10 days, the level should be building up to 0.8 to 1.2 mEq/L. It is important to monitor clinically for toxic signs during the buildup period; the serum levels act as a further guide and check. Signs of toxicity may arise during intervals between laboratory checks. Toxicity should be expected, if levels have reached more than 2 mEq/L. It is quite well known that more of the drug is needed and tolerated during the acute phase. Reduction in dosage to maintenance levels should be accomplished as soon as there is clinical improvement.

Lithium prophylaxis and maintenance. Bipolar affective disorder—that form of manic depressive illness in which there has been at least one clinical attack of mania or hypomania—has always been marked by recurrences of greater or lesser frequency. Until the advent of lithium, no adequate prophylaxis was available. The use of lithium has reduced considerably, and in some cases completely, the serious ravages of this illness on affected individuals and their families, by preventing, or allowing early and rapid treatment of recurrences. (So to speak " a floor and ceiling" are provided.)

The effective level for prophylaxis is 0.8 to 1.2 mEq/L. Monitoring of serum level should occur monthly, but once a steady state has been achieved, less frequent estimations of serum lithium level are necessary. Random checks, however, are a means of determining compliance, especially in situations where the clinical picture changes.

Side effects and toxic effects. The early side effects seen with lithium parallel the biological effects. These are nausea, diarrhea, and fine hand tremor. These usually disappear with continued use. Their recurrence, later on in treatment, with any intensity can be seen as a possible indication of impending toxicity, and the lithium levels should be checked. Particularly in elderly patients, hand tremor may be quite disturbing and, if necessary, can be checked by the use of propranolol, 10 to 40 mg per day. Occasionally, diarrhea remains a chronic and persistent side effect and may require treatment with suitable doses of loperimide.

CARDIAC SIDE EFFECTS. Lithium invariably produces T-wave flattening and inversion in the ECG. It also has effects on electrolyte and catecholamine metabolism. There is, therefore, concern of continuing cardiac toxicity in patients on lithium who develop coronary illness. In therapeutic doses it is probably safe to continue lithium following the healing of the acute disease. However, both cardiac state and lithium levels must be followed closely. In the absence of pre-existing cardiac disease cardio-toxic manifestations rarely occur with lithium at therapeutic levels. As with any potent therapy, using lithium must be measured against the risk of recurrent illness.

THYROID. Lithium therapy may be associated with a diffuse, non-tender thyroid enlargement, hypothyroidism, or both. The occurrence of goiter is about 4%. Treatment may be effective by discontinuation of the drug, or, more usefully, by the administration of exogenous thyroid.

LITHIUM AND PREGNANCY. Animal studies have long shown that lithium is potentially teratogenic. Therefore, a number of registries of lithium-treated, pregnant women have been set up to monitor such cases. Preliminary results indicate that the incidence of congenital abnormalities is no greater than in the general population. However, unless extremely strongly indicated, and the risks thoroughly understood, lithium should not be administered to pregnant women, particularly during the first trimester. As with many drugs, lithium is present in plasma-like concentration in breast milk and, therefore, breast feeding of infants should be avoided by mothers taking lithium. Women during child-bearing age taking lithium should be aware of these potential dangers.

LITHIUM AND THE KIDNEY. Polydypsia, polyuria and lithium induced diabetes insipidus are the three most common effects of lithium on the renal system. The first two are not uncommon initially and usually disappear after a few weeks but in some patients reappear often to a troublesome degree. These symptoms are benign and respond to lowering the dose of lithium. Tolerance of these side effects is almost always preferable to risk of relapse.

Lithium induced diabetes insipidus is unresponsive to the administration of exogenous anti-diuretic hormone (ADH). Lowering the dose of lithium almost always reverses the syndrome. However, there is a risk of relapse. Thiazide diuretics are known to increase the serum levels of lithium and constitute the treatment of choice in lithium induced diabetes insipidus. This paradoxical effect is believed to occur as a result of compensatory proximal tubular reabsorption of sodium and water along with lithium, counteracting the thiazide-induced decrease in distal tubular sodium reabsorption. Because of the increased serum level of lithium, the use of thiazide and other diuretics in patients taking lithium requires a serum level to be monitored very closely.

Lithium is clearly a drug not only with great effectiveness but with numerous actions throughout the body, many of which are still being elaborated. Thus placing a patient on lithium requires considerable evaluation of the risks and benefits, cannot be done lightly and requires close monitoring, particularly in cases of prophylaxis and where an extended period of time must be allowed before an evaluation can be made.

Antidepressant Medication

Antidepressant medications, essentially tricyclic compounds and monoamine oxidase inhibitors, were discovered and introduced into clinical practice early in the modern psychopharmacological era. These drugs have given rise to a tremendous interest into the study of the chemical basis of psychiatric illness and, to a large extent, the search for an understanding of the chemical mechanism underlying normal behavior. It has occurred largely because of the fact that depression and its

counterpart, elation, are universally understood and experienced emotions, and become illness and pathological often only when they exist in excessive amounts, and over long periods of time. A prime example of the important work stimulated by these drugs was the elaboration of the catecholamine hypothesis as a basis for understanding the mechanisms of actions of antidepressant medication and, also, the pathochemistry of depression. This hypothesis fits in with some of the known facts of drug action, for example, the inhibition of catecholamine reuptake at synaptic clefts, and its destruction intracellularly.

Indications and use. One of the great problems in the use of drugs in the treatment of depression has to do with being able to select those depressive entities which are responsive to pharmacotherapy. In the estimation of the effect of treatment on depression, utilizing biological and physical methods, whether pharmacological or physical (ECT) it is vital to have placebo control groups. The following compares the generally accepted effectiveness in depression of different treatments.

Treatment	Efficacy (%)
ECT	80–100
TCA	60–80
MAOI	40–60
Placebo	0–40

Time lag. The onset of action of antidepressant drugs as measured in vitro is rapid, whereas, when used in patients, effects are not seen for 10–14 days. These drugs, therefore, should not be given to patients unless there is a reasonable indication that the illness will not remit without the use of specific antidepressant medication. Mild reactive depressions usually improve using psychological approaches, or with the help of antianxiety "minor tranquilizers."

A key point is the existence of a previous episode which responded to antidepressant medication. Generally, it is agreed that those depressions, which show considerable biological or autonomic involvement, respond best to antidepressants, most often tricyclic medication. Some of the features denoting this type of depression, in addition to sadness of mood, are psychomotor retardation, loss of interest in food, loss of libido, loss of weight and difficulty in concentration.

The presence in patients of significant amounts of anxiety, agitation or psychotic thinking will require adjustment in the therapeutic approach. In the first instance, antianxiety compounds may suffice, and in the second, phenothiazines may be required.

Selection of drug. As previously mentioned, antianxiety agents and antipsychotic agents have a place in the treatment of certain kinds of depression. Lithium carbonate is often used as an antidepressant in bipolar depressions.

sant. The student and/or practitioner should become familiar with the categories of these agents and know in some detail the usefulness and activity of one from each category. These drugs, in addition to their effect on catecholamines, also have profound anticholinergic effects which may or may not be necessary for their mediation of the antidepressant effect. In view of the side effects they produce, the difficulty in obtaining patients' compliance, and concern for patients' safety in suicidally prone patients, speed of action is an important consideration. Part of the reason for the proliferation of these drugs has been an attempt to find an agent which would have a minimum number of side effects and a speedy onset of action. In these critical areas no differentiation between these compounds has as yet emerged. They can, however, be categorized in terms of degrees of sedative activity:

Sedative Activity	Generic Name	Trade Name	Average Daily Dose
Greatest	Trimipramine	Surmontil	150–300 mg
	Doxepin	Sinequan	150–300 mg
	Amitriptyline	Elavil	150–300 mg
Middle Range	Chlorimipramine	Anafranil	150–300 mg
	Maprotiline	Ludiomil	150–300 mg
	Imipramine	Tofranil	150–300 mg
Least	Protriptyline	Triptil	15–60 mg
	Nortriptyline	Aventyl	75–150 mg
	Desipramine	Norpramine	
		Pertofrane	100–250 mg

Tricyclic Antidepressants

The majority of patients selected for treatment with antidepressant medication receive tricyclic antidepressants. A much smaller number receive monoamine oxidase inhibitors. This latter category of drug is rarely used initially, unless there is a history of previous response.

As with the phenothiazines, none of the tricyclic antidepressants has been shown to be superior to any of the others. It is, therefore, often difficult to choose one when starting a patient on an antidepres-

Method of treatment. Even in properly selected cases which will respond positively to tricyclic antidepressants, a good deal of individual variation exists in terms of the eventual therapeutic dose and time of response. The basic principles, therefore, include the build up to an adequate, that is to say maximal, dose, and exposure of the patient to this level for adequate lengths of time. The usual minimum dosage, at which any effect can be expected to take place, is 75 mg a day. It is, therefore, usual to start with this dose. Initially, this is given in divided doses, but can also be given once a day, usually at night. This is often preferable, as many of the unpleasant side effects, particularly sedation, are minimized during waking hours. Biological half-life of these compounds allows once a day dosage to be given without affecting plasma levels. No clearcut dosage routine exists for increasing medication and this is, therefore, worthwhile to consider. One suggestion is to start at 75 mg a day, and increasing by 75 mg every week until improvement exists, or a dose of 300 mg has been reached and maintained for one month. Depending on the patient's tolerance and circumstances, that is to say, hospitalization versus out-patient locale, merit dosage can be reached sooner. It is not advised to proceed beyond the maximum average dose of 300 mg a day. Most investigators believe that going higher than this does not markedly increase the rate of response, but merely intensifies and increases the incidence of side effects.

If a patient has previously responded to a certain dosage, it is worth continuing with the drug beyond the four week period. Should there not be the presence of this positive history, then the switching to a drug in a different category of the tricyclics is warranted. There still might not be any response, and most clinicians would, at this point, seriously consider the use of ECT. If this is decided upon, then it is not necessary to discontinue the use of tricyclics, merely to lower their dosage to the expected maintenance amount.

Maintenance treatment. Maintenance dosage should be approximately one-half the dosage required to produce improvement. This dosage should be maintained for some six months to a year. In patients who have recurrent attacks of depression, the use of the maintenance amount as a prophylactic agent should be tried, although it is not always successful. Recurrent depression is still an unresolved therapeutic problem. Other approaches involve the use of lithium. In certain vulnerable individuals, no prophylactic approach is effective, and treatment with adequate doses of tricyclics, other antidepressants, or ECT must still be utilized.

Side effects and toxic reactions of tricyclics. Tricyclic antidepressants produce many different side effects, often to an uncomfortable degree, resulting in noncompliance of medication intake, unless considerable guidance and encouragement is given by the physician. These side effects are an outgrowth of one of the essential characteristics of the drugs, namely, their anticholinergic effect. Major side effects and their management are as follows:

ANTICHOLINERGIC EFFECTS (PERIPHERAL). These are the most common and consist of, in order of frequency, dry mouth, blurring of vision, and constipation. Because they are anticholinergic, they can, therefore, exacerbate narrow-angle glaucoma, produce urinary retention, and, on rare occasions and mainly when excessive kinds of additional anticholinergic medication is given, paralytic ileus. The latter situation has occurred in the past when patients were given, in combination, tricyclics, phenothiazines and antiparkinsonian agents. Patients should be prepared for these side effects. Constipation can become a problem, particularly in the elderly, and is best dealt with by adequate nutrition and food intake, and the use of gentle laxatives if necessary. If these side effects, particularly dry mouth, become severe or uncomfortable, it is possible to recommend taking a cholinergic agonist, such as Bethanechol 25 mg, three times a day. If the side effects are severe, the drug should immediately be discontinued and reintroduced, if necessary, at a lower dose.

CENTRAL NERVOUS SYSTEM EFFECTS. Drowsiness, or severe sedation, particularly at the onset of treatment, may occur in susceptible individuals, even in low doses and, particularly, when highly sedative forms of tricyclics are taken, such as amitriptyline. In high doses these drugs produce a fine tremor, not related to parkinsonism, and responding only to diminution of the drug itself.

CARDIOVASCULAR TOXICITY. Orthostatic hypotension is quite frequent and patients should be warned about this. Frequently, changes in the ECG occur, with main features being prolonged QT interval, depressed ST segment, and flattened T wave. This possibility may produce problems in patients with pre-existing cardiac disease. Therefore, it is a wise precaution to have an ECG before starting with tricyclics. Many clinicians would consider ECT safer than tricyclic antidepressants in these cases.

OTHER SIDE EFFECTS. Excessive sweating is often complained about. Infrequent allergic skin reactions occur and these can be treated with antihistamines. If tricyclics are suddenly withdrawn, then withdrawal syndromes can occur. Nausea and vomiting are the major symptoms.

Interactions and incompatibilities. Other anticholinergic agents should be used cautiously because of the danger of the development of paralytic ileus. MAO inhibitors, in combination with tricyclics, may, on occasion, produce severe hypertensive reactions. It is important to note that the antihypertensive action of guanethidine is interfered with and prevented by tricyclics.

Overdosage of tricyclics. This is a severe problem for two major reasons. Many physicians are unaware of the danger and prescribe, for suicidal patients, excessive amounts. Potential cardiac toxicity of these drugs, in the high doses taken during suicidal attempts, is not as well known as should be. The major syndrome following an overdose is characterized by restlessness, agitation, and delirium which may progress into coma. Cardiac problems may ensue. Certain general principles in the treatment of the overdosage need to be understood and followed.

The delirium is, usually, short-lived because of the rapid detoxification of the drug by the liver. However, many side effects are longer lasting inasmuch as significant amounts of the drug are bound to the plasma. Cardiac problems should be managed. Cardiac symptoms caused by the anticholinergic effect of the drug are best treated by the use of physostigmine, given intravenously and slowly, in doses of 1–3 mg. Cardiac monitors should be used.

Clearly, prevention is a preferable route and this can often be dealt with in cases where suicide attempts are suspected. When hospitalization is neither indicated nor possible, then supplies of medication, given to the patient directly, should be kept to a minimum—no more than one week's supply.

Monoamine Oxidase Inhibitors

Historically, the drug marsilid was used clinically prior to the introduction of tricyclics. Despite its therapeutic potency, cases of severe hepatic toxicity (acute yellow atrophy) occurred, and led to its complete withdrawal from clinical use. New drugs in this family are generally available for use. They are phenelzine (nardil), available in 15 mg tablets; isocarboxazid (marplan), available in 10 mg tablets; both the latter are hydrazine derivatives. There is one non-hydrazine derivative used clinically, and this is tranylcypromine (parnate) available in 10 mg tablets. Parnate is considered to be the most effective of the MAO inhibitors and has, in addition, a mild stimulant effect. Phenelzine (nardil) is generally considered to be next in effectiveness. These drugs, usually given in divided doses, should not be used in high doses, unless the patient is hospitalized, or there has been a previous positive experience with the medication. As with the tricyclics, there is a delay of 10 to 14 days before improvement can be expected, provided adequate dose levels have been achieved. These have to be developed individually and it is unlikely that more than 5 to 6 tablets a day are indicated. Serious side effects are most apparent at high dose levels. Following two weeks at maximal dose levels, if no improvement has been achieved, the medication should be discontinued. However, if there has been improvement, then maintenance should be arranged at somewhat less than half the maximum dosage.

SELECTION OF PATIENTS. These drugs are used clinically only under special circumstances:

1. Where the patient has a history of responsiveness to these agents.
2. Where a patient has been unresponsive to tricyclics, and, especially where a relative has a history of responsiveness to an MAO inhibitor.
3. In exceptional cases in combination with tricyclics. The MAOI drugs should only be commenced in patients who are under the care of a psychiatrist. Since a fair number of people fall into the aforementioned categories, it will not be unusual to encounter patients who are taking monoamine oxidase inhibitors. These drugs have interesting and unusual side effects and interactions, which must be kept in mind.

Side effects and toxic reactions. MAO inhibitors, on occasion, can produce insomnia. This is an extension of the central stimulating effect and, on occasion, restlessness and agitation may also be seen.

AUTONOMIC SIDE EFFECTS. These are not as severe or frequent as with the tricyclics. Orthostatic hypotension can be a problem.

Interaction effects. These, usually, refer to the production of a hypertensive crisis characterized by a severe headache of sudden onset, usually occipital in location, a few hours in duration, and, usually, without after-effects. However, in some cases intracranial bleeding may occur which can be fatal. Where the hypertension is deemed to be severe, then antihypertensive agents, such as phentolamine, must be used.

These interactions are usually the result of the following situations:

1. Medication containing sympathomimetics, as are used in cold tablets.
2. In connection with anesthesia:
   (a) Some local anesthetics contain epinephrine;
   (b) Intravenous barbiturates produce interaction with MAOI.
3. When tyramine containing foods are eaten. The best known example is the "tyramine-cheese" reaction. The ingestion of foods with a high tyramine content, while an individual has been taking monoamine oxidase inhibitors, may result, in vulnerable patients, in a severe hypertensive crisis. Patients must be cautioned about potential interactions. The following are some foods which have produced the hypertensive syndrome: aged cheeses, Chianti wine, chicken livers, and yeast products.

Overdosage of MAOI. Monoamine oxidase inhibitors should not be used in seriously suicidal patients, because of the risk of ingestion of excessive amounts of the drug, as well as the unreliability of such patients to comply with the rigid dietary restrictions.

Future Directions of Antidepressants

The ideal antidepressant has still not been discovered, particularly in view of the large number of side effects, the considerable lag time prior to any effective action, and the fact that the drug works in a maximum of 80% of patients.

Inasmuch as a considerable amount of biochemistry of depression and affective disorders is known, it is possible in the future that measurements of various metabolites in the blood will enable the clinician more accurately to match antidepressant drug and antidepressant syndrome. While the depressive syndrome is a final common pathway, the underlying disturbances are in all probability quite varied. It is not surprising, therefore, that a medication will work in one patient, but a different medication, albeit with similar properties, will be required for another.

It is generally agreed that the neurotransmitter substances affected in depression are the catecholamines, norepinephrine and serotonin. Their chief metabolites MHPG (3-methoxy-hydroxyphenyl glycol) of the former and 5-HIAA (5-hydroxyindoleacetic acid) of the latter have been shown to exist in differing concentrations in some cases of depression. It is possible that some cases with low urinary MHPG levels will correlate with low CNS norepinephrine and will respond to tricyclic anti-depressants having a potent inhibitory effect on norepinephrine re-uptake. Drugs which are potent inhibitors of serotonin re-uptake may indeed be particularly effective in those patients who have a low 5-HIAA urinary level correlating with low CNS serotonin. Amitriptyline is said to be particularly effective in those cases of depression marked by a low 5-HT. Desipramine is believed to have reverse indications and imipramine to be equally effective in cases with either low 5-HT or MHPG urinary levels. These trends still require further clinical testing.

Plasma levels can be measured for nearly all available antidepressants. Each antidepressant medication requires its own specialized test, thus making it difficult, at the moment, for these tests to be widely available. Until now, measuring plasma levels of various antidepressants has indicated considerable variability in the dosage required to produce equivalent plasma levels. While not yet available for widespread use, in many difficult cases such measurements can be helpful, particularly to determine whether nonresponse is due to inadequate absorption. In addition the measurement of plasma levels may be important to determine compliance, to pre-vent impending toxicity in the elderly, and in patients with liver disease.

The measurement of plasma levels has given rise to the term "therapeutic window" which has been most carefully worked out for nortriptyline the ranges being 50 nanograms per milliliter to 75 mg/ml. Initially it was believed that levels below 50 mg/ml were ineffective; this no longer is believed to be so. Of greater interest, however, are the upper limits of the so-called therapeutic window: some patients who seem refractory will respond if their levels are lowered.

ANTIANXIETY AGENTS (MINOR TRANQUILIZERS)

The antianxiety drugs generally available, that is to say members of the benzodiazepine family, are the most widely prescribed drugs in North America. This widespread use has produced alarm in many quarters, particularly the fear that these drugs will be used as a substitute for learning to cope with difficulties in life. As has been stressed on many occasions, drugs per se do not alleviate personal conflicts. However, used judiciously, they do not interfere with psychotherapy or problem solving, and, in fact, in many cases, by reducing anxiety to a tolerable level, they actually enhance the ability of most people to come to terms with difficult situations. In fact, it has been the experience of most practising clinicians that, except in certain cases, the majority of patients who take antianxiety drugs cease to do so as soon as they find themselves able to tolerate the level of distress they are encountering.

The reason for this is that most bouts of anxiety are shortlived, although often recurrent in nature. Therefore, for the majority of patients who require this medication, it can be prescribed and is usually taken to deal with situations as they arise.

This medication should not be prescribed casually for simple situations resulting in tension and anxiety, nor for those individuals who have chronic cases of anxiety. Unlike with antidepressants and antipsychotic compounds, benzodiazepines and other antianxiety agents are adjunctive treatments, and appropriate psychotherapeutic approaches and methods must be used to deal with the underlying situation.

However, it must be remembered that these drugs are among the safest available to physicians for use by patients. Relatively rapid in action, effective in reducing feelings of panic, fear and tension, they also serve as hypnotic agents. For these and other reasons the drugs are widely prescribed and used.

The availability of these agents has made it unnecessary, except in extremely exceptional cases, to utilize barbiturates. As is well known the barbiturates produce serious syndromes of tolerance. The amount needed to deal with insomnia for even a short period—say, one to two weeks—is enough, if taken at one time, to produce a lethal overdose. This is not the case with benzodiazepines.

Mechanism of action. Although these drugs are the most widely prescribed in medicine and have been available for some 20 years, it is only very recently that progress has been made in elucidating the mechanism of action. It is generally believed that the drugs exert their effect through activity on GABA-ergic systems.

Indications and use. ACUTE ANXIETY. Parenteral Use—diazepam, particularly, may be used intravenously, and is particularly useful in states of agitation, confusion, especially when associated with toxic and/or delirious states.

Five to twenty mg may be given intramuscularly or intravenously, and the dose repeated if initially inadequate effect was obtained. Cases of severe anxiety, and particularly for initial treatment, the drug is usually taken in divided doses. Most often for moderate problems of anxiety and tension, diazepam, in amounts of five mg tid and five to ten mg at bedtime, initially,

can be considered to be close—a standard dose. More than with any other category of compounds, individual consideration is vital and the physician must educate the patient according to the needs that the patient has at any given time. This form of discontinuous use of the drug will help to ensure that the medication is taken only when absolutely needed. Patients should be encouraged to cope with as much anxiety and tension as possible and to take medication only when necessary. Maintenance treatment should be recommended only following careful investigation, with frequent checking of the patient's condition and medication intake, and therapy aimed at modification of intra- or interpersonal environment.

SELECTION OF DRUGS. There is a wide variety of antianxiety benzodiazepine compounds available. The older variety of drugs, now available as generic products, are much less costly to the patient. At the moment, these drugs are chlordiazepoxide and diazepam. The facing table lists the various benzodiazepines available and the average daily dose. Clinical tests have not demonstrated any difference among these drugs in the treatment of anxiety. Pharmacological differences however are known, particularly as regards the duration of the drug in the body. This phenomenon is dependent on the half-life of the drug and is related to the presence or absence of active intermediate metabolites which have some of the same characteristics as the parent compound. It should be noted that chlordiazepoxide, diazepam, chlorapate and prazepam are all converted into the active metabolite desmethyldiazepam, a drug which is just as effective as a tranquillizer as chlordiazepoxide or diazepam. Oxazepam, lorazepam and triazolam are the three benzodiazepines currently available which have no active metabolites and have considerably shorter half-lives than the other compounds used.

Therefore drugs with longer half-life, that is, those with active metabolites, reach steady state in one or two days, and can thereafter be given once daily. Shorter acting drugs such as oxazepam and lorazepam need to be given in divided doses, three times daily, in order to maintain a full therapeutic level.

In terms of outcome, studies in anxious patients, all benzodiazepines have been equally effective. In practice and in general this group of drugs has been a satisfactory substitute for the much more potentially toxic barbiturates.

scribed for more than a few nights at a time. Caution in the prescription of hypnotic agents should be observed in patients with respiratory impairment, mental depression or problems of substance abuse such as alcoholism.

All benzodiazepines in adequate dosage provide reasonable sedative effect. The most popular hypnotic, flurazepam has a half-life of nearly two days and slowly accumulates in the blood. This phenomenon may be responsible for the report that sleep

Benzodiazepines

Generic Name	Trade Name	Usual Adult Dosage	Half-life (hrs.)
Diazepam	Valium	5–10 mg BID–QID	36
Chlordiazepoxide	Librium	10–25 mg BID–QID	30
Oxazepam	Serax	15–30 mg BID–QID	8
Chlorazepate	Tranxene	7.5–15 mg BID–QID	
Lorazepam	Ativan	1–2 mg BID–QID	12
Flurazepam	Dalmane	Insomnia–15–30 mg	48
Triazolam	Halcion	0.5–1 mg–Insomnia	3

Side effects of antianxiety drugs. The most common ones are drowsiness, ataxia, and dizziness, or vertigo. Drowsiness is, by far, the most common and usually subsides with continued use.

Because these drugs are used so widely it is important to caution patients about the effect of these drugs on psychomotor skills, for example car driving, working with heavy duty machinery, etc.

Overdoses are frequently attempted with benzodiazepines, but unless these attempts are accompanied by significant abuse of other medication such as barbiturates, antidepressants and alcohol, they are rarely serious and almost never fatal.

THE TREATMENT OF INSOMNIA

Many patients seeking medical advice complain of insomnia. The most important aspect of the treatment of insomnia is the development of a diagnosis and therefore the treatment of the underlying condition. Insomnia, as such, is occasionally due to stress-related situations and is almost always of a short duration. Therefore, as a general rule hypnotics should not be pre-

in the second or third night on flurazepam therapy is better than the first. When this drug is used, attempts should be made to maintain as low level of intake as possible, that is 15 mg a day. Recently a new hypnotic has become available, namely, triazolam, with the shortest half-life of all benzodiazepines. It can be used in doses of 0.5 or 1 mg per night.

Use of Drugs in the Elderly

The subjects of geriatrics and gerontology are increasingly receiving intensive study. By and large, the same indications exist in the elderly, as in other age groups for the use of psychotropic medication. Some principles should, however, be followed:

1. Tolerance to large amounts of medication in the elderly is reduced. Therefore, drugs should be given in smaller quantities and at longer intervals than in the younger patients.
2. Physiological changes which accompany the aging process essen-

tially extend the biological activity of any given drug and lower the threshold for toxic side effects.

3. Monitor vital signs often.

Psychopharmacology is a field which is expanding rapidly. The increase of knowledge in psychopharmacology increases the effectiveness of the physician in utilizing pharmacotherapy. As always in psychiatry good treatment demands attention to the patient as a whole. No amount of medication will substitute for a good patient-doctor relationship which will, in itself, enhance the therapeutic effect of drugs (placebo effect), establish good lines of communication so that compliance to drug intake can occur, and discussion and prevention of side effects can take place. In this way, the psyche and the anatomical and biochemical substrate can be treated and the therapeutic effect maximized.

FURTHER READINGS

Relating to Electroconvulsive Therapy:

Blachly, P.H. and Gowing, D. (1966): Multiple monitored electroconvulsive treatment. *Compr. Psychiatry 7*:100.

Blachly, P.H. (1977): Attitudes, data, and technological promise of ECT. *Psychiatr. Opin. 14*:9.

Friedberg, J. (1977): ECT as a neurologic injury. *Psychiatr. Opin. 14*:16.

Blachly's contribution is an up-to-date account of modern views of ECT. Friedberg's is an article by a neurologist who is concerned about the negative aspects of ECT.

Furlong, F.W. (1972): The mythology of electroconvulsive therapy. *Compr. Psychiatry. 13*:235.

An attempt to account for and explain the anti-ECT articles which exist in the scientific literature.

Lancaster, N.P., Steinert, R.R., and Frost, L. (1958): Unilateral electro-convulsive therapy. *J. Ment. Sci. 104*:221.

Kalinowsky, L.B. (1975): Electric and other convulsive treatments. In *American Handbook of Psychiatry*. 2d ed. Vol. 5. Edited by S. Arieti. New York, Basic Books.

This is a good account with adequate detail of the use of electroconvulsive therapy in psychiatry. The author has been studying this modality of treatment and has written about it for a good many years.

Relating to Drugs:

Appleton, W.S. and David, J.M. (1973):*Practical Clinical Psychopharmacology*. Baltimore, Williams & Wilkins.

Bassuk, E.L. and Schoonover, S.C. (1976): *The Practitioner's Guide to Psychoactive Drugs*. New York, Plenum.

Shader, R.I. (1975):*Manual of Psychiatric Therapies: Practical Psychopharmacology and Psychiatry*. Boston, Little Brown.

Much of the structure, activity and relationships have become extremely complex and to detail them would require a comprehensive report. It is therefore necessary for companion reading with and/or reference to at least one of the above. These are issued as relatively small manuals with both theoretical and practical information in them. They will serve as excellent handbooks for the student and the practitioner.

Arieti, S. (1975): *American Handbook of Psychiatry* Vol. 5. New York, Basic Books.

Baldessarini, R.J. (1978): Chemotherapy. In *The Harvard Guide to Modern Psychiatry*. Edited by A. M. Nicholi. Cambridge, Mass., Harvard University Press.

Barchas, J.D., Berger, P.A., Ciaranello, R.D., et al. (1977): *Psychopharmacology: From Theory to Practice*. New York, Oxford University Press.

This is an excellent textbook on the principles of both pharmacotherapy and psychopharmacology and is a good introduction for those who are interested in the field.

Freedman, A.M., Kaplan, H.I., and Sadock, B.J. (1975): *Comprehensive Textbook of Psychiatry*. Baltimore, Williams & Wilkins.

Lipton, N.A., DiMascio, A., and Killam, K.F. (1978): *Psychopharmacology A Generation of Progress*. New York, Raven Press.

An encyclopedic compendium and textbook. Currently the definitive work in the field of psychopharmacology and the use of psychotropic drugs.

Solomon, F., White, C.C., Parron, B.L., et al. (1979): Sleeping pills, insomnia and medical practice. *New Engl. J. Med. 300*:803.

Current concepts of insomnia and appropriate methods of treatment.

The author wishes to acknowledge the help he received fom T. R. Einarson, Pharmacist, DMPH Wing, G. and M. Hospital, Owen Sound, Ontario in reviewing and revising this chapter for publication.

35

Treatment: Hospital

George Voineskos

Hospital treatment may be offered on an emergency, inpatient, part-time or outpatient basis. In addition most psychiatric units offer consultation services to other medical and surgical units in the general hospital and to the various health and social agencies in the community. Emergency, inpatient, part-time hospitalization, outpatient, and consultation and educational services, constitute the five essential services that should be provided by psychiatric facilities of general and psychiatric hospitals. In some instances, as for example in the U.S.A. and Ontario, Canada, legislation has been enacted to declare these services "essential."

EMERGENCY SERVICES

Many patients enter psychiatric care through emergency consultation. The emergency room of the general hospital is the primary site of emergency psychiatric services in most communities (Glick et al., 1976). The emergency room is open 24 hours a day and available when private practitioners' offices and agencies are closed. In addition to psychosocial problems, many people come to the emergency room with physical problems such as headache, pain, insomnia, and self-injuries which necessitate psychiatric evaluation. The general nurse, the intern, the medical resident and the non-psychiatric physician are the primary health professionals operating the emergency room. Whether the patient will have a psychiatric evaluation depends on the level of awareness of the manifestations of psychiatric disorders and of psychological accompaniments of physical disorders of the personnel in the emergency clinic.

Accessibility and availability on a round-the-clock basis are the governing principles of emergency services. Twenty-four hour emergency psychiatric consultation is now available in the hospital emergency rooms of most cities in North America. The fundamental working unit of a psychiatric emergency service is a multidisciplinary team consisting of a psychiatrist, a social worker, and a nurse. Rapid assessment of the emergency patient and his family, and mobilization and linkage with community agencies are essential components of the crisis intervention approach employed by the team. A small back-up emergency or crisis ward (Voineskos, 1974) should be an integral part of the psychiatric emergency service. Fortunately, this has become a standard facility in most hospitals. The number of emergency beds varies from 4 to 14. The beds may be in the emergency room or in the psychiatric unit. In a few hospitals the psychiatric emergency ward is self-contained; a desirable organization but one that space limitations often do not permit. A common feature of the operation of the emergency ward is the time-limited stay. The maximum stay varies from 24 hours to 21 days; the shorter period is characteristic of general hospitals. The function of the inpatient component also varies. Some operate merely as "holding" units, where assessment and disposition occurs the day after admission, while other units operate as fully fledged crisis intervention or brief therapy units offering an organized treatment program.

The thorough evaluation of the therapeutic efficacy of brief hospitalization is yet to come; however, the few studies available indicate that brief hospitalization and crisis intervention are therapeutically promising in the treatment of psychiatric emergencies.

INPATIENT SERVICES

Admission to the inpatient service used to be the rule in the mental hospital since there was little else to offer. Such admission would usually take place under some form of compulsory order and patients were hospitalized for very long periods. In the last twenty years, however, this situation has changed dramatically. The emphasis has shifted from inpatient treatment to outpatient care as a result of the early discharge policy of the psychiatric hospitals, changes in mental health legislation, the introduction of modern psychotropic medication, and the development of psychiatric units in general hospitals. Today inpatient treatment is only one phase in the total treatment program of most psychiatric patients. The optimum size of the psychiatric ward, whether of a general or psychiatric hospital, is 25 to 30 beds.

Facilities for relatively unobtrusive observation for disturbed patients should be available. The design of the ward should be simple and easily identifiable and the decoration and furnishings attractive. Facilities should be available for interviewing, and for small and large group therapy meetings.

The most frequent reasons for inpatient treatment (Tucker and Maxmen, 1973) are one or more of the following:

1. Increased symptoms or maladaptive behavior to a disabling level, despite all other interventions.
2. Failure to clarify a diagnostic problem.
3. Inability of the environment (therapist, family, work) to further tolerate the patient's behavior, or its persistent reinforcement of the previous maladaptive behavior.
4. The need to institute a form of treatment that requires careful medical supervision and monitoring.
5. Violent or destructive behavior to self or others.

The primary goal of hospitalization is at least to alleviate, if not eliminate, the reasons for which hospitalization became necessary, and thereby to enable the individual to return to community living. The objectives of hospitalization therefore focus on attaining a level of functioning compatible with living in the community.

The goals of inpatient and outpatient treatment differ most in their emphasis on the ability to function rather than the resolution of lifelong residual symptoms or psychodynamic conflicts. A second difference arises from the fact that during hospitalization the patient is present for observation, treatment, and intervention 24 hours a day. The social milieu of the hospital should be structured to provide ample opportunities for interactions, initiative, responsible behavior, and activities. In these situations the patients are likely to recreate typical interactions characteristic of their daily life outside the hospital, inasmuch as they tend to use the same ways of dealing with other people in group therapy and other therapeutic activities as they use in their private lives. These interactions are available for discussion and more adaptive skills may be taught.

John and Elaine Cumming (1962) in their influential book *Ego and Milieu* put together the best account available of milieu therapy. They link theories of psychological functioning with the attempts to structure and utilize the hospital environment for therapeutic change.

Further discussion of the therapeutic milieu and the negative effects of hospitalization will be found in the chapter on social treatment. At this point, we might draw attention to the interruptions that hospitalization creates on the individual's life and his family. In addition to interruptions of the patient's life caused by pathological or destructive patterns of behavior, hospitalization itself interrupts most of the ordinary social roles people perform. Admission to a hospital, for any reason, means that the individual can no longer effectively perform the role of father, provider, mother, worker, husband, or neighbor. Furthermore, as an inpatient, the individual has to depend on others for food and shelter and others regulate ordinary daily activities such as time of shaving, or taking a bath, which in ordinary life are taken for granted but which involve the exercise of initiative, responsibility, and social role performance. Social roles that are not practised over a long period of time tend to atrophy from disuse, and some people are more vulnerable to this than others. And dependency on the hospital environment can develop. Many patients experience an exacerbation of symptoms when preparation for discharge begins and occasionally the anxiety provoked by impending discharge is so severe that it can jeopardize the therapeutic result of the entire stay in hospital.

The usual psychiatric ward is of the general type. It accepts patients suffering from all forms of psychiatric disorders. Particular attention is paid to the therapeutic milieu of the ward since it has been recognized that the events of the entire day can have therapeutic influences on the patient. The program usually includes individual therapy, group therapy, occupational and recreational therapy, as well as pharmacotherapy and other physical forms of treatment. The program is operated by a multidisciplinary team consisting of one or more psychiatrists, social workers, nurses, an occupational therapist, and a psychologist.

In addition to general units there exist *specialist* ones. The specialist inpatient units are organized on the basis of a common characteristic of the patients, either age group or a particular psychiatric problem. Illustrations of the latter include forensic units, units for the treatment of alcoholism or drug addiction, or special research units, e.g., for affective disorders. The advantages of having such units relate to the special space or equipment needs for some, and they allow the development of the required expertise by the staff of the treatment team. Research is also facilitated in such units.

Inpatient units for longer term patients, particularly those requiring prolonged rehabilitation, are usually located in mental hospitals, partly because of space requirements and partly because of historical reasons. The therapeutic milieu on these wards is usually based on group therapy or token economy or a combination of these two. These programs have a strong element of work therapy, in the form of occupational therapy or more often industrial therapy.

PART-TIME HOSPITALIZATION

Part-time hospitalization includes day, night, and weekend hospital programs.

A day hospital developed in Moscow in 1933 had little or no effect on later developments in the Western world. Canada has the distinction of having the first organized day hospital in the Western world; this was established at the Allan Memorial Institute, Montreal, in 1946, by D. Ewen Cameron.

In a day hospital, full hospital treatment is given under medical supervision to patients who return to their homes at night. Day hospital programs have one or more of the following functions (Voineskos, 1976):

1. They serve as an alternative to inpatient treatment. Studies have demonstrated that up to two thirds of those requiring inpatient treatment can be treated just as well in a day hospital. While the diagnoses of patients vary, those who benefit most are patients suffering from depression, personality disorders, psychosomatic illness, and schizophrenia. Serious suicidal risk or homicidal risk, severe sociopathy, alcoholism or drug addiction, and severe brain damage are associated with an unfavorable outcome in day hospital treatment. The availability of a supportive family, or ability to arrange accommodation for the patient, and access to an inpatient ward for crisis hospitalization are essential for the operation of these programs.

2. These programs serve as a transition from inpatient to outpatient treatment for those whose symptoms are exacerbated by the anxiety provoked by impending discharge. Transitional programs also facilitate the patient's gradual reintegration into the community.

3. They may be used for rehabilitation of long-term patients and maintenance of severely disabled patients. The majority of these programs have been developed by psychiatric hospitals for patients who suffer from the social and vocational deficits associated with chronic psychiatric disorder. Most of the patients suffer from chronic schizophrenia and have often spent many years as inpatients, either continuously or intermittently. These programs focus on work therapy and supervision of medication.

4. As an alternative to, or extension of outpatient treatment, these programs are useful for patients requiring more intensive treatment than can be offered on an outpatient basis and for those who require a milieu emphasizing interpersonal relations and social factors.

Day hospitals for specific age groups. They are often utilized in psychiatric services for children. During day hospitalization, while the child and the family are engaged in treatment, the child's parents continue their parental and nurturing role and the child maintains his family status. Day hospitals for the elderly are set up in association with psychiatric or more often geriatric hospitals or units. Organization of transportation between home and hospital is important, for many elderly patients may be unable to use public vehicles. Many patients who might otherwise be in psychiatric wards or in nursing homes are able to be in the community because of their attendance at the day hospital.

The night hospital. These are particularly useful for people who need intensive psychiatric treatment without interrupting their work or studies, and for inpatients who are able to resume their usual daily work but require continuing therapy (Voineskos, 1976). However, night hospitals are difficult to administer and part-time hospitalization is largely limited to day programs.

Economic aspects. Escalating costs of health services and fiscal restraints place increasing demands on today's physicians to be aware of the relative costs of treatment modalities and to consider the cost in seeking the best treatment for their patients. For instance, inpatient treatment is the most expensive modality of care; the cost per bed often exceeds $200 per day and this sum does not include medical and special investigative procedures. By contrast day hospital treatment is much more economical in both capital and operating costs (Voineskos, 1976). Existing buildings can easily be adapted for day care and the space required for day patients is much smaller than that for an equal number of inpatients. One nursing shift is required rather than three, and kitchen and domestic staff are needed for less time each day for only five days a week. The operating cost of day hospital treatment is estimated at approximately one third to one half the cost of inpatient treatment.

OUTPATIENT SERVICES

In the past twenty years there has been an enormous growth of outpatient therapy. A major reason for this growth has been the development of psychiatric units in general hospitals. Most of these units started on an outpatient basis and the inpatient component developed later.

Outpatient departments offer consultation to family practitioners and other physicians for their patients. Outpatient departments also accept patients from the inpatient services, the emergency department, and agencies in the community.

Individual, group and family therapy are practised in outpatient departments. However, individual psychotherapy is the most frequent mode of outpatient therapy in North America. Group therapy, despite its documented merits for selected groups of patients, is less often practised.

Many hospitals operate special clinics for certain kinds of patients. Prominent among these are clinics for patients suffering from chronic schizophrenia and for those suffering from affective disorders. There are many merits to such clinics. Most important is the monitoring of medication. For schizophrenic patients, the clinic affords the opportunity of sociotherapy by a small team of staff which in combination with medication has proven effective in the prevention of relapse and in posthospital adjustment. Other specialized clinics such as for behavior therapy or clinics for sexual or addiction

problems allow the concentration of professional skills and necessary equipment. As well, electroconvulsive therapy can be administered to outpatients, if the procedure is carefully monitored, and good recovery facilities are available.

CONSULTATION AND EDUCATION SERVICES

Consultation and education services are offered to various community health and social agencies. The consultee-centered case consultation is the most favored approach to consultation. Here the responsibility for the patient remains with the professional who has requested the consultation (Caplan, 1964). The same approach is also applied in the consultation and liaison service of the general hospital (Khantzian and Mack, 1970), though at times it becomes necessary for the psychiatrist to take over the responsibility for the management of the patient and effect transfer to the psychiatric unit.

The consultation and liaison service is one of the most important psychiatric services the general hospital offers. The chief objectives of this service are (a) the detection, diagnosis and treatment of frank psychiatric disorders and detection and treatment of the psychosocial complications or accompaniments of physical illness, and (b) the education of the medical and nursing staff concerning the emotional needs of their patients. Of the several models of organization of the liaison service, the most successful and commonly practiced is the one where each psychiatrist works consistently with one or more services, for example the medical, the obstetrical-gynecological services, etc., while one psychiatrist coordinates the entire liaison service. This model permits the psychiatrist to get to know and become known by the nonpsychiatric physicians and the nursing staff of the service(s), and it facilitates education and encourages research.

Several authors (Hackett and Weisman, 1960; Khantzian and Mack, 1970) have emphasized that noninterpretative intervention is the preferred approach in the liaison service of the general hospital. It is of course important for the psychiatrist to appreciate the dynamic determinants of a particular emotional reaction, whether in a patient or in a member of staff. However, the level of psychological sophistication of the staff is a compelling reason for the psychiatrist to deal with the reality aspects of the situation by suggesting common-sense pragmatic approaches and clarifications in the management of the patient. Similarly, the psychiatric consultation report should be written in a language which does not contain psychiatric jargon and which can be readily understood by physicians of other disciplines.

REFERENCES

Caplan, G. (1964): *Principles of Preventive Psychiatry*. New York, Basic Books.

Cumming, J. and Cumming, E. (1962): *Ego and Milieu: Theory and Practice of Environmental Therapy*. New York, Atherton Press.

Glick, R.A., Meyerson, A.T., Robins, E., et al. (1976): *Psychiatric Emergencies*. New York, Grune and Stratton.

Hackett, T.P. and Weisman, A.D. (1960): Psychiatric management of operative syndromes: the therapeutic consultation and the effect of noninterpretive intervention. *Psychosom. Med.* 22:267.

Khantzian, E.J. and Mack, J.E. (1970): The initiation and practice of psychiatric consultation in the general hospital. In *The Practice of Community Mental Health*. Edited by H. Grunebaum. Boston, Little, Brown.

Tucker, M.J. and Maxmen, J.S. (1973): The practice of hospital psychiatry: a formulation. *Am. J. Psychiatry. 130*:887.

Voineskos, G. (1974): Psychiatric emergencies: the crisis intervention approach. *Univer. Tor. Med. J. 51*:85.

Voineskos, G. (1976): Part-time hospitalization programs: the neglected field of community psychiatry. *Can. Med. Assoc. J.* 114:320.

36

Treatment: Social-Environmental

George Voineskos

During the first half of this century mental hospitals were large and overcrowded, most of the wards being occupied by chronic, long-stay patients who led restricted and inactive lives. The major concern was the safe custody of the patients. Little or no attention was paid to the social environment, or milieu, of the institutions in which the patients would spend many years. With isolated exceptions, such as the unit for schizophrenic patients organized by Harry Stack Sullivan in the late 1920's, and Rowland's studies of the mental hospital (1938) it was only after the second World War and in particular in the 1950's that explicit attention began to be paid to the milieu in which treatment was given (Clark, 1964).

An impetus for that attention was provided in the 1950's by social scientists who studied psychiatric institutions and the roles of the staff and patients. Belknap (1956), a sociologist, studied a large mental hospital that had been "reformed" several times. He found that the doctors and the administrative nurses were transient members of the staff. Doctors stayed on the average a little over two years and were ineffectual in bringing about any change. The "culture" of the institution was perpetuated by a small group of attendants and maintenance staff who stayed in the hospital their entire working lives. These staff members had developed their own way of coping with troublesome or rebellious patients by denying them access to the doctors or reporting them as disturbed or paranoid. Indeed these staff members controlled the wards and the details of the patients' daily lives. They were, in fact, the carriers of the enduring life of the institution. Belknap found in the hospital a stratified society with six layers: the doctors, the charge attendant and his deputies, the attendants, the worker-patients, the limited-privilege patients, and the patients with no privileges. Everyone, however psychotic, knew where he stood on this scale and showed an awareness of his rights and obligations. While head nurses, medical directors, nursing supervisors, occupational therapists, and others came and went, the long-stay attendants and long-stay patients made up the enduring reality of the mental hospital.

Goffman (1961), a sociologist, reporting on St. Elizabeth's hospital in Washington, D.C., drew attention to the common characteristics of "total institutions," including monasteries, prisons, and similar places. He described the "stripping process" in which the individual is deprived of all the things that gave him his identity and individuality, including clothes, money, and personal belongings. In total institutions a peculiar system of rewards and punishments develops for actions not regarded as exceptional in the outside world. This system is designed to teach the individual his place in the institution. Withdrawal, rebellion, passive compliance, or overcompliance were some of the ways in which the patients reacted to the institutional system and way of life.

Caudill (1958), a social anthropologist, reported on the patient culture which he observed while disguised as an "inpatient" and, later, as a social scientist-observer at the Yale Psychiatric Institute. He described how the other patients taught him his role (such as how he should behave to get a weekend pass or permission to shave) and the sort of fantasies each doctor liked to hear during psychotherapy.

Stanton, a psychiatrist, and Schwartz, a sociologist, studied, over a three year period, Chestnut Lodge in Maryland, a small and expensive private hospital for the psycho-analytic treatment of psychotic patients (1954). They pointed out that beyond the daily hour of analytic treatment, many events of the rest of the day influenced the patient's therapy. In addition, disagreements among the staff, such as the "triangular conflict," in which two staff differ about the management of a patient, when unresolved culminated in a serious crisis in which the patient's clinical condition worsened.

These earlier studies demonstrate the unwanted powerful influences upon a person who lives in an institution for a long time. Inflexibility of routine, regimentation, social distance, loss of contact with the outside world, loss of personal friends and possessions, lack of opportunity to practise ordinary social roles, and inactivity led to "institutionalism" or the "social breakdown syndrome." Barton suggested that many of the "signs" of chronic schizophrenia were in effect the product of long

years of this type of regimented institutional living (Clark, 1964). The "signs" he referred to include apathy, lack of initiative, loss of interest, and deterioration in personal habits. He also described a characteristic posture, with hands held across the body or behind an apron, drooped shoulders, head forward, and a shuffling gait. Many of the negative features of "total institutions" had been present in mental hospitals, at least until the early 1960's, and patients who had been residents in mental hospitals for two years continuously in 1960 would have been exposed to them (Wing and Brown, 1970).

THERAPEUTIC MILIEU AND MILIEU THERAPY

Paul Sivadon (1957) suggested that a psychiatric hospital, in order to fulfill its role as a therapeutic milieu, should do three things: first, offer to the new patient, whatever the nature of his illness, living conditions suited to his present level of functioning; second, provide for him those circumstances which will permit him to establish satisfactory relationships with his physical and social environments, and progressively perfect his ways of relating to them. Finally, furnish, at all times, to the largest possible number of patients, the opportunity and means of developing social behavior approximating the normal.

Clearly, therefore, the hospital milieu has to be deliberately organized in order to be therapeutic. Cumming and Cumming (1962) delineated the characteristics of the milieu which can promote a wide range of competence in the individual patient. Such a milieu must offer a clear, organized, and unambiguous social structure, a variety of settings with problems to solve in a protected situation, a peer group, a helpful and encouraging staff, assisting the patient to act in clearly defined roles and to live more effectively. Cumming and Cumming also pointed out the importance of the physical aspects of the milieu and how these in turn can aid the social structure of the hospital and ward environment.

Cumming and Cumming (1962) defined *milieu therapy* as a scientific manipulation of the environment aimed at producing changes in the personality of the patient. Drawing on the work of many authors in the field of personality theory, especially ego psychology, they formulated a theoretical framework of milieu therapy. This they then integrated with their rich experience from organizing therapeutic milieux and from visiting rehabilitation hospitals. They put together clear recommendations for the organization of a therapeutic milieu that could result in "ego restitution" of the damaged self.

A specific kind of therapeutic milieu is the therapeutic community. In the later years of the Second World War British psychiatrists and psychoanalysts experimented with the application of social factors in the treatment of soldiers who were psychiatric casualties. The "Northfield (hospital) Experiment" was an attempt to use the organizational and social structure of the hospital as a therapeutic instrument in the treatment of the patients. The main pioneer of the therapeutic community as a technique was Maxwell Jones, who set out to restructure the entire social organization of hospitals and individual wards on both sides of the Atlantic. In his words "a therapeutic community is distinctive amongst other comparable treatment centers in the way the institution's total resoures, both staff and patients, are self-consciously pooled in furthering treatment" (Clark, 1977). In the therapeutic community the structure of the day varies a great deal, but community meetings, in which all staff and patients attend, are held frequently, often daily. The development of the therapeutic community entails freeing of communication, flattening of the authority pyramid and decision making at all levels so that patients and staff can participate freely. It also provides learning experiences particularly of "social learn-ing," role examination of all members of the community and social analysis of all events in order to understand individual and interpersonal dynamics. Crisis situations and what Jones has called "living-learning" situations arising from the daily living on the ward and the hospital are opportunities for practising these principles (Jones, 1968).

REHABILITATION

Aims and disabilities. Psychiatric rehabilitation is aimed at reducing the social and vocational deficits which often accompany psychiatric illness so that the individual can resume his life in the community.

Most of the rehabilitative work in psychiatry has focused on patients suffering from schizophrenic disorders, because the early onset and chronic course of schizophrenia often have a crippling effect upon the vocational and social abilities of those afflicted. Four major aspects of rehabilitation will be discussed, characterized more by overlap than demarcation, namely: the social environment, accommodation, leisure time, and work. While schizophrenia is used as the paradigm, much is applicable to other psychiatric disorders.

The factors which hinder the community resettlement of the schizophrenic patient have been classified by Wing (1963) into three large groups:

"Premorbid" disabilities which are present before the overt onset of the illness, and are due to persisting deficiencies of personality, education, social competence or occupational skill.

"Primary" disabilities which are basically part of the illness and can be conveniently classified into negative and florid symptoms. The negative symptoms include social withdrawal, flatness of affect, poverty of speech, slowness, under-activity and a low level of motivation. The florid symptoms include delusions, hallucinations, incoherent thought and speech, overactivity, and various forms of odd behavior.

"Secondary" disabilities which are not part

of the illness but arise as a result of the patient's personal reaction to being ill or of the reaction of the social groups in which the patient lives, exists or interacts and upon whose goodwill his conditions of life may depend. These secondary disabilities are liable to occur in many forms of prolonged illness, including physical ones.

The premorbid disabilities and the early onset of schizophrenia result in an individual who is poorly equipped with the vocational and social skills required in life. The negative primary disabilities, e.g., social withdrawal and lack of motivation, are among the major persistent obstacles in rehabilitation; the florid ones on the other hand can seriously interrupt the already precarious work and social relations. Finally, the secondary disabilities may confirm the stamp of invalidism on the individual.

The social environment. In any one individual the three types of disability described above blend together to give one clinical picture, but in planning for a course of rehabilitation it is helpful to separate the various elements and to be aware of the different kinds of environmental factors which can cause deterioration or improvement in them.

An understimulating environment tends to increase the negative symptoms such as social withdrawal, passivity, inertia and lack of initiative (Wing and Brown, 1970). This process is seen best in a patient who has been on a ward which does not have an adequate therapeutic program for a long time. On such an inpatient ward, the attitudes and expectations of staff and other patients can have a great influence on the secondary disabilities. Prolonged stay in hospital, inactivity, lack of opportunity to practise social roles, and therapeutic pessimism gradually push the individual towards passivity, apathy and acceptance of himself as invalid. While these conditions used to be found in the old-fashioned mental hospital, they have also been described in foster homes for discharged patients in Canada in a penetrating report (Murphy et al., 1972).

On the other hand, under conditions of social overstimulation there is a tendency for florid symptoms to reappear or become worse. This process is most frequently seen outside the hospital but it can certainly also be seen within it. The onset of florid symptoms is often preceded in the previous three weeks by a significant change in the patient's social environment (Wing and Brown, 1970).

Brown et al. (1958) have shown that schizophrenic patients were more likely to relapse if they returned to live with their parents or wives after discharge than if they went to a hostel, rooming accommodation, or lived with siblings. Brown and his associates (1972) later showed that the important factor contributing to relapse was not the type of relative but rather a high degree of what they termed the "expressed emotion" shown by the relative. This "expressed emotion" consisted of three components, the most important of which was the "critical comments" made by the relative, the other two being "emotional over-involvement" and "hostility." This contributory factor to relapse was independent of other factors such as length of history, type of symptomatology, or severity of previous disturbance. Furthermore they found that social withdrawal of the patient from his relatives could be a protective factor and that 35 hours per week of exposure to relatives was the critical period beyond which the chances of relapse were greatly increased. Brown et al. (1972) have suggested that reduction of the hours of contact with these relatives such as would occur if the relative or patient went out to work, or if the patient attended day hospital, or simply allowing the patient to withdraw can act preventively. The work of Brown and his associates has provided us with a theoretical framework and guidelines for family therapy or counselling for schizophrenic patients who return to live with their family, and for the optimum social environment, whether the patient is in the hospital or in the community. According to Brown et al. (1972) the desirable social environment is a structured one, with clear cut roles, only as much complexity as any given individual can cope with, and with neutral but active supervision to keep up standards of appearance, work and behavior. Most of these guidelines are also applicable and have been applied empirically in the organization of housing alternatives for patients who have no family to return to.

Accommodation. Many psychiatric patients have few environmental supports, and often no family to return to. In addition, as suggested above, for some patients it may not be therapeutic to return to their families after discharge. The available housing for these patients ranges along a continuum from transitional to more permanent sheltered housing and ultimately to competitive housing in the community. The housing alternatives include:

HALFWAY HOUSES. These have a stay ranging from a few days to six months, and there is usually a house staff member living-in.

COOPERATIVE HOUSING. There is less supervision in this type of housing, and residents often undertake some house work such as cooking.

APARTMENTS. Some agencies have purchased a building and have converted it to small apartments which are rented by former psychiatric patients. On other occasions agencies rent apartments under their own name and then sublet them to patients.

BOARDING HOMES. Some hospitals and agencies have delveloped a relationship with privately owned boarding homes in which they basically offer social services or psychiatric liaison but do not operate the home itself.

FOSTER HOMES. Canada pioneered a foster homes program for psychiatric patients in the 1960's. Many patients were discharged from psychiatric hospitals to foster homes. However, the hope of integrating these patients into the families they lived with was not realized.

A basic assumption in the operation of these housing facilities has been that the patients will be better integrated in the community in which they live. While there are bright examples of this, such as Fountain House or Horizon House in the United States, a survey of foster homes in Canada by Murphy et al. (1972) revealed that residents can be just as isolated in foster homes, as they can be in the "back wards" of a barren mental hospital.

Leisure time. The mastery of leisure time has been the stimulus to the growth of a multi-billion dollar industry, and is still a problem to many people in contemporary society, even to those not afflicted by a psychiatric illness.

To patients with a chronic psychiatric illness such as schizophrenia, leisure time is the period when their isolated state is at its clearest. With few or no family supports, scarce friends, poor interpersonal skills, and meager financial resources the chronic schizophrenic patient is likely to spend the weekend sleeping in his rooming place, watching television, or walking in the downtown streets, or a nearby park. Teaching effective use of leisure time has been increasingly recognized as a very important aspect of rehabilitation. To this effect social and recreational clubs in the community have been utilized, and some hospitals have evening social groups for discharged psychiatric patients. However, of the several goals of rehabilitation the most difficult and elusive one seems to be the effective use of leisure time. Among the reasons that could be postulated for this difficulty include: the disabilities of the patient, the nature of recreational activities in present day society, and the approach taken by most mental health professionals in organizing social and recreational activities exclusively for psychiatric patients rather than fostering the patients' integration with non-patient groups.

Work. Rehabilitation requires not only that an overall plan be made but also that great attention be paid to seemingly trivial details of the patient's adjustment. This applies both to the living situation and to work. Work alone is not enough. It must be varied and in keeping with the patient's capabilities. As his capabilities increase, the patient can be moved, by gradual steps, through a series of more complex and demanding tasks.

The importance of work in rehabilitation was recognized during the nineteenth century. However, modern industrial therapy and training in hospital workshops and community-based sheltered workshops were started in Britain barely four decades ago following the example of the Netherlands. Subsequently, workshops were introduced in psychiatric hospitals in North America. During the last twenty years community-based rehabilitation workshops for former psychiatric patients, operating as non-profit community agencies, have been in existence in Canada and the U.S. Black (1964) writing about the Altro Workshops, which was the first community sheltered workshop in the U.S. to offer programs to psychiatric patients, described the fundamentals involved in sheltered work. The structure and support provided by a supervised, sheltered work situation allow for reality testing in an environment where there are no immediate consequences for such instances as there would be in competitive employment; the learning and mastery of reality tasks help to encourage ego strengths so that progress instead of avoidance or regression becomes the pattern. Realistic behavior is facilitated, work skills and habits are reinstated or acquired which are crucial in effecting the patient's transition back to the community and in maintaining him there.

Several experiments have shown that goal-setting and knowledge of results, which improve the performance of most people, failed to improve the performance of the schizophrenic patient. In contrast, social pressure brought to bear by familiar staff-nurse supervisors increased the workshop output of schizophrenic patients. This increase was accompanied by a significant decrease in the patient's abnormal behavior in the workshop. However, the decrease in abnormal behavior in the workshop was not necessarily reflected in improvement in the behavior on the ward (Wing and Brown, 1970).

Goldberg (1974), in discussing work rehabilitation, suggests that the working patient by virtue of his job has a defined role or position beyond the patient role. Work reduces his sense of social incompetence by providing an opportunity for socially productive behavior, by developing his skills and applying his aptitudes, by fostering social interaction, and by helping to structure his time usefully.

Conclusion. In psychiatric rehabilitation a social situation must be provided which enables the patient to overcome difficulties in communication, in making decisions, in mastering his emotional and affective states, in controlling his behavior and in the performance of social roles. Thus, the ward or sheltered housing in which the patient lives should approximate as far as possible everyday life, not only in its physical, but in its social structure. Treatment of the illness also includes provision of social opportunities which foster social adaptation. It is clear that treatment and rehabilitation in psychiatry overlap, and sometimes they are indistinguishable. Naturally, this attracts the attention of critics of psychiatry because the model of rehabilitation is not directed at treating the causes of illness. However, Tucker and Maxmen (1973) have drawn a suitable analogy in suggesting that, while no one has ever believed that the techniques of speech therapy or physiotherapy are suitable for removing the vascular lesion responsible for a stroke, or that they would be effective in preventing further cerebral vascular accidents, nobody doubts the value of such treatments.

REFERENCES

Belknap, I. (1956): *Human Problems of a State Mental Hospital.* New York, McGraw-Hill.

Black, B.J. (1964): Psychiatric rehabilitation in the community. In *Handbook of Community Psychiatry and Community Mental Health.* Edited by L. Bellack. New York, Grune & Stratton.

Brown, G.W., Carstairs, G.M., and Topping, G. (1958): The post-hospital adjustment of chronic mental patients. *Lancet.* 2:685.

Brown, G.W., Birley, S.L.T., and Wing, J.K. (1972): Influence of family life on the course of schizophrenic disorders: a replication. *Br. J. Psychiatry.* 121:241.

Caudill, W.A. (1958): *The Psychiatric Hospital as a Small Society.* Cambridge, Mass., Harvard University Press.

Clark, D.H. (1964): *Administrative Therapy.* London, Tavistock.

Clark, D.H. (1977): The therapeutic community. *Br. J. Psychiatry.* 131:553.

Cumming, J. and Cumming, E. (1962): *Ego and Milieu: Theory and Practice of Environmental Therapy.* New York, Atherton Press.

Goffman, E. (1961): *Asylums: Essays on the Social Situation of Mental Patients and Other Inmates.* Garden City, N.Y., Anchor Books.

Goldberg, D. (1974): Principles of rehabilitation. *Compr. Psychiatry.* 15:237.

Jones, M. (1968): *Beyond the Therapeutic Community.* New Haven, Yale University Press.

Murphy, H.B.M., Pennee, B., and Luchins, D. (1972): Foster homes: the new back wards? *Canada's Ment. Health.* 20:1.

Sivadon, P.D. (1957): Techniques of Sociotherapy. *Psychiatry.* 20:205.

Stanton, A. and Schwartz, M. (1954): *The Mental Hospital.* New York, Basic Books.

Tucker, G.J. and Maxmen, J.S. (1973): Practice of hospital psychiatry: a formulation. *Am. J. Psychiatry.* 130:887.

Wing, J.K. (1963): Rehabilitation of psychiatric patients. *Br. J. Psychiatry.* 109:635.

Wing, J.K. and Brown, G.W. (1970): *Institutionalism and Schizophrenia: A Comparative Study of Three Mental Hospitals, 1960—1968.* London, Cambridge University Press.

CHAPTER **37**

Difficult Challenges in
Medical Practice

Stanley E. Greben

The physician, as he engages in medical practice, meets a spectrum of patients, insofar as their response to his therapeutic efforts is concerned. At the one end are those who respond quickly, favorably, and completely. At the other end are those who respond slowly, or unfavorably, or incompletely, or not at all. This spectrum confronts the practitioner in family practice, as well as in any specialty, including psychiatry. And so one way of addressing the difficulty of treating certain patients is to look at the problem of their relative lack of response to our therapeutic efforts.

Psychiatrists are especially interested in feelings, and this interest includes not only the feelings of patients, but also the feelings of the physician. As indicated above, a "difficult challenge" can be assessed by objective response or lack of response to therapy. But "difficulty" may also be measured in terms of the feelings which dealing with the patient generates in the physician. We will pay particular attention to this.

In order to understand the negative feelings which are generated within physicians in their treatment of patients, we have to first consider some of the expecta-

tions which most doctors bring to their work. Candidates for medical school are usually assessed with regard to their interest in helping others and in making ill people well. Medical school attempts to enlarge such motivations, in order to produce practitioners who will work principally to help the ill and disadvantaged. Such expectation of the physician is evident in his traditional credo, the Hippocratic Oath.

There are numerous reasons for wanting to help others. Some are creative, and arise out of the good feelings and basic endowment of the physician as a person. Some arise out of conflict, and are unwitting attempts to resolve something out of the physician's past. For example a very deprived or abused child might want to be a doctor and help eliminate deprivation or abuse of others. A child who has experienced serious illness himself, or in his immediate family, may be strongly motivated to cure illness in others.

The typical medical student will approach his future profession with a considerable degree of idealization. During the course of his training, he will learn to use those many potent tools of medicine and surgery, and be impressed with their effectiveness. Concurrently, however, he will be seeing the limits of the potency of those tools. These limits will at least frustrate him, and perhaps even worry and anger him.

There are two elements to this frustration. The first is unavoidable, and is based on the fact that his wish to help and to cure, the origins of which are briefly referred to above, is blocked from being realized. When the need to cure is excessive in degree the physician may be said to exhibit "therapeutic zeal," and, as a result, has an overwhelming need always to be successful in his efforts to help his patients. The second frustrating element is based upon the idealization of his chosen profession. He had expected Medicine to be greater than it *can* be, and this leads to some degree of disillusionment.

If the medical student or resident is fortunate, he will have teachers who are not only able to teach him the scope of what he will be able to accomplish, but who will also teach him how to live realistically with the limits of what he can achieve. He should be helped, as he proceeds through his training, to continue to see Medicine as a far from perfect, yet at the same time as a very satisfying and effective profession. If his ability to see his chosen field realistically is too long postponed, if he does not begin early enough to see that many can be helped considerably but some will be beyond his powers to change very much, then when he enters practice he will be in great danger of disillusionment. This can in turn lead to dissatisfaction in his work, something which, in most instances, should be avoidable.

All brances of Medicine have their limits. This, of course, includes Psychiatry. All branches of Medicine have patients who die suddenly; in Psychiatry this largely includes those who die by suicide. All branches of Medicine have their chronic patients: for instance medical cardiac patients whose organs will always remain impaired to a significant degree; or psychiatric patients in whom there will be some permanent residue of disorder because of genetic, social or emotional damaging factors. The physician is required to come to terms, in regard to these chronic patients, with the fact that they will always be with him, they will never be entirely well; on the other hand, there will usually be some ways, however modest, in which he will be able to make them more comfortable.

The usual view of the physician is that of one devoted to the care of his patient. Further, the physician is expected to have principally, or even exclusively, positive feelings for his patient. This expectation is one which the young medical student or physician has of himself, or at least he has it as an ideal conception of how he should be. But, of course, physicians also have negative feelings towards their patients. It is the "difficult" patients towards whom they principally have these feelings. And it is important for physicians to accept that they will sometimes have such feelings. In some instances the physician's anger towards or dislike of the patient will be entirely within the bounds of an appropriate response. In other instances, the patient's demands evoke disproportionate anger and dislike on the physician's part which usually arises out of the physician's idiosyncratic and personal sensitivities; the anger is a reflection of the doctor's personality, and is not completely defined by the patient and his illness. This latter situation would be called negative countertransference. Winnicott (1949) has written clearly on this subject within the context of psychotherapy.

VARIOUS TYPES OF DIFFICULT CHALLENGES

Having said that subjective difficulty might be measured by the feelings which the patient gives rise to in the physician, we can now consider the usual effects of certain categories of patients in terms of physician response.

The patient who does not improve. If much of our motivation for being physicians (including psychiatrists) is based on the wish to help or cure people, then our patients who do not improve threaten our sense of effectiveness or usefulness, and this produces negative feeling in us. An example is patients who, despite our best efforts, are dying. It is commonly observed that, in a hospital, unless special efforts are made to prevent this, physicians and other professional personnel tend to avoid the dying patient. One reason for this is to avoid confronting approaching death, which inescapably reminds us of our own mortality.

The patient with physical symptoms of emotional origin. As physicians we are generally more comfortable with symptoms which are clearly of physical organic origin. When painful emotions are converted into disruptions of physical well-being, we easily assume the position that there is something fraudulent going on. This is unreasonable, as the patient may be entirely unaware of the emotional sources of his symptoms, which are experienced as quite real by him. We may say he has "functional" disease, or that it is "all in his mind," or that it is "supratentorial." Each of these terms has some degree of derogation of the patient included in it, a derogation which arises out of our fear that the patient will "fool" us or "deceive" us. It is also a reflection of our greater comfort with clear, proven, organic etiologies, and our discomfort with less precise, more vague, emotional etiologies. It may help the physician to remember that the most concrete physical events and the most subtle emotions become "real" to the sufferer through the same mental and psychological mechanisms; the pain produced by fear is as disabling as the pain produced by fire.

The patient with multiple social and medical difficulties. Many patients come to the physician, particularly those from deprived backgrounds, with a multiplicity of family, personal, and medical problems. Many professional people, including physicians and social workers may be involved. Many institutions, including hospitals and social and government agencies may have a connection to the case. Since the causes are so multiple, and the scars are so numerous, the physician comes to feel helpless in the morass of problems. There are crossed lines of communication. The physician feels that his best efforts are of little or no avail. He feels that efforts are overlapping, duplicating and unproductive. He is afraid that some other professional will shirk his responsibility, and the other professional in turn feels that *he* will have someone else's impossible problem dropped in his lap.

Such problems, difficult at best, will show limited results from the therapeutic efforts invested. It is especially important to avoid duplication of effort and interprofessional rivalry and resentment.

The excessively dependent patient. Most physicians enjoy the natural dependency which their patients exhibit towards them. The gratitude and the expectations are a significant component of the physician's rewards for his work.

But some patients develop an excessive dependence upon the physician. The hypochondriacal patient may require the constant repetition of reassurance by the doctor. The patient may transfer to the physician those dependent longings which have previously been directed towards parents, or teachers, older siblings or loved ones. When the dependency becomes very great, the physician may feel smothered and confined, and become resentful. This is turn may lead him to avoid contacts with the patient. Somehow he must find a reasonable balance between responding to the patient's real needs and being drawn too much into constant contact with the patient.

If the patient's dependent demands become too great, and the physician becomes too resentful, the system may break down and, angry and disillusioned, the patient may, to the physician's possible relief, seek the help of another doctor.

The hopeless, helpless patient. Medical practice, especially in traditional hospital or clinic settings, has as one of its greatest challenges the repeated, frustrating contacts with markedly damaged patients. Such patients thwart the physician's desire to be of evident assistance. These hurt and scarred individuals whose bodies and lives cannot be repaired constantly confront him with the limits of his effectiveness. Such derogating terms as "crocks" may be used as a way of venting one's anger at the impossible task one is asked to perform (Lipsitt, 1970, Adler, 1972).

The demanding, suspicious, or paranoid patient. The large majority of the physician's patients treat him with respect and gratitude. A few patients have become so suspicious of the world, even to the point of an irrational paranoid attitude, that the physician may become the object of such feelings. He may then find himself having to justify whatever he does and whatever he advises. He finds that his efforts are not appreciated, but disparaged and resented, since he has not been able to bring the patient to the desired state of comfort. Fortunately such situations are rare, because they are distressing and wearying. The family physician may need to refer such a patient to a psychiatrist. The psychiatrist, in turn, tries to support the patient and, at the same time, to find and alleviate the emotional pain that lies behind the aggressive accusatory stance.

The sexually seductive patient. Aggressive, angry and hating feelings between patient and physician are, as has been said, real challenges to the physician. As difficult on occasion are another set of feelings, those of sexual attraction which pose another kind of challenge.

In the course of work with patients, the physician will from time to time experience some feelings of sexual attraction. Ordinarily this poses no problem, as such feelings, just as when they occur in the course of any kind of work, can be blended into the general matrix of a positive working relationship.

Part of the professional set of the physician is to maintain a friendly and supportive attitude without being excessively intimate or seductive. A few patients, who are frankly sexually inviting in the consulting room, may create a difficult situation for the physician, who finds himself torn between his own emotions and the requirements of his professional role.

THE MANAGEMENT OF SUCH CHALLENGES

Traditionally, textbooks of medicine and psychiatry have not entered into a discussion of the negative and difficult feelings a physician may have for a patient. This has been based upon the attitude that physicians experience only positive or benign feelings towards their patients. Such an unrealistic attitude does not assist the physician in managing the problems that arise.

There are no *specific* guidelines for specific patients. But it is likely useful to put forward some *general* principles which might be of assistance in such instances. They are as follows:

It is easier to manage feelings of which one is aware, than feelings which one avoids or denies. If the physician will let himself know more of the attitudes he really does have toward certain patients, there is less likelihood that they will be unmanageable;

Physicians should be taught that such feelings are unavoidable in dealing with some of their patients, and that just to experience such feelings is not in itself unusual or wrong;

The responsibility for especially demanding patients should be *shared*, whenever possible, rather than being carried by one physician alone. This is often automatic in clinic practice, where the patient will be known to more than one doctor, and where, as a result, the pressure on the individual doctor is lessened;

The physician must realize that whereas a supportive and positive attitude towards most of his patients most of the time is the best possible attitude, it is important that he not be positive to a fault. All human beings, in their dealings with others, require limits. If the physician never sets limits on the demands of his patients, he will not be doing them a favor, and certainly will not be doing himself a favor. Young physicians must be helped to realize when to say "no" to the excessive demands of patients or of their families: not unkindly, not destructively, but very firmly. In this way the physician will use those finite energies which he has available to him in reasonably economic ways.

When one suffers from difficult feelings about a patient, it is helpful to share these feelings with a colleague. This does not imply that one should air such emotions in a social setting. It means, rather, the serious discussion of problem cases with a respected colleague. This can be done: informally, as part of a brief professional discussion of cases which everyone finds difficult, or; through a formally requested consultation with a colleague. This latter may bring to light some other way of dealing with the patient, or, as useful, that there is no other way, and that one has a right to continue with what one has in fact been doing.

At times the feelings on the part of the physician will be so strong as to interfere with adequate management, and in this case the patient should be transferred to a colleague. Often such a transfer will occur as the result of the rejection of the physi-cian by the patient. At other times it may follow a consultation, initiated by the physician.

SUMMARY AND CONCLUSIONS

The very largest part of medical (including psychiatric) practice takes place within the context of positive, mutually-supportive feelings between the patient and the physician. In a few instances this is not the case. These may be due to the chronic nature of the patient's complaints, the demanding or seductive nature of his personality, or idiosyncratic sensitivities on the part of the physician.

An awareness of these feelings on the part of the physician will help, as will the knowledge that one may share responsibility for such patients. In a few instances, it is best for the physician and the patient not to continue together, and the patient should be referred to a colleague for treatment.

REFERENCES

Adler, G. (1972): Helplessness in the helper. Br. J. Med. Psychol. 45:315.
Lipsitt, D.R. (1970): Medical and psychological characteristics of "crocks". Int. J. of Psychiatry in Medicine. 1:15.
Winnicott, D. W. (1949): Hate in the countertransference. Int. J. Psychoanal. 30:69.

FURTHER READING

Bibring, B.L. (1956): Psychiatry and medical practice in a general hospital. N. Engl. J. Med. 254:366.
Groves, J.E. (1978): Taking care of the hateful patient. N. Engl. J. Med. 298:883.
Negative reactions of physicians to several categories of very difficult medical patients.
Martin, P.A. (1955): The obnoxious patient. In Tactics and Techniques in Psychotherapy. Vol. 2. Countertransference. Giovacchini, P. (Ed.) New York, Jason Aronson, pp. 196–204.

CHAPTER 38

Referral to the Psychiatrist

Frederick H. Lowy

Most patients are best managed by the physician who is able to provide comprehensive care yet willing to consult specialists when they are needed. The physician who calls on specialists for help when he is unsure of the diagnosis or the treatment is not only following sound medical practice but also being prudent from the medicolegal point of view. Sometimes patients or their families request a consultation with a specialist; the physician should not disregard such a request.

Unfortunately, psychiatric consultation and referral are not always the smooth processes they should be. Some physicians are reluctant to refer patients to a psychiatrist; or they do so when it is too late, or they do so inappropriately, when the psychiatrist is not able to help. The following pages discuss relevant aspects of the referral, giving information that might help make the referral process easier for all involved.

WHAT THE PSYCHIATRIST CAN OFFER

Help in assessing the patient. Comprehensive assessment of the patient involves more than assigning a diagnostic label to his disorder. It involves identifying the factors that have predisposed the patient to the illness, that have precipitated the development of the illness, or that may be perpetuating it. Those factors can be biological, psychological and/or social. Some of the factors may be amenable to change but others may not be.

When the physician suspects that the patient has a psychiatric disorder or when the patient's medical or surgical illness seems to be complicated by psychosocial factors, it may be appropriate to refer the patient to a psychiatrist for a comprehensive assessment.

Although family practitioners, non psychiatric specialists, and mental health workers may be aware of the physical manifestations of psychiatric disorders and the psychological presentation of physical disorders, the psychiatrist, by virtue of his training, is the person best qualified to assess the patient.

Help in managing the patient. The family physician is often best equipped to manage the patient who has a psychiatric disorder or who has marital or other family problems—especially if the physician can consult with a psychiatrist. The psychiatrist can help the family physician choose a psychotherapeutic approach and can advise him about the use of psychotropic drugs and about how members of the patient's family can be included in the treat-

339

ment. The consultant usually is familiar with community mental health resources, which may be helpful. Help in managing the patient can take one of two forms. Depending on the situation, the consultant can simply give an opinion about the case and then withdraw from it, or he can continue to guide the treatment through repeat consultations, either seeing the patient each time or meeting with the referring physician to discuss the treatment.

Help with the legal aspects. Non psychiatric physicians are often not sure about such matters as how to deal with patients who are not mentally competent to manage their affairs, how to arrange for a patient's involuntary admission to a psychiatric facility, or how to determine whether the patient has the capacity to make a will. The psychiatrist can usually advise the physician about such matters.

Taking over the complete management of the patient. Sometimes the family physician or the non psychiatric specialist refers a patient to a psychiatrist with the intention of transferring the patient to his care. The patient should be transferred if he requires a kind of treatment that the psychiatrist can best carry out and if he is likely to respond to this. However, after the psychiatric consultant has made a comprehensive assessment of the patient, he may conclude that the patient is not likely to respond to the treatment he was referred for (such as psychotherapy, behavior modification therapy, or electroconvulsive therapy) and/or that the family physician is better able to manage the problem. The situation calls for a full and frank discussion between the referring physician and the psychiatrist to insure that the care of the patient does not fall between two stools.

Help in improving the family physician's psychiatric skills. Besides helping the patient, the psychiatric consultant is at times able to help the referring physician update his knowledge and skills. Since it is impossible for anyone to keep on top of developments in all fields of medicine, opportunities to update knowledge are welcome, and consultation with a specialist often provides this. In the consultation process the psychiatrist can make his colleague aware of new drugs and of new techniques of prescribing familiar drugs; he can help the referring physician sharpen his skills in individual counseling and in family interviewing; and he can advise on techniques useful in treating difficult patients.

WHEN TO CONSULT WITH A PSYCHIATRIST

As in other types of consultations, the family physician should consider consulting a psychiatrist whenever he thinks he needs help. Usually he needs help in one of the following circumstances.

When he suspects that the patient has an undiagnosed psychiatric disorder. The family physician may suspect that a particular patient has a primary psychiatric disorder even though the patient's presenting symptoms are physical. Psychiatric illness cannot be diagnosed accurately by exclusion. The lack of a satisfactory diagnosis after thorough investigation does not necessarily mean that the patient's illness is psychogenic, though of course it could mean this. The diagnosis of a psychiatric disorder must be based on positive evidence, and when that is hard to obtain, a psychiatric consultation is indicated. A psychiatric consultation is indicated also when the physician suspects that the patient's physical disorder is complicated or perpetuated by psychosocial factors. Occasionally, the psychiatric consultant can help diagnose a previously undetected physical illness on mental status examination, much as the ophthalmologist can sometimes help diagnose diabetes or hypertension.

When the condition of the patient with a known psychiatric disorder worsens. Obviously the family physician need not consult a psychiatrist about every patient who has a psychiatric disorder. But a psychiatrist should be consulted when the physician notes a deterioration in the condition of a psychiatric patient who is under his care. The treatment may need to be changed (perhaps the patient should be hospitalized) or other aspects of the patient's social system may need attention.

When the patient's self-defeating life patterns become apparent. The physician often becomes aware that the patient has recurrent maladaptive behavior patterns that he and his family do not see or have ignored. Those patterns may arise from a recurrent mood disorder, a neurotic conflict, or a personality disorder that might respond to treatment. Such a patient is often helped by psychotherapy or, if he has a mood disorder, by long-term treatment with lithium. Unfortunately these behavior patterns may not be amenable to change but the patient deserves a diagnostic consultation.

Sometimes psychological or social factors contribute heavily to the patient's problems in his marriage or at school or work. Again a consultation with a psychiatrist may lead to successful treatment and a far-reaching improvement in the quality of life of the patient and his family.

When the patient first has a psychotic episode. A psychiatric consultation and a comprehensive assessment of the patient are indicated when the presence of a psychosis is first recognized. Usually the patient is hospitalized so that an accurate diagnosis can be made and both short-term and long-term treatment programs can be initiated.

When it is suspected that the patient has a primary affective disorder. Almost every day the family physician encounters a patient who has a reactive depression. The family physician is the best person to treat such a patient. It is important that he distinguish a reactive depression from a severe affective disorder. The extreme manifestations of a primary affective disorder are recurrent, severe manic or depressive psychoses. The full-blown syndrome is easy to diagnose, but it is not always easy to distinguish milder forms of a primary affective disorder from the mood changes that are a part of everyday life. Today most primary affective disorders respond well to medication (the tricyclic antidepressants for depression; phenothiazines, haloperidol, or lithium for mania) and many patients can be protected against future attacks by the long-term administration of lithium. Thus it is important to identify patients who will respond to such a drug regime and the consultant can help with that.

HOW TO—AND HOW NOT TO— CONSULT A PSYCHIATRIST

To derive maximum benefit from a psychiatric consultation the physician should be guided by the following rules:

Prepare the patient. Prepare the patient for the referral. The patient and sometimes his family should be prepared for the psychiatric consultation. Usually it is best that the physician tell the patient why he considers a psychiatric consultation desirable, perhaps explaining that he has asked the psychiatrist to help him assess and manage the patient's problem. A psychiatric consultation should almost never be arranged without the patient's knowledge and the fact that the consultant is a psychiatrist should not be concealed. If the family physician does not explain why he thinks the psychiatric consultation would be helpful and if he does not try to enlist the patient's cooperation, the consultant will have to spend considerable time doing just those things, and perhaps never achieve a working alliance with the patient.

Before he tells the patient about the psychiatric consultation the family physician should consider why the patient might resent having the consultation. Psychiatric disorders still can carry a stigma. That is especially true in some subcultures, among whom referral to a psychiatrist is seen as an indication of insanity and a prelude to long-term hospitalization. Some employers discriminate against people who have had psychiatric treatment, and many patients are understandably concerned about this.

The patient may have more subtle concerns. He might think that a psychiatric consultation indicates that his family physician no longer believes in him or that he considers the patient's symptoms to be imaginary and invalid. The patient might also feel that his family physician, whom he trusted, has rejected or betrayed him by calling in a psychiatrist. Or the patient might feel that if he goes to a psychiatrist he will lose his status with his family or that he will be regarded as weak, silly or irrational.

Finally, the patient might resist a psychiatric consultation because he is afraid to look into himself or to reveal himself to others or because he is afraid that his confidence will be betrayed.

Don't wait. Do not wait to refer the patient. Usually there is no merit in postponing the referral until further investigations are done or other consultants are heard from. If there are indications for a psychiatric consultation, it should be had in any event, and the sooner the better. With patients who somatize, that is, who experience and report intrapsychic distress as physical symptoms, it is particularly important for the psychiatrist to be called in early in the treatment—before the patient undergoes uncomfortable or even mutilating procedures, and before the patient becomes unalterably convinced that his problem is a physical one.

Don't arouse unrealistic hopes. Do not arouse unrealistic hopes for a cure. Unrealistic expectations about a cure can be a problem, especially in a patient who has a severe personality disorder that has led to failure in school or at work, or to marital problems, or to trouble with the law. The physician who first realizes that the pa-

tient may have a psychological disorder may be excused for being optimistic about psychiatric help. But the patient and his family can easily build up false hopes; not all patients can be helped by currently available methods.

Choose the right consultant. Not all psychiatrists are interested in, or skilled in, treating all the kinds of problems mentioned above. When the physician is in a position to choose from a number of psychiatrists, he should find out who is skilled in what kinds of therapy. The consultant who is best able to arrive at an accurate diagnosis of a disorder that is complicated by interdependent physical, psychological, and social factors may not be the best one to conduct psychotherapy or to treat a child. In large general hospitals, organized consultation-liaison services are often available and they usually provide a wide range of services, including advice about further referrals if psychiatric treatment is required.

A point to note is that the working day is often highly structured for many psychiatrists, particularly those who do intensive psychotherapy, which requires that blocks of uninterrupted time be set aside. These psychiatrists can only be reached between appointments or in the evening, and may not be able to comply immediately with an urgent request for consultation. In such a case, the hospital consultation-liaison service, which provides 24-hour service, can help.

Prepare the psychiatric consultant for the referral. When the family physician is setting up a psychiatric consultation, by telephone or using a hospital request form, he should tell the psychiatrist exactly what kind of help is being asked for. The psychiatrist should be told whether the referring physician wants the psychiatrist to take over the complete care of the patient, or whether he is asking only for his opinion.

The psychiatrist should be told whether the patient must be seen immediately, whether the family suggested the consulta-

tion, who will prescribe any medications, and what the patient expects.

If the patient is especially concerned about privacy and confidentiality, the psychiatrist should know that. It should be made clear to the psychiatrist whether the results of the consultation are to be given to the patient and his family by the psychiatrist or by the referring physician.

FURTHER READINGS

Abram, H.S. (1971): Interpersonal aspects of psychiatric consultations in a general hospital. *Psychiatry Med.* 2:321.

Lipowski, Z.J. (1974): Consultation-liaison psychiatry: an overview. *Am. J. Psychiat.* 131:623.

Schwab, J.J. and Brown, J. (1968): Uses and abuses of psychiatric consultation. *J. A. M. A.* 205:65.

39
Mental Retardation
Joseph M. Berg

The topic of mental retardation, with its seemingly endless ramifications, embraces a wide range of problems often falling within the orbit of psychiatrists. Thus, for example, the psychiatrist may be called upon: to recognize the disability and associated manifestations, to establish its degree of severity, to explain its nature and origin, to differentiate it from other conditions such as various forms of mental illness and specific learning disorders, to initiate preventive procedures, to institute medical, educational, social and other rehabilitative therapeutic measures, to provide guidance on prognosis, and to deal with the anxieties, emotional stresses, and misconceptions which frequently arise in the minds of relatives of affected persons and even the general public. The subject matter is enormous. A brief and broad outline of various of its facets is presented here.

ON DESIGNATING INDIVIDUALS AS RETARDED

Deficiency in mental ability, as deficiency in bodily height, is a clinical sign and not a disease entity as such. A diagnosis of intellectual deficit is thus as imprecise as a diagnosis of short physical stature. Precision is added by delineating the severity of the impairment, by ascertaining the presence of concomitant features which may enable recognition of a specific syndrome, and by making an attempt to determine the etiology.

Intelligence or intellectual capacity, though a very difficult concept to define and delineate accurately, is, of course, not an all-or-none phenomenon. In a general population it ranges as a continuum, along a normal distribution curve, from the extremes of grave impairment on the one hand, to marked superiority on the other. Hence the dividing line between those considered to be mentally retarded and those not is an arbitrary one. Depending on how and where the dividing line is drawn, opinions differ as to what proportion of the population can be reasonably designated as mentally retarded; but approximately 3% is usually regarded as appropriate, with the large majority of individuals labelled as retarded falling within the mildly or moderately retarded range.

In practice, various criteria are used in different circumstances for designating a person as retarded. These criteria include biomedical, social, educational, vocational, and psychological considerations. Thus, the recognition of a distinct syndrome such as that of Down, the presence of social incompetence, scholastic inadequacy or vocational incapacity, and the demonstration of a reduced developmental or intelligence quotient can be, each by itself or in combination, the basis for a diagnosis of mental retardation. It may be useful to highlight some pitfalls in each of these respects.

At or soon after birth, the recognition of certain syndromes by clinical, cytogenetic, chemical, or other means indicates a prospect of mental retardation which will become apparent later in the overwhelming majority, or even in practically all, cases. Examples are the syndromes of Apert and of Down and such metabolic disorders as classical phenylketonuria and certain mucopolysaccharidoses. Because retardation associated with such conditions varies considerably in severity, it is unwise to make premature predictions, on the basis of preconceived stereotypes, of the degree of mental deficit which will occur. Statements such as "Your baby will not progress beyond a one-year level or will be able to do hardly anything for himself" are still made with astonishing frequency in circumstances where retardation is likely or certain, but where its level could be determined only by careful follow-up assessment of the patient.

Later on, lack of social, scholastic, and vocational competence certainly can be indications of mental retardation (and, indeed, often are) but are not, by themselves, proof of intellectual deficit. The ineptitude referred to may have its origin in a particular problem of a different kind. Included in this differential diagnosis are auditory, visual, or motor defects, a specific learning disability associated with conditions such as dyslexia and dysphasia, and emotional disturbance related to adverse home or neighborhood environment or other factors. Circumstances of these kinds may be readily apparent; however, they also can be hidden, in which case awareness of their possible existence significantly in-

creases the prospect that they will be uncovered. It must be remembered that such conditions frequently also co-exist with, and exacerbate, mental retardation.

Developmental and psychometric intelligence tests have been widely used for many years as a means of establishing or confirming the presence and degree of mental retardation. These procedures attempt to measure the developmental or intellectual capacities of individuals in comparison with norms derived from general population groups of like age. Such formal tests are undoubtedly useful, but they too can be misleading. For instance the time for individual signs of developmental progress, such as smiling, walking, or talking, has a fair degree of normal variation and a child may be advanced in some and delayed in others. In general, a suspicion of mental retardation is most likely to prove correct if all, or nearly all, "milestones," rather than individual ones, are reached late. Psychometric tests of intelligence also should be interpreted with caution. They are imperfect, and inappropriate tests, as well as such factors as disinterest and unsatisfactory rapport in the test situation, can lead to invalid scores and erroneous conclusions.

Despite imperfections, intelligence tests, when suitably chosen and undertaken, provide a convenient numerical representation of intellectual level. The intelligence quotient (I.Q.) is calculated from this formula: mental age over chronologi-

TABLE 17   ONE SUBDIVISION OF DEGREES OF RETARDATION ON BASIS OF I.Q. SCORES*

Degree of Retardation	I.Q. Range
Mild	50–70
Moderate	35–49
Severe	20–34
Profound	<20

* Source: Manual of the International Statistical Classification of Diseases, Injuries, and Causes of Death. 9th Revision, Vol. 1, Pp. 212–3. World Health Organization, Geneva, 1977.

cal age × 100. The upper limit for chronological age is usually 16 years. In some tests, alternative calculation procedures are used. Most persons considered to be retarded have I.Q.s below 70, and the degree of retardation can be subdivided into categories, on the basis of scores down the I.Q. scale. In the example quoted, the range of I.Q.s for each category is based on a test, such as the Wechsler, with a mean of 100 and a standard deviation of 15. However, there is no indisputable, intrinsic rationale for a given number of subdivisions or for placing their cut-off points in one set of positions on the I.Q. scale rather than another. The 8th revision (World Health Organization, Geneva, 1967) of the manual quoted in the table, for example, had slightly different I.Q. divisions and included an additional category, called borderline retardation, with an I.Q. range of 68–85.

In the final analysis, no single criterion is entirely satisfactory for a designation of mental retardation and for an adequate conclusion as to its severity. Each has its place in particular circumstances and several together often are necessary to make an accurate judgement of the individual's capacities and potential.

ETIOLOGICAL CONSIDERATIONS

The causal factors responsible for mental deficit are so wide ranging and numerous that an attempt to list them comprehensively results in an extensive catalogue which can be perplexing and formidable to assimilate. It is best, in considering these causal factors, to classify them in groups. Different classifications have been proposed from time to time, some of which unfortunately confuse the issues by not distinguishing between causes and effects. Microcephaly, for instance, is not an etiological designation but a consequence of some underlying cause which can result both in the small head size and in cerebral pathology connected with mental retardation. The deficiency in both head size and intellect can be due to a variety of causes as diverse as, for example, autosomal recessive transmission of a harmful gene by each of the heterozygous parents, or intra-uterine cytomegalovirus infection during pregnancy. Clearly, the gene or the virus concerned is the basic cause of the retardation and not the small head.

Bearing this in mind, it is best to think of the causes of mental retardation as being predominantly either genetic or environmental. On this basis, an etiological classification can be made (Table 18).

The table is oversimplified, in that nature and nurture are not mutually exclusive and are closely interlinked in producing mental and somatic consequences; for instance, radiation may result in disadvantageous gene mutations or chromosomal errors, and genetic constitution can modify the response to environmental influences such as hazardous drugs or social adversity. Furthermore, attributing a clinical state to a genetic or environmental cause may depend upon timing. For instance, a phenylketonuric mother owes her

TABLE 18 ETIOLOGICAL CLASSIFICATION OF MENTAL RETARDATION

Etiological Factors	Specific	General
Genetic	Harmful specific genes and aberrant chromosomes	Deleterious polygenic influences
Environmental	Particular physical hazards before, during and after birth	Adverse domestic and social circumstances

defect to harmful genes as a consequence of which her child can be retarded because he or she was exposed to the environmental hazard of maternal hyperphenylalaninemia in utero.

Harmful specific genes are usually transmitted in an autosomal recessive, autosomal dominant or X-linked recessive manner, resulting in mathematically exact expectations for the occurrence or recurrence of the genetic syndromes or phenotypes in question. Among the mentally retarded, autosomal recessive transmission is the commonest of these characteristic mendelian patterns of inheritance; most inborn metabolic errors associated with retardation, for example, are transmitted in this way. *Chromosomal aberrations*, which are nearly always connected with mental deficit and occasionally with mental disorder, involve the autosomes or sex chromosomes and sometimes both. They consist primarily of excess or loss of chromosome material through a variety of mechanisms which are often not clearly understood. Recent developments in chromosomal banding procedures and other staining techniques facilitate the recognition of small duplications and deletions which can have mental and somatic consequences as serious as morphologically grosser aberrations. *Particular physical hazards* of environmental origin are many. Chemical and infectious agents of various kinds are among the commoner ones pre- and post-natally, and circumstances involving hypoxia or physical trauma to the central nervous system are important at or near the time of birth. Growing concern about teratogens, and environmental pollutants operating postnatally, as well as advancing obstetrical sophistication, has focussed attention on these hazards.

The "general" etiological factors mentioned in Table 18 are, on the whole, more subtle and interrelated and hence more difficult to pinpoint and differentiate precisely, than the "specific" ones. *Multiple*

genes contribute to intellectual level and (leaving aside the specific causes of mental retardation discussed above) to producing some correlation between the average intelligence of close blood relatives, as parents and their children. Particular combinations of polygenic influences may be responsible for some degree of intellectual deficit just as other combinations lead to higher levels of intelligence. Hand in hand with these effects, domestic and social adversity, and other disruptive or unstimulating circumstances, can impair intellectual function as well as cause additional disturbing mental consequences. In these contexts, the extent of the respective roles of genetic and environmental factors in producing mental deficit, and the exact relationship of these factors, are not yet convincingly resolved. The debate continues, often with strong emotional and ideological overtones which lead rather frequently to a blurring, or even erasure, of the distinction between fact and fiction.

A further significant consideration with respect to Table 18 is that the "specific" etiological factors usually tend to produce relatively marked mental retardation, whereas the "general" ones are more likely to be connected with retardation of milder degree. Also, definite morphological cerebral pathology is very frequently detectable in markedly retarded persons (I.Q. below 50), but in only a small proportion of those with mild retardation (I.Q. above 50). These findings lend considerable weight to the argument that marked intellectual deficit is generally a consequence of recognizable cerebral maldevelopment or organic damage due to specific circumscribed physical causes, whereas mild deficit often results from the same kind of multifactorial biological and social influences that create the difference between those of average and those of superior intellect. Further evidence favoring this proposition, in general populations, is an excess of persons with I.Q.s below 50 compared with the normal Gaussian expectation; by contrast, the numbers of those with I.Q.s above 50 approximate more closely to the expected Gaussian distribution.

The establishment of the underlying cause in a given instance of mental retardation, as with other conditions, is facilitated by eliciting a detailed personal and family history, by careful clinical examination, and by relevant specific investigations such as biochemical, cytogenetic, and radiological ones. No matter how carefully these procedures are undertaken, etiology remains unclear in many retarded persons in the present state of knowledge. Even the recognition of distinct syndromes, of characteristic combinations of phenotypic manifestations, may not be etiologically informative (examples of such causally obscure mental retardation syndromes are those of Sturge and Weber, of de Lange, and of Rubinstein and Taybi). Nevertheless, etiological clarity is often more readily attained among the retarded than among those with other kinds of mental disabilities or disorders.

Elucidation of etiology in the contexts discussed is, of course, not merely an academic exercise for its own sake. It has significant practical implications in regard to prevention, and to prognosis and treatment of those already affected. These aspects are considered in the following sections.

PREVENTION

Prevention is a primary objective for all forms of mental retardation because curative treatment, in the sense of restoration to intellectual "normality", is an unrealistic prospect for most cases in the foreseeable future. Despite uncertainty about various facets of etiology and the existence of many retarded individuals in whom causation is entirely obscure, important advances in understanding the causes of mental retardation have been made. In this regard, it is a matter for concern that, in

addition to gaps in knowledge, another substantial gap exists between what is known and what is generally applied in practice for purposes of prevention. A short discussion of various available measures bearing on prevention of mental defect, follows.

Genetic aspects. Genetic counselling is of value when there is anxiety, for whatever reason, that mental retardation may occur or recur in a particular family. Most often, it is sought by parents or other relatives after an affected child is born. In these circumstances, clarifying the etiological basis for the retardation is the crucial prerequisite for accurate prediction of recurrence. For instance, if the disability or syndrome in question is autosomal recessive in nature, the heterozygous parents for the gene concerned have a one in four chance that each child of theirs would have the condition. Similarly, precise risks can be calculated for specific gene defects with other mendelian patterns of transmission. These risks also are often high for close relatives. By contrast, chromosomal disorders usually are sporadic with a relatively low recurrence risk, with the important exception of a parent who is a translocation carrier. A helpful clue regarding the odds of having certain types of chromosomally and phenotypically abnormal children is maternal age. Down's syndrome is the most striking example. The chances of a child being born with standard (regular) trisomy 21 is 25 to 50 times greater from maternal ages under 20 years or over 40 years. When causation is unknown, risk figures have to be based on empirical data. Non-specific mental retardation of marked degree, for instance, has been found empirically to recur in between 3 to 6 per cent of siblings of affected individuals.

The genetic counselling approach to psychiatric disorder in general is similar to that outlined above. When etiology is known, as in the autosomal dominant disease Huntington's chorea, the chances of recurrence often are clearly apparent. When etiology is obscure, as in schizophrenia, recurrence risks have to be estimated empirically.

A point worth stressing, regarding concerns about retarded individuals themselves having retarded children, is that many persons with specific genetic types of mental retardation (involving high risks of transmission) are infertile or even sterile. No fully affected Down's syndrome male, for example, is recorded to have been a father and only a few dozen Down's syndrome mothers have been reported. The mildly retarded, by contrast, are often fertile and, if they reproduce, tend to have children of below average intellect, though these children frequently are more intelligent than their retarded parent or parents. These considerations should be borne in mind in contemplating the issue of sterilization of retarded persons. To many, including the present writer, sterilization of the retarded, on a group basis, is unacceptable. In particular individual instances of retardation, however, it can be a reasonable and appropriate undertaking, more often on what may broadly be called social, rather than biological, grounds.

Connected with genetic counselling are procedures for recognition of potential parents at increased risk of having affected children before they are conceived. There are also prenatal diagnostic techniques for use during pregnancy. An example of the former is screening, usually biochemical, for a heterozygous carrier state in clinically normal persons. Such procedures are not realistic at present for use on a large scale, but can be applied effectively to circumscribed identifiable groups within the population who may be at special risk. Successful programs for detecting carriers of the gene for Tay-Sachs disease in Jewish communities of Eastern and Central European origin is a good example. With regard to prenatal diagnosis, there have been rapid and dramatic advances in recognizing distinct types of retardation during gestation, with the option of terminating the pregnancy if the fetus is found to be affected. Fetal cells from an amniotic fluid sample can be examined cytogenetically and biochemically. Chemical characteristics of the fluid itself can be determined. This is useful when there is an increased likelihood of occurrence of abnormalities detectable in these ways, for example in Down's syndrome or an open neural tube defect. Ultrasonography has also become advantageous, both as a precaution prior to amniocentesis and as a prenatal diagnostic technique. Direct fetal visualization with fibre optic devices is a method of recognizing external morphological abnormalities, e.g., in the Laurence-Moon-Biedl syndrome. Further, fetoscopy opens up the prospect of sampling fetal tissues, such as blood, for diagnostic purposes. All these measures have major, if sometimes controversial, preventive implications for various types of mental retardation.

Environmental aspects. Prevention of recognizable environmentally determined mental deficit should be attainable. In principle, this is so. In practice, all too many hazards persist even in affluent, technologically advanced, and relatively well-informed societies. The individual physician may be able to protect individuals or small groups, but protection of the population as a whole often depends on intervention by state or regional authorities who may not do so for a variety of economic, sociological, and political reasons.

Known environmental dangers to normal mental and physical development which can be counteracted, removed or decreased occur at various times before conception, during pregnancy and delivery, and after birth. Some, like exposure to excessive irradiation, certain chemicals, and infectious agents, are potentially damaging in more than one of these periods. Prior to conception, protection against possible mutagens (e.g., radiation) and harmful infections (such as the rubella virus in non-immune women) are examples of preventive measures. During gestation, especially in the first trimester, the fetus is remarkably sensitive to disadvantageous environmental agents of many kinds. In addition to the most widely known teratogens, including radiation and the rubella virus mentioned above, increasing attention is being paid to less apparent, potentially deleterious, influences. These include the general state of health and nutrition of the pregnant woman and the effects on the pregnancy of alcohol and tobacco. Adequate obstetric care, both during pregnancy and at birth, also contributes to reducing the toll of mental and physical abnormality. Postnatally, damage to the central nervous system such as poisoning by heavy metals, and physical injury to the unprotected head are preventable.

More complex, in terms of preventive action, are the problems of counteracting adverse psychological and socio-cultural stresses on the growing child. They are of many kinds and originate in homes, and in the wider environmental milieu. Such adversity can make the difference between reasonable, and substantially impaired, intellectual progress and adaptive behavior.

TREATMENT

It is unrealistic to expect that mental deficit in general will be prevented on a large scale in the near future, though one can speculate that in a more distant brave new era a combination of dramatic genetic and environmental achievements may lead to great advances. At present, treatment remains an undiminished major need. The term, treatment, is used here not just in its narrower medical sense, but to include also the large array of multidisciplinary pursuits necessary for improving the prospects of the mentally retarded and easing the emotional strains in their families.

Medical and related measures. In a sphere where anxious relatives are inclined to clutch at therapeutic straws, there is ample scope for superficially attractive, ill-founded, claims that particular medications will help mental retardation, without regard to basic underlying pathology. Glutamic acid, for example, was at one time recommended as a panacea for mental retardation, and chemical cocktails, of various composition, have been touted periodically as helpful in Down's syndrome. It is wise to be extremely cautious about such claims and to avoid using medications of dubious value.

Medication of a more specific kind is, of course, another matter. Examples of appropriate treatment are thyroid hormone replacement therapy in congenital hypothyroidism and dietary restriction of galactose and phenylalanine in, respectively, galactosemia and phenylketonuria. Symptomatic medication for symptoms often accompanying mental retardation, such as appropriate anticonvulsants for epilepsy and psychopharmacological agents for emotional and behavior disturbances, obviously are important. So too are surgical procedures, including cerebrospinal fluid shunt operations in certain types of hydrocephaly and corrective surgery in some forms of craniosynostosis.

Clearly, other treatments as well are widely applicable in conditions frequently associated with mental retardation. Illustrations are auditory and visual aids for impairments of hearing and sight, physiotherapy for abnormalities of tone and posture, and psychotherapy (individually or in groups) for personality and related problems.

Educational and vocational concerns. The increasing emphasis on the potential capacities of retarded persons, rather than on their limitations, has led to a number of new programs designed to allow the retarded to reach their full potential. Early on, infant stimulation programs, showing the parents how best to encourage developmental progress, can be advantageous. In nursery schools also, relatively simple self-help and other skills can be taught effectively even to severely retarded youngsters. Later, the children can benefit substantially from special education classes geared to their levels of intellectual functioning. The educational diet offered and the techniques used vary in these settings, but generally they are concerned with imparting useful knowledge and practices and fostering appropriate adaptive behavior.

Still later, vocational training and opportunities become important. In sheltered workshops and suitably selected training and job placements (both urban and rural) in the community at large, many retarded individuals can find a niche as reasonably contented and productive members of the population. There is a view expressed sometimes that, as society becomes technologically more advanced, the vocational scope for those who have intellectual limitations will decline. Be that as it may, even in a comparatively complex industrialized society there remain many useful occupations in which retarded individuals do very well. Visits to settings in which the retarded are gainfully employed in manufacturing, assembly, and service pursuits will prove the point.

Social issues. Retarded individuals, like others, benefit from home conditions and a social environment which provides concerned interest and opportunities for their well-being, and in which such disruptive influences as cruelty, abuse, and neglect are not tolerated. Reasonable conditions prevail for many retarded persons in the homes of their families, and there has been a growing inclination in many countries to provide such arrangements where they are lacking. Small group homes, operated on family-like patterns, for example, have increased in numbers in general communities, as have programs designed to provide opportunities for social contacts and leisure-time pursuits similar to those

considered suitable for the population as a whole. Such developments have enriched the outlook of significant numbers of retarded citizens by enhancing their chances of leading relatively "normal" lives and by enabling them to contribute to society in accordance with their capabilities. Fears, in some quarters, that this kind of integration would lead to eugenic disaster, burgeoning crime and other such horrors have not materialized. It seems appropriate, therefore, to recommend that physicians and other professionals concerned with the retarded lend their support to such programs. They are likely to serve not only the interests of the handicapped themselves, but also of society in general.

CONCLUSION

An attempt has been made in this chapter to focus on principles with illustrative examples rather than on details, with an appended bibliography as a suggested source for elaboration in each of these areas. Perhaps enough has been written here, however, to demonstrate that the problems of mental retardation impinge on many branches of learning and professional endeavor (including biology, medicine, psychology, sociology and education), and that psychiatry is not least among the disciplines involved. The chapter deliberately has touched on various facets not usually occupying much attention of psychiatrists in clinical practice. This has been done in the belief that current trends towards integrating the mentally retarded into the general community, as opposed to relative isolation in sometimes remote institutions, will continue and perhaps accelerate. If so, the practising psychiatrist is likely increasingly to be called upon to apply his or her own skills, and to provide informed guidance about other undertakings, for the well-being of the mentally handicapped and their families.

FURTHER READINGS

Other relevant and meritorious texts could be added, of course, to the bibliography below. However, the short selection listed provides a reasonably comprehensive picture of current knowledge, philosophies and practices concerned with mental retardation. Readers with an inclination to delve even further into particular issues will find almost limitless scope in the references contained in each volume.

Begab, M.J. and Richardson, S.A. (1975): *The Mentally Retarded and Society: A Social Science Perspective*. Baltimore, University Park Press.
A timely, wide-ranging presentation, by 27 contributors, on social aspects of mental retardation.

Bernstein, N.R. (1970): *Diminished People: Problems and Care of the Mentally Retarded*. Boston, Little, Brown.
A helpful commentary on social and clinical issues presented by 15 authors with professional backgrounds in spheres which include psychiatry, psychology, social work, special education, and law.

Clarke, A.M. and Clarke, A.D.B. (1974): *Mental Deficiency—The Changing Outlook*. 3rd ed. London, Methuen.
An important, clearly formulated volume, by 18 contributors, dealing with biosocial, behavioral, assessment, ameliorative and service aspects of mental retardation. An abridged paperback edition entitled *Readings from Mental Deficiency—The Changing Outlook* was published in 1978.

Crome, L. and Stern, J. (1972): *Pathology of Mental Retardation*. 2nd ed. Edinburgh, Churchill Livingstone.
An erudite and well-written text by two authors with much experience in, respectively, the neuropathology and biochemistry of mental retardation.

Holmes, L.B., Moser, H.W., Halldórsson, S., et al. (1972): *Mental Retardation—An Atlas of Diseases with Associated Physical Abnormalities*. New York, The Macmillan Co.
A very well illustrated pictorial atlas with a summary of the conditions depicted.

Johnston, R.B. and Magrab, P.R. (1976): *Professional Guide to Developmental Disorders*: Baltimore, University Park Press.
A praiseworthy multi-disciplinary undertaking by 20 authors on the themes indicated in the title.

Kanner, L. (1964): *A History of the Care and Study of the Mentally Retarded*. Springfield, Ill. Charles C Thomas.
A scholarly and fascinating historical survey by a psychiatrist of great distinction. Remarkably comprehensive despite the relative brevity (150 pages).

Kirman, B.H. (1975): *Mental Handicap*. London, Crosby Lockwood Staples.
A brief and lucid practical guide by a British psychiatrist who has devoted almost all his professional life to work with the retarded.

Menolascino, F.J. (1970): *Psychiatric Approaches to Mental Retardation*. New York, Basic Books.
An instructive overview by 32 contributors of, in the editor's words, major areas of psychiatric involvement in mental retardation.

Menolascino, F.J. and Egger, M.L. (1978): *Medical Dimensions of Mental Retardation*. Lincoln, University of Nebraska Press.
A substantial recent focus on medical aspects of mental retardation with particular reference to causes and their consequences, and including material on treatment and management.

Milunsky, A. (1975): *The Prevention of Genetic Disease and Mental Retardation*. Philadelphia, W. B. Saunders Co.
A commendable review, by 24 contributors, of a substantial amount of current knowledge bearing on the themes indicated in the title.

Mittler, P. (1977): *Research to Practice in Mental Retardation*. Baltimore, University Park Press.
The proceedings of a major congress with international contributions in 3 volumes, each respectively concerned with care and intervention, education and training, and biomedical aspects.

Penrose, L.S. (1972): *The Biology of Mental Defect*. 4th ed. London, Sidgwick and Jackson.
A classic textbook on the subject of the title by a deservedly renowned pioneer of the scientific study of mental retardation.

Robinson, N.M. and Robinson, H.B. (1976): *The Mentally Retarded Child—A Psychological Approach*. 2nd Ed. New York, McGraw-Hill.
A scholarly, exceptionally well-documented book reasonably designated, with admiration, by one reviewer as a Baedeker on mental retardation.

A Short Glossary of
Psychiatric Terms

A

Acting out: The physical expression of unconscious conflict in the patient's real life, as contrasted with the verbal expression of such conflicts within the psychotherapeutic situation.

Affect: Mood, emotional state.

Affective disorders: Diseases of mood disturbance: depression and mania.

Ambivalence: The simultaneous experience of opposing feelings, e.g., love and hate.

Anaclitic: Intense dependency. Often used to describe inappropriately childish or infantile behavior.

Analysand: A patient in psycho-analysis.

Anankastic: Rigid and obsessional as in Anankastic personality.

Anhedonia: The inability to experience pleasure.

Anomie: The sensation of detachment from personal goals, and society in general. Disconnectedness. Alienation.

Apperception: The subjective perception and interpretation of stimuli.

B

Bisexuality: Sexual responsiveness to members of both sexes. Also Freud's view that people are fundamentally bisexual in nature.

Borderline state: An often confused diagnostic label used to denote severely disturbed individuals who are not typically psychotic, but who manifest severe unstable disorders of mood, behavior and socialization.

C

Catharsis: Originally the term used by Aristotle to describe the relief experienced on watching a tragedy; the experience of being purged by "pity and terror," now used to describe the relief felt after giving expression to strong feelings.

Cathexis: The investment or attachment of emotion to people or objects.

Clang association: The symptom of uttering rhyming words found in some manic or schizophrenic conditions.

Cognitive: The mental process of thinking, remembering and reasoning.

Compulsion: The symptom of an unwanted urge to act or think.

Conative: Pertaining to will or volition.

Confabulation: Lying to fill gaps in memory, e.g., in Korsakoff's syndrome.

Conversion: The unconscious defense mechanism whereby unconscious conflicts are expressed in physical symptoms either in the voluntary musculature or the special senses.

Counterphobic (behavior): Seeking out experiences which are consciously or unconsciously feared.

Countertransference: The conscious or unconscious feelings of the psychotherapist towards the patient.

Cyclothymic personality: The non-psychotic innate tendency to cyclic severe mood change.

D

Defense mechanism: The unconscious modes of preventing unacceptable thoughts and feelings emerging into consciousness.

Delirium: A reversible state of psychic disorganization characterized by disturbance of mood, perception, consciousness and activity.

Delusion: A strongly-held false belief, resistent to logic and persuasion.

Dementia: An irreversible state of psychic disorganization characterized by loss of intellectual capacity.

Depersonalisation: A symptom of many psychiatric disorders, most commonly reported in schizophrenia. A feeling of strangeness either of the patient or the environment.

Derealisation: The symptom of feeling that the world around one is unreal.

E

Ego-alien: Seeming foreign or unacceptable to the person.

Ego-syntonic: Seeming natural or acceptable to the person.

F

Flexibilitas cerea: Waxy flexibility: A condition in which it is possible to move a patient's limbs into positions which will then be sustained. Found in some cases of catatonic schizophrenia.

Flight of ideas: The symptom of excessively rapid thought and speech, characterized by moving from one idea to another through associations which may or may not be apparent to the observer. Most often seen in manic and hypomanic states.

Fugue: A flight from the usual environment, during which the patient is usually amnesic.

H

Hallucination: A false perception without an object: Visual, auditory, olfactory, gustatory or tactile.

I

Ideas of reference: The symptom of perceiving personal significance in objective data which in fact are totally unrelated to the subject. E.g., the belief that newspaper headlines refer to oneself. Commonly present in paranoid conditions.

Illusion: The misinterpretation of experience. E.g., believing that a coat hanging on a chair is an intruder.

L

La belle indifference: The symptom of apparent lack of distress in the face of severe disability. Seen in hysterical conversion.

M

Malingering: Pretending to a non-existent illness or exaggerating an existing one to gain some benefit.

Mania: Mood disorder characterized by hyperactivity, euphoria; elation, irritability. (When moderate referred to as hypomania.)

N

Neologism: Literally, a new word. Words coined by patients characteristically suffering from schizophrenia or organic brain syndrome.

O

Obsession: The symptom of intrusive, unwanted thoughts.

P

Parapraxis: Slips of the tongue or mistakes in behavior arising out of unconscious conflict.

Phobias: Persistent, abnormal dread or fear.
Some relatively common phobias are:
  Acrophobia—Fear of heights.
  Agoraphobia—Fear of open public places.
  Claustrophobia—Fear of enclosed spaces.

R

Repression: The unconscious mechanism of defense whereby painful or unacceptable thoughts or memories are rendered inaccessible to consciousness.

Resistance: The conscious or unconscious prevention of the emergence of painful or unacceptable thoughts or feelings in the course of psychotherapy.

S

Secondary gain: The advantage deriving from a disability.

Stupor: A state of unresponsiveness to the environment while the patient is conscious.

Suppression: The conscious mechanism of attempting to block unwanted thoughts, feelings or impulses.

T

Transference: The conscious or unconscious feelings of the patient for the psychotherapist.

Index

Page numbers in *italics* refer to illustrations; page numbers followed by t refer to tables.

Abstract thinking, 11
Acceptance, 64
Accidents, 59
Accommodations during rehabilitation, 329
Acting-out, 41
Action as feelings, 249–250
Activity, in aging, 45
  in stress, 65
Adaptation, coping and, 64–66. See also *Adjustment*
    and *Coping*.
  defensive, 64
  definition of, 56
  in aging, 47
  regressive, 64
Addiction, drug. See *Drug addiction*.
Addison's disease, 244–245
Adjustment, convalescence and, 64. See also *Adapta-*
    tion and *Coping*.
  in crisis, 64
  to life events, 62
Adjustment phase reactions, 63–64
Adolescence, biological development in, 33–35
  career choice in, 251
  choice in, 36
  clinical problem areas of, 40–41
  cognitive development in, 35–36
  conceptual problem areas of, 40–41
  definition of, 33
  dependency in, 40–41
  disorders of. See *Childhood disorders*.
  early, 37–39
  emancipation from family in, 251
  empathy in, 36
  identity in, 36, 37, 251
  ideologies and, 39
  independence during, 36–37
  integration of sexual drive in, 251
  late, 40
  loneliness of, 33
  nostalgia in, 33
  psychological development in, 36–37
  psychopathology in, 41
  relationship intimacy in, 37
  self-consciousness in, 38
  sexual conflicts of, 36
  sexual interest during, 38
  social development in, 37
  society and, 36

suicide in, 263–264
  task of, 33, 36
  young adulthood and, 33–41
Adrenal insufficiency, 244–245
Adrenal overactivity, 239
Adrenaline, 60
Adrenaline-noradrenaline dissociation, 60
Adulthood, adjustment to, 65
  young, 40. See also *Adolescence*.
"Aesculapian authority," 6
Affect, 92–93
  meaning of, 171
Affective disorders, 171–183
  biological factors in, 174–175
  catecholamine theory of, 74
  complications of, 178
  course of, 178
  diagnosis of, 179
  differential diagnosis of, 179
  electroconvulsive therapy for, 298
  epidemiology of, 173
  etiology of, 173–176
  genetic factors in, 173–174
  history of, 171–173
  lithium and, 309
  monoamines and, 74
Age, development and, 27–30t
  learning and, 51
Aged, 51–53
  confusional states in, 52
  depressive illnesses of, 52
  drug treatment for, 52
  psychotherapy for, 46, 52–53
  societies' reactions to, 45
  use of drugs by, 317–318
Aging, activity in, 45
  adaptation in, 47
  biologic clock mechanism of, 44
  collagen and, 44
  "composite" theory of, 44
  connective tissue and, 44
  creativity and, 45–46
  development during, 46–47
  disengagement theory of, 45
  error theory of, 44
  extracellular theories of, 44–45
  feelings of worthiness and, 53
  immunoprotein theory of, 44

Aging, *cont.*
 isolation in, 45
 male potency in, 49–50
 medical profession and, 46
 mental functioning and, 43
 mutations versus longevity in, 44
 neuronal degeneration in, 43
 physical changes in, 43–45
 self-esteem in, 47
 sexuality and, 48–50
 society and, 45
 stresses of, 51
 theories of, 44–45
Aging concept, 43
Aging process, 43–45
Aging profiles, 43
Aggression, in attention disorders, 259
 limbic system and, 72
Agranulocytosis, 307
Akathisia, 305
Alcohol, cross-tolerance with other drugs of, 240–241
 psychological effects of, 240–241
 suicide and, 276, 277
Alcohol abuse, biological factors in, 222–223
 psychological factors in, 223
 social factors in, 223
Alcoholics, hallucinosis of, 226
 personality characteristics of, 223
Alcoholism, diagnosis of, 225–226
 disruption of needs and, 3
 memory disorders in, 225
 syndromes associated with, 225–226
 treatment of, 228
 withdrawal in, 225
Alexander's Holy Seven, 149
Alexithymia, 136, 155
Alliance, therapeutic, 77, 282–283
 working, 77
Alzheimer's disease, 43–44, 234
Amitriptyline, 314
Amnesia, after electroconvulsive therapy, 298
 as dissociative disorder, 131–132
Amniocentesis, 350
Amphetamines, effects of, 227, 242
Anal personality, 127
Analysand, 4
Analysis, behavioral, 294. See also *Psychoanalysis.*
Anancastic personality, 127
Anemia, 105
Anesthesia, glove, 139
Anger, disaster and, 57
 grief and, 64
"Anger-in vs. anger-out" studies, 60
Anomie, 204
Anorexia, 177
Anorexia nervosa, as psychosomatic disorder, 151–152
 body weight and, 152
 clinical features of, 152
 differential diagnosis of, 152
 electroconvulsive therapy for, 298
 identity and, 152
Anorgasmia, 214
Anoxia, brain disorder from, 238–239
 hyperventilation and, 239

Korsakov's psychosis and, 239
 symptoms of, 238
Antianxiety agents, 124, 127, 315–317
Antibiotics, 243
Anticonvulsants, 243
Antidepressants, 180, 310–311
 future directions of, 314–315
 indications for, 310
 psychological effects of, 241
 selection of, 311
 time lag for, 310–311
 use of, 310
Antihypertensives, 243
Antiparkinsonian agents, 306
Antipsychotic drugs, 300–307, 302t, 304t
 acute dystonic reaction and, 306
 agranulocytosis and, 307
 akathisia and, 305
 dose of, 303–305
 dose range of, 303–305
 for schizophrenia, 303–305
 indications for, 303–305
 Parkinsonian-like syndrome and, 305
 pharmacology of, 301–303
 side effects of, 305–307
 tardive dyskinesia and, 306–307
 use of, 303–305
Antipyretics, 243
Anxiety, 121–130
 as a psychoanalytic concept, 122
 as a psychopathological condition, 121–122
 as an everyday occurrence, 121
 defense mechanisms and, 15
 description of, 121
 disruption of needs and, 3
 forbidden wish and, 123–124
 from sensory deprivation, 246
 in dissociative disorders, 131
 learning theory and, 124
 mastery versus, 12
 performance, 212
 physical disorders associated with, 6
 preschool, 25
 psychoanalytic theory of, 123–124
 thought content and, 94
 unconscious, 122
 unconscious conflicts in, 124–125
Anxiety attack, 122, 123–124
Anxiety disorder, 122–125
 biological determinants of, 123
 case report of, 123
 causes of, 123–124
 incidence of, 122
 repression in, 123
 treatment of, 124–125
Anxiety neurosis, 239
Anxiolytics, 124, 127, 315–317
Aphasia, motor, 93
Aphonia, hysteric, 139
Aptitude tests, 109
Arousal, 72
Arthritis, 149
Aspirin, 243
Associative connections, 93
Astasia-abasia, 138

Asthma, as psychosomatic disorder, 149, 150
  bronchospasm in, 150
  emotions and, 150
  mother separation and, 150
  personality type, 150
  psychiatric disorder and, 102
  social supports and, 67
Attachment, 20
  lack of, 21
  love and, 21
  separation and, 21
  to object, 22
Attention, deviations of, 258–260
  reticular activating system and, 72–73
  testing of, 96
Attention disorders, aggression in, 259
  hyperactivity in, 258–259
Autism, 11, 258, 262–263
Avoidance, 125, 126

Babcock sentences, 96
Barbiturates, 226–227, 241
Bargaining behavior, 64
Bedwetting, 167
Behavior. See also specific types.
  bargaining, 64
  biology and, 71–75
  chromosomal abnormalities and, 71
  deviant illness, 101
  examination of, 92
  innate, 18
  mental functioning and, 71–75
  of coping, 65
  subcortical structures and, 71
Behavior modification, in sexual responses, 215
  indications for, 295–296
Behavior therapy, 293–296
Behavioral analysis, 294
Belle indifference, 137
Bender Visual Motor Gestalt test, 108
Benzodiazepines, 315–317
  for insomnia, 317
  indications for, 316
  mechanism of action, 316
  selection of, 316–317
  side effects of, 317
  use of, 316
Bereaved. See Grief.
Beri-beri, 244
Biologic clock mechanism of aging, 44
Biological development, 12, 13. See also Develop-
    ment or specific period such as Adolescence.
Biology, behavior and, 71–75
  mental functioning and, 71–75
  of depression, 74
Biopsychosocial model of disease, 149
Birth of first child, 17–18
Blocking, at development crises, 12
  thought, 93
Body image, 102, 103
  anorexia and, 151
  pain and, 160
Body versus mind, 1
Bonding, 20

Brain disorders, endocrine overactivity and, 239
  extracerebral causes of, 238–248
  from anoxia, 238–239
  from hypothermia, 238
  intoxication and, 239–244
  temperature change and, 238
  tests for, 97–98, 108–109
"Brain failure," 52
Brain function, 73–74
Brain syndrome, acute, 63
  organic. See Organic brain syndrome.
Breathlessness, 137
Bromide, 243
Bromism, 243
Bronchospasm, 150
Buffalo Creek syndrome, 56–57
Buffer role of support systems, 66

Cancer as psychosomatic condition, 154
Cannabis, 242–243
Carbon dioxide, 243
Carbon monoxide, 243
Cardiovascular system, 103
Career choice in adolescence, 251
Caregivers, 66–67
Caretaker, primary. See Mother.
Case report, anxiety disorder, 123
  catatonic schizophrenia, 93–94
  conversion disorder, 140
  formulation, 114–115
  language development, 20
  middle childhood, 31
  obsessive-compulsive disorder, 127, 129
  organic brain dysfunction test, 108–109
  personality development, 17
  phobia, 126
  preschool years, 25
  projective tests, 109
  reformulation, 115–116
  temperament of child versus needs of parents, 10
  thought processes, 93–94
  toddler phase, 23
Catastrophic reaction, 98
Catecholamine response dissociation, 60
Catecholamine theory of affective disorders, 74
Catharsis, 140
Cephalization index, 44–45
Cerebral cortex, 71
Cerebral disorder. See Brain disorder and Organic
    brain syndrome.
Change, grief and, 58
  units of, 59
Change of life, 46–47
Character, 203
Child, development of. See Development, child, and
    specific aspects of development.
  parents' disappointment with, 17
  relationship to mother, 10, 13
Child-parent interaction, 252–253
Child-parent mismatch, 10
Childhood, infancy and, 9–31. See also specific as-
    pects.
  middle, 25–26, 31
  separation in, 251–252

Childhood disorders, 249–266
    action as communication of, 249–250
    classification of, 253–265
    developmental considerations in, 249
Children, aggressive, 250–251
    depression in, 263–265
    divorce and, 252
    quiet, 251
    reasons for psychiatric referral of, 250
Chlorpromazine, 307
Chromosomal abnormalities, 71, 348
Clang associations, 93
Climacteric, 46–47, 48
Clinics, 323
Clouding, 98
Cocaine, 242
Cognition, deviations of, 256–258
    restructuring of, 294
Cognitive development, 12, 13, 14–15
    by age, 27–30t
    in adolescence, 35–36
    play in, 21
    preschool, 24
    toddler, 21
Cognitive set, 19
Cognitive skills, 12
Colitis, as psychosomatic disorder, 149, 153–154
Collagen in aging, 44
Compensation neurosis, 235
Competence testing, 97
Complaint, history of, 78
    in history taking, 85–86
"Composite" theory of aging, 44
Compromise formation, 126
Compulsion, 127. See also Obsession; Obsessive-
        compulsive.
Concentration span testing, 96
Concept testing, 97
Concrete operations stage, 26, 35
Conduct disorder, 261–262
Confabulation, 96, 226
Confidant, 68
Conflict, disease and, 143. See also specific problem
        or condition.
    in anxiety, 124–125
Confrontation, 26, 292
Confusional states in the aged, 51–52
Connections, associative, 93
    in new experiences, 11
Connective tissue in aging, 44
Conscience, 15
Consciousness, disorders of, 73
    reticular activating system and, 72–73
    testing of level of, 98
Consultation services, 323–324
Continuous–discontinuous theories of child devel-
        opment, 11–13
Contraceptives, oral, 243
Contract, 294
Controls, 23
Convalescence, 64
Conversion, 135
    hypochondriasis versus, 141
    psychoanalytic model and, 140
    repression in, 137

secondary gain from, 138
    symbolism and, 143
Conversion disorders, 136–141
    abnormal movements in, 138
    case report of, 140
    causes of, 140
    clinical manifestations of, 138–139
    conflict and, 137
    differential diagnosis of, 140–141
    epidemiology of, 139–140
    forbidden wish in, 137
    hysteria and, 136
    repression in, 140
    somatization and, 135
    treatment of, 140
Conversion mechanism, 137
Conversion reactions, 131
Conversion symptoms, as stereotype of a disorder,
        139
    description of, 136–137
    malingering and, 141
Conversion syndromes, 160
Convulsions, 238
Convulsive therapy. See Electroconvulsive therapy.
Coping, adaptation and, 64–66. See also Adjustment.
    behavior and, 65
    definition of, 56
Coping mechanisms, 65
Coping skills, 66
    job change and, 63
Coping tasks, 64
Counterirritation, 158
Counterphobia, 125
Countertransference, 334
Courtship behavior anomalies, 218
Creativity in old age, 45–46
Crib death, 168
Crisis, 55
    adjustment in, 64
    as transition state, 63
    definition of, 55–56
    denial and, 65
    description of, 62
    developmental, 12
    effects on outcome of, 66
    factors of, 68
    help and, 62
    information seeking in, 65
    lack of resolution of, 62
    life cycle and, 62–63
    occurrence of, 62
    phases of, 63
    psychiatric emergencies and, 268–269
    resolution of, 62, 64
Crisis intervention, 270, 319–320
    definition of, 62
    grief counseling and, 58
Crisis theory, 62–64
    of psychiatric emergencies, 269–270
    role transitions and, 63
Crisis ward, 319–320
Cross-gender identity, 217
Cross-tolerance with drugs, 240–241
"Crushes," 38–39

Death, depression and, 151
 facing, 51
Decompensation, 48
 grief and, 61
 psychic, 40
Defense mechanisms, 15, 65
Defensiveness in crisis, 64
Deficiency disorders, 244–245
Déjà vu phenomenon, 94, 134
Delusions, definition of, 95
 of paranoid conditions, 187–188
 somatic, 135
Dementia. See also specific organic disorders that
   may precipitate this condition.
 cerebrovascular, 233
 clinical forms of, 232–233
 from organic disorders, 237–238
 in old age, 233–234
 of diabetic ketosis, 239
 presenile, 234
 renal dialysis and, 240
 senile, 232
 treatment of, 234
Denial, acceptance and, 64
 anticipatory mourning and, 65
 in crisis, 65
Dependency, 38
 duodenal ulcers and, 152
 in adolescence, 40–41
Depersonalization, 94, 134
Depression, amitriptyline for, 314
 anorexia in, 177
 biological basis of, 74
 clinical aspects of, 176–177
 disruption of needs and, 3
 heart disease and, 151
 in childhood, 263–265
 indoleamine hypothesis of, 74
 insomnia in, 177
 life events and, 59
 management of, 179–181
 MHPG test and, 175
 monoamine oxidase inhibitors in, 174
 neuroleptics for, 182
 pain in, 177
 presentation of, 176
 psychosocial factors in, 175–176
 relapses of, 59
 self-esteem and, 175
 separation and, 176
 signs of, 176–177
 sudden death and, 151
 symptoms, 176–171
 tricyclics for, 180–297, 298, 311–313
Depressive illnesses of aged, 52
Derealization, 94, 134
Dermatological system, 103
Desensitization therapy, 124, 216, 295
Desipramine, 314
Development, age and, 46–47
 as integrated process, 11. See also specific areas.
 biological, by age, 27–30t
  in adolescence, 33–35
 by age, 27–30t
 child, arrest of, 11

basic parameters of, 13–16
 biological aspects of, 12, 13
 choices necessary in, 11–12
 cognitive skill deprivation, 12
 crises of, 12
 critical stage of, 12
 emotional deprivation in, 12
 disorders and, 249
 epigenetic theories of, 13–14
 general principles of, 9–13
 in utero experience in, 17–18
 lack of predictability of, 11–12
 principles of, 9–13. See also specific areas under
    Development.
 cognitive. See Cognitive development.
 deviations of, 253–256
 emotional, 14–16
 first year, 18–21
 in body control, 18
 in motor skills, 18–19
 in utero, 17–18
 intrapsychic, 14
 language. See Language development.
 middle childhood, 25–26, 31
 moral, middle childhood, 31
  of toddler, 23
 normal, 16–31, 27–30t
 one to three years, 21–23
 personal/social, emotional versus, 16
  role models and, 16
 prenatal, 17–18
 preschool years, 24–25
 psychological, 36–37
 sensory, 18
 smile and, 19
 social, 37
 stages of, 37–41
 survival mechanisms in, 18
Diabetes, as psychosomatic disorder, 153
 lithium induced, 310
Diagnosis, after mental state examination, 99. See
    also specific conditions.
 treatment and, 281
Diagnostic Statistical Manual of Mental Disorders,
    206
Digit span, 96
Digitalis, 243
Disabilities, premorbid, 327, 328
Disaster, anger and, 57
 definition of, 56
 guilt and, 57
 impact phase of, 57
 panic and, 57
 post-traumatic phase of, 57
 reactions to, 56–58
 recoil phase of, 57
 requisite aspects of, 57
 specific reactions to, 57
Disease, emotional conflict and, 143. See also Illness.
 in pregnancy, 18
 life events and, 145
 personality structure and, 143
 psychosocial effects of, 146
 stress and, 144–145
Disengagement theory of aging, 45

Disequilibrium, 55–56, 62
Disorder. See also specific conditions.
　affective. See *Affective disorders.*
　anxiety. See *Anxiety* and *Anxiety disorders.*
　gastrointestinal, 61
　mother-child relationship and, 61–62
　obsessive-compulsive, 127–130
　personality, 118
　physical, emotions and, studies of, 1–2
　　personality types and, 61
　physical-psychological, studies of, 1
　psychiatric, common, 117–119. See also specific
　　disorders.
　　diagnosis of, 117
　　intelligence tests and, 108
　　physical disorder and, 102–103
　　psychological, life events and, 59
　　physician consultation for, 2
　psychosomatic. See *Psychosomatic disorders.*
　stress-related, 61
Dissociation of catecholamine responses, 60
Dissociative disorders, 131–134
　anxiety and, 131
　causes of, 132–133
　description of, 127
　differential diagnosis of, 133–134
　hysteria and, 136
　kinds of, 131–132
　repression in, 133
　treatment of, 133
Distress, complexity of, 3
　situational, 144
Divorce, 252
Dols of pain, 157
Dopamine, 74
"Double-bind" communication, 192
Doubling, 134
Down's syndrome, 256, 349, 350
Dreams, 94
Drives, 15
Drugs, categories of, 300–301. See also *Treatment*
　　under specific disorders and specific types
　　of drugs.
　for elderly, 52
　impairment of sexual function by, 213–214
　neurotransmitters and, 73
　pregnancy and, 18
　psychoactive, 300
　psychotropic, cardiac side effects of, 103
　　classification of, 222
　　psychological effects of, 241
　　side effects of, 104–105
　sedative, 241
　use by the elderly, 317–318
Drug abuse, definition of, 221
Drug abuse syndromes, 222–225
　etiology of, 222–224
　specific, 224–225
Drug addiction, 221
　enkephalins and, 74–75
　opiate peptide hypothesis of, 75
Drug dependence, diagnosis of, 226–228
　syndromes associated with, 226–228
　treatment of, 228
Drug dose, 149. See also specific drugs and types of
　　pharmaceuticals.

Drug habituation, 221
Drug intoxications, 241–244
Drug therapy, 300–315, 302t, 304t
Drug tolerance, 75
Drug use disorders, 221–228
Drug withdrawal, 75
Drunkenness, 225
Dysfunction. See specific types.
Dyskinesia, overt, 306–307
　tardive, 52–53
　　antipsychotic drugs and, 306–307
　　withdrawal, 306–307
Dyspareunia, in men, 211
　in women, 214–215
Dystonic reaction to antipsychotic drugs, 306

Earthquake neurosis, 55
Echolalia, 94
Ecological unit, 250
ECT. See *Electroconvulsive therapy.*
Education services, 323–324
Ego alien, 118, 127
"Ego integrity" concept, 47
Ego mechanisms of defense, 65
"Ego restitution," 327
Ego syntonic, 118
Ejaculation, premature, 211
　　treatment of, 215–216
Ejaculatory incompetence, 211
　treatment of, 216
Elderly. See *Aged* and *Aging.*
Electroconvulsive therapy, 53, 297–300
　amnesia and, 298
　contraindications for, 299
　criticisms of, 297
　electrode placement for, 299
　for affective disorders, 298
　for anorexia nervosa, 298
　for depression, 180, 297, 298
　for hypomania, 298
　for mania, 298
　for schizophrenia, 298
　in outpatient departments, 323
　indications for, 298
　numbers of treatments by, 299–300
　procedures for, 299–300
　technique of, 299–300
Electroencephalography, 103–104
Electrolyte disturbances, 245
Emergency(ies), psychiatric, 267–273
　assessment of, 270–272
　case report of, 269, 271–272
　case report on management of, 272–273
　channels of referral of, 267–268
　common, 268t
　crisis situations and, 268–269
　crisis theory of, 269–270
　current problems of, 272
　definition of, 267
　definition of problem of, 272
　demographic characteristics of, 268
　diagnostic categories of, 268
　ecological group approach to, 272
　goals of treatment of, 272
　hours of referral of, 267–268
　incidence of, 267

management of, 272–273
medication for, 273
neuroleptics for, 273
presenting behavior in, 268–269
prevalence of previous treatment of, 268
systems approach to, 272
task mastery and, 272
techniques of, 272
timing of therapy for, 272
social, 269
"Emergency" reaction, 60
Emergency services, 319–320
Emergency ward back-up, 319–320
Emotions, adrenaline-noradrenaline levels and, 60
deprivation, in child development, 12
duodenal ulcers and, 152
expressed, 328
heart disease and, 151
hormone levels and, 60
in asthma, 150
limbic system and, 72
paradoxical, 146
synchronous, 146
toddler development of, 22
Emotional development, 14–16
in adolescence, 36–37
Emotional turbulence, 41
Empathy, 36
Encephalopathy, hepatic, flapping tremor and, 240
Korsakov's syndrome in, 240
psychological effects of, 240
uremic, 239–240
Encopresis, in Hirschsprung's disease, 255
treatment of, 255–256
Endocrine hyperactivity, 239
Endocrine hypoactivity, 244–245
Endocrine system, 103
Endorphins, 74
Enkephalins, 74–75
Enuresis, 254–255
treatment of, 255
Environment, constant internal physiological concept of, 60
disruption of, 55
in mental retardation, 350–351
influence on child development, 9
Epigenetic theories of child development, 11, 13–14
Erectile reflex activation, 213
Erikson, on adolescence, 251
on "ego integrity," 47
on identity, 36, 37, 39
on life crises classification, 62–63
Erotic preferences, anomalous, 216–219
Error theory of aging, 44
Ethology in infant relationships, 3
Evasion, 62
Events. See *Life events.*
Examination, by psychological testing, 107–111
for psychological complaints, 105
formulation and, 113–116
history, 81–89
mental state, 78–79, 91–99
abnormal perceptual experiences, 95
affect, 92–93
appearance, 92

behavior, 92
congruence of interviewer observation and patient's subjective experience, 92
ending of, 99
mood, 92–93
organic cerebral disorder, 97–98
sensorium, 95–97
speech, 93–94
thought content, 93–95
verbal/nonverbal behavior, 91
notes on, 91
of mental processes, 91
physical, 101–105
Excitement phase of sexual response, 214
Exhibitionism, 218
Expectations of parents, 252–253
Experience, life, 46–47
"Expressed emotion," 328
Extracellular theories of aging, 44–45
Eye convergence, 19

Factual information testing, 97
Failure to thrive, 13
Family, child and, 250
history taking of, 87, 88, 89
illness and, 101
patient treatment and, 282
Fears. See *Phobias.*
Feedback, 56
Fetishism, 217
Fetoscopy, 350
Fight or flight, 145
"Fix," 242
Flapping tremor, 240
"Flashbacks," 227, 242
Flight of ideas, 93
Flooding therapy, 295
Flurazepam, 317
Folic acid deficiency, 244
Forbidden wish, 128
anxiety and, 123–124
in conversion disorders, 137
Formal operations, 11
Formal operations stage, 26, 31, 35–36
"Formication," 242
Formulation, case report of, 114–115
following examination, 113–116
in mental state examination, 99
steps of, 113–114
Freud, Anna, on defense mechanisms, 65
on dependency, 36–37
Freud, Sigmund, impact on psychiatry, 291
on psychoanalytic aspects of child development, 11
Frotteurism, 218
Fugue, 132, 133
Functioning, mental. See *Mental functioning.*

Gases, 243–244
Gastrointestinal disorders, 61. See also specific disorders.
Gastrointestinal system, 102–103
Gender-identity, 31
General adaptation syndrome, 144
General paralysis of the insane, 6

Generalists, 66–67
Generation gap, 251
Generativity versus stagnation, 50
Genes in mental retardation, 348, 349
Genetics, influence on child development, 9
Gerontophilia, 217
Gesell on developmental skills, 27–30t
Gestalt, 19
Gilles de la Tourette syndrome, 256
"Giving-up–given up" reaction, 61
    in psychosomatic conditions, 144
"Giving up reaction," 1, 153, 154
Glossary of psychiatric terms, 355–357
Glove anesthesia, 139
Glucocorticoid excess, 239
Glutethimide, 241
G.P.I., 6
Grief, anger and, 64
    change and, 58
    decompensation and, 61
    description of, 58
    inadequate, 58
    stress and, 61
Grief counseling, 58
"Grief work," 58
Guilt, disaster and, 57. See also specific disorders.

Habituation, 73
Hallucinations, 95
Hallucinogens, 242
Heart disease, as psychosomatic disorder, 150–151
    depression and, 151
    emotions and, 151
    Type A personality and, 151
Hebephilia, 217
Hematological system, 103
Hepatolenticular degeneration, 245
Heredity in psychopathology, 71
Hero worship, 38–39
Hippocrates, 172
Hirschsprung's disease, 255
History taking, 55, 78, 81–89
    family history, 87. See also Interview.
    identifying data, 84–85
    mental and physical history of previous illness,
        86–87
    organization of, 84–89
    personal history, 87–89
    personality, 89
    presenting complaint, 85–86
    referral aspects of, 85
    reliability of information, 85
    symptomatology of complaint, 86
Histrionic personality, 204
Homeostasis in crisis resolution, 62
Homosexuality, 216–217
Hormones, female, psychological effects of, 243
    levels of, emotions and, 60
Hospital, day, 321–322
        economic aspects of, 322–323
        for specific age groups, 322
        functions of, 322
    mental, study of, 325
    night, 322
Hospital treatment. See Treatment, hospital.

Hospitalization, part-time, 321–323
"Host factors," 281–282
Hostility of paranoia, 185
Housing during rehabilitation, 329–330
Huntington's chorea, 234
Hyperactivity in attention disorders, 258–259
Hypercalcemia, 239
Hyperdominance, erotic, 219
Hyperesthesia, glove, 139
Hyperparathyroidism, 239
Hypersexuality, 211
Hypersomnia, 167
Hypertension, 149
Hyperthyroidism, 239
Hyperventilation, anoxia and, 239
    psychological effects of, 243
Hypnosis for conversion symptoms, 140
Hypnotics, for insomnia, 317
    psychological effects of, 241
Hypochondriasis, 135, 140, 141–142
    conversion versus, 141
    definition of, 141
    disorders involving, 141
    nosophobia in, 135
    sense of self in, 141
Hypoglycemia, 244
Hypomania, 298
Hypoparathyroidism, 245
Hyposexuality, 211
Hypothermia, 238
Hypothesis. See Formulation.
Hypothyroidism, 244
Hysteria, 136

Ideas of influence, 94
Ideas of reference, 94
Identity, 36, 37, 39
    anorexia nervosa and, 152
    in adolescence, 36, 251
Ideologies in adolescence, 39
Illness, attitude to, 101
    attitude to family during, 101
    attitude to medical personnel during, 101
    deviant behavior during, 101
    fatal, reaction to, 64
    hidden psychiatric, 2
    isolation and, 145
    life events and, 55–68
    models of, 4, 135
    pain in, 102
    physical, as conversion symptom, 139
        life event and, 59, 60–62
        psychological disorders in, 6
    physical-psychological, 1–2
    psychological, physical disorders in, 6
        treatment of, 6
    psychosocial effects of, 146
    psychosocial life events and, 102
    secondary gain from, 101–102
    social status incongruence and, 145
    stress related, 1–2
Illness-prone, 2
Illusions, 95
Imagination in middle childhood, 31
Immunoprotein theory of aging, 44
Impact phase, 57

Impact phase reactions, 63
"Impaired role," 4
Implosion therapy, 295
Impotence, 211
    post-myocardial infarction and, 49–50
    situational, 212
    treatment of, 215
    vascular, 212
In utero experience in development of child, 17–18
Incidence, 173
Independence in adolescence, 36–37
"Individuation," 11, 47
Indoleamine hypothesis of depression, 74
Infancy, childhood and, 9–31. See also *Development, child.*
Information seeking, in crisis, 65
    in interview, 81
Inpatient services, 320–321
Inpatient treatment, 320
Inpatient units, 321
Insight testing, 97
Insomnia, 165–166
    benzodiazepines for, 317
    causes of, 166
    in depression, 177
    psychological effects of, 245
    treatment of, 317–318
Instincts, 72
Institution, influences on life in, 325–326
    study of, 325–326
"Institutionalism," 326
Insulin coma, 300
Integrity, 3
Intellectual development, 12, 13–14
Intelligence, assessment of, 97–98
    influences on, 10
Intelligence tests, 108
    mental retardation and, 346
Interpretation, 292
Intervention, 324
Interview, as intrusion, 81
    ending of, 99
    evaluative, 78. See also *History.*
    information seeking in, 81
    observation in, 82
    purposes of, 81–82
    sodium amytal, 140
    structured, 81
    therapeutic, 78–79, 82
    unstructured, 81
Interviewing, alertness to patient, 83
    assumption avoidance, 83
    basic rules of, 82–84
    communication problems, 84
    language difficulties, 84
    patient ease, 82–83
    patient uniqueness, 83
    record making and, 83
    social class modifiers, 83–84
    termination of, 84
    time allotment, 83
Intimacy, in adolescence, 37
    in late adolescence, 40
    life events and, 68
Intoxication, 239–244

Intracellular theory of aging, 44
Investigations after interview, 99, 101–105
Isolation, illness and, 145
    in aging, 45
    obsesssive-compulsive disorder and, 128

Jealousy, 226
Job change reactions, 58
Job depression, 171–172
Judgment testing, 97

Ketosis, 239
Kidney, lithium and, 309–310
Kleine-Levin syndrome, 167
Korsakoff syndrome, 225, 231
Korsakov's psychosis, 239
Korsakov's syndrome, 240
Krafft-Ebing, on sadism, 218–219

Language, in preschool years, 24
    of play, 250
    sense of self and, 22
Language development, 16
    by age, 27–30t
    first year, 20
    second year, 21
Language function testing for cerebral defects, 98
Latency stage, 25
LCU, 59
L-Dihydroxyphenylalanine, 243
L-Dopa, 243
Lead intoxication, 244
Learning, age and, 51
    needs and, 3
Learning disabilities, 257–258
Learning theory, anxiety and, 124
    on obsession, 129
Leisure time use, 329
Liaison service, 323
Life change units, 59
Life chart, 55
Life cycle crises, 62–63
Life events, accidents and, 59
    adjustment to, 62
    cumulative effects of, 58–60
    definition of, 55
    depression and, 59
    disease and, 145
    evasion of, 62
    growth and, 62
    illness and, 55–68
    independent, 59–60
    intimacy and, 68
    patients and, 55
    physical illness and, 59, 60–62
    "private," 58
    psychologic disorders and, 59
    schizophrenia and, 59–60
    social supports and, 67
    stress of, 145
    suicide and, 59
    threatening, 59, 62
Life experience, 46–47
Life review, 44
Limbic system, 72

Limits, 23, 39
Lithium, 307–310
    bipolar affective disorder and, 309
    cardiac side effects of, 309
    in mania, 181
    indications for, 308
    initiation of treatment with, 308–309
    kidney and, 309–310
    mania and, 307–310
    pharmacology of, 307–308
    polydipsia and, 309–310
    polyuria and, 309–310
    pregnancy and, 309
    psychological effects of, 243
    side effects of, 309
    toxic effects of, 309
    use of, 308
Lithium-induced diabetes, 310
Lithium maintenance, 309
Lithium prophylaxis, 309
Lithium therapy, 105, 309
Logoclonia, 94
Loneliness, 31, 45
Longevity. See also Aging.
    cephalization index and, 44–45
    mutations versus, 44
Loss, dynamics of, 64
    reactions to, 58
    stress and, 61
Love, attachment and, 21
    in late adolescence, 40
LSD, 227
Lying, pathological, in somatization, 136
"Lytic cocktail," 301

"Mad Hatter syndrome," 244
Magician healer, 5–6
Malarial fever, 300
Malingering, 108, 136, 141
Mania, clinical aspects of, 177–178
    delirious, 178
    electroconvulsive therapy for, 298
    lithium and, 307–310
    management of, 181–183, 182t
    use of lithium in, 181
"Manifest aging," 47
MAOI. See Monoamine oxidase inhibitors.
Marijuana, 242–243
Masochism, 219
Masters and Johnson technique, 296
Mastery, 12
Masturbation, 38
Maturity, 43–53
Mechanisms. See specific type.
Medical practice challenges, 333–337
    management of, 336–337
    types of, 334–336
Medical science progress, 5
Medication. See Drugs.
Megalomania, 187
Melancholia, involutional, 177
    mourning and, 172
Mellaril, 105
Memory, limbic system and, 72
    organic cerebral disorder and, 98
    testing of, 96

Memory disorders, in alcoholism, 225
Mental functioning, behavior and, 71–75
    biology and, 71–75
    neurotransmitters and, 71–72
Mental retardation. See Retardation, mental.
Mental state examination. See Examination, mental
    state.
Mercury intoxication, 244
Metabolic disorders, 239
Metabolism disorder, 103
Metals, heavy, 244
Metaphors, somatic, 136
Methaqualone, 241
Methylphenidate, 259, 260
MHPG, 175
Microcephaly, 347
Mid-adolescence, 39–40
Middle age, 43–53
Middle childhood, 25–26, 31
"Middle" generation, 50–51
Milieu therapy, 321, 326–327
Mineral disturbances, 245
Minnesota Multiphasic Personality Inventory, 109
M.M.P.I., 109
Model(s), of illness, 4
    role, 16
    somatopsychic-psychosomatic, 61
Molidone, 307
Monoamine theory, 74
Monoamine oxidase inhibitors, 174, 313–314
    autonomic side effects of, 314
    in depression, 174, 180
    interaction effects, 314
    overdosage of, 314
    selection of patients for, 314
    side effects of, 314
    toxic reactions to, 314
Mood, 92–93, 171
Mood disorders, 40
Moral development, during preschool years, 24
    middle childhood, 31
Morphine, 241–242
Mother, age of, 349
    relationship to child, 10, 13
    responsiveness of, 18
    "schizophrenogenic," 192
    separation from, 150
Mother-child relationship, bonding in, 20. See also
                specific aspects such as Oedipal period.
    genetic disorder and, 61–62
    object permanence and, 19
    primary caretaker and, 20
    separation and, 21
    toilet training and, 23
Motor aphasia, 93
Motor behavior, 72
Motor development deviations, 253–254
Motor skills, first year, 18–19
    preschool, 24
    toddler, 21
Motor tic disorders, 256
Mourning, anticipatory, 65
    melancholia and, 172
Mourning period, 64
Musculoskeletal system, 103

Mutations, 44
Mutism, elective, 254
Myocardial infarction, 49–50
"Myxedema madness," 244

Narcolepsy, 168
Narcoleptic tetrad, 168
Narcotherapy, 293
Narcotics, 158
Nature-nurture theories of child development, 10–11
Necrophilia, 218
"Need to exercise" concept, 45
Needs, 2–3
Neologisms, 94
Neurasthenia, 141
Neurodermatitis, 149
Neuroleptics, for depression, 182
  for psychiatric emergencies, 273
  in schizophrenia, 74, 198
Neurological investigation, 103–104
Neurological system, 102
Neuronal degeneration in aging, 43
Neurosis, definition of, 118
  earthquake, 55
Neurotransmitters, action of, 73
  anatomic locations of, 73–74
  brain function and, 73–74
  drugs and, 73
  mental health and, 71–72
  names of, 73
  receptors for, 73
Night terror, 167–168
Nonsadistic hyperdominance pattern, 219
Nonspecificity, 144
Noradrenaline, 60
Norm-bearers, 50
Nosophobia, 135
Nostalgia, 33
Note taking, 79
NREM sleep, 163–165
  disorders of, 167–168

Object permanence, 11, 19
Obsession, definition of, 127
  learning theory on, 129
Obsessional character, 127
Obsessive-compulsive disorders, 127–130
  case report of, 127, 129
  causes of, 128–129
  defense mechanisms of, 128–129
  ego alien act and, 127
  incidence of, 128
  omnipotence in, 127
  personality traits of, 127–128
  psychoanalytic theory of, 128
  treatment of, 130
Obsessive-compulsive idea, 125
Oculogyric crisis, 306
Oedipal period, 24
Office setting, 79
Old age. See *Aged* and *Aging*.
Operant conditioning techniques, 295
Opiates, 227–228, 241–242
Opiate peptide hypothesis of drug addiction, 75
Opiate receptors, 74–75

Opisthotonus, 306
Oral needs, 152
Organic brain disorder, clinical presentation of, 229–230
  dementia and, 237–238
  examination for, 97–98
  extracerebral causes of, 237–248
  intracerebral causes of, 229–236
  psychological symptoms of, 237–238
Organic brain syndrome, acute, 230–231
  differential diagnosis of, 230–231
  drugs for, 231
  treatment of, 231
  chronic, 231–232
  subacute, 231
Organic psychiatric syndrome, 229
Organic view of physician-scientist, 6
Orgasmic dysfunction, 216
Orgasmic phase of sexual response, 214
Orientation testing, 96
Outpatient services, 323
Oxygen intoxication, 243

Pain, 157–161
  body/environment and, 159
  body image and, 160
  clinical, 158
  diversion and, 158
  dols of, 157
  experimental, 158
  in conversion syndromes, 160
  in depression, 177
  intensity of, 159
  narcotics and, 158
  perception of, 158
  placebos and, 158
  psychological reaction component of, 159–161
  social responses and, 160
  specificity theory of, 157
  theories of, 157–158
  view of, 102
Pain asymbolia, 159
Palimpsests, 225
Panic, 57
Paradoxical emotional responses to illness, 146
Paranoia. See *Paranoid disorders*.
Paranoid disorders, 185–188
  hostility in, 185
  psychotic, 186–187
  treatment of, 188
  types of delusions in, 187–188
Paranoid psychosis, 187
Paraphrenia, 187
Paralysis in conversion disorders, 138–139
Parents, dependency on, 38
  disappointment with child, 17
  expectations of, 24, 25
    effect on children of, 252–253
  limit setting by, 39
  reaction to retardation by, 257
Parent-child mismatch, 10
Paresis in conversion disorders, 138–139
Parkinsonian-like syndrome, 305
Passivity feelings, 94
Patient, analysand versus, 4
  behavior of, 3–4

Patient, *cont.*
  challenging types of, 334–336
  common characteristics of, 4
  compartmentalizing of, 1
  history of, 81–89
  interruption of life of, 320
  life events and, 55
  needs of, 2–3
  physician and, 1–7
  physician's approach to, 78–79
  relapse of, 328
  role of, 3–4
Patient culture, 325–326
Patient-physician relationship. See *Physician-patient relationship.*
Pedophilia, 217
Peers, competition with, 26
  in mid-adolescence, 39
  in preschool years, 24
  influence of, 31
Pellagra, 244
Perception, 95
"Performance," 47
Performance anxiety, 212
Performance skills in middle age, 50
Perseveration, 93
Personal/social development, 16
Personality, coronary artery disease and, 61
  definition of, 203
  disease and, 143
  disorders of. See *Personality disorders.*
  history taking of, 89
  histrionic, 204
  hysterical, 207
  multiple, 132
  physical disorders and, 61
  psychopathic, 206
  Type A, 61
Personality disorders, 118, 203–209
  anankastic, 207–208
  antisocial, 207
  asocial, 207
  avoidant, 207
  classification of, 206–208
  compulsive, 207–208
  dependent, 207
  diagnosis of, 208
  epidemiology of, 204–205
  etiology of, 205–206
  high-level, 203
  histrionic, 207
  low-level, 204
  narcissistic, 207
  paranoid, 206–207
  schizoid, 207
  schizotypal, 207
  treatment of, 208–209
    case report, 208–209
  unstable, 207
Personality inventories, 109
Phenothiazines, 301
Phenylketonuria, 256
Pheochromocytoma, 239
Phobias, 125–127
  avoidance and, 125, 126

case report of, 126
causes of, 126
description of, 125
incidence of, 125
influence of, 94
preschool, 25
psychoanalytic theory of, 126
trauma and, 126
treatment of, 126–127
Photosensitivity, 307
Phrenologists, 71
Physical defect, 102
Physical examination, 101–105
Physician, approach to patient, 78–79
  as magician, 5–6
  as scientist, 5
  frustrations of, 333–334
  history taking by, 78
  negative feelings of, 333–334
  nonjudgmental, 80
  patient and, 1–7
  priest versus, 6
  role of, 4–7
  supportiveness of, 283
  techniques for, 283–284
  therapeutic qualities of, 79–80
  training for, 5
  treatment of psychologic illness by, 6
Physician-patient relationship, 77–80
  therapeutic aspects of, 79–80
Piaget, cognitive theory of child development of, 11
  concrete operations stage of, 26, 35
  formal operations concept of, 11
  formal operations stage of, 26, 31, 35–36
  operational period concept of, 21
Pick's disease, 234
Pickwickian syndrome, 167
Pituitary insufficiency, 245
Pituitary overactivity, 239
Placebos, 158
Plateau phase of sexual response, 214
Play, language of, 250
  role of, 23
  toddler, 21
Play therapy, 250
Playmate, imaginary, 23
Polydipsia, 309–310
Polyuria, 309–310
Porphyria, 240
"Postpartum blues," 246–248
Post-traumatic disorder, 235
Post-traumatic phase, 57
Potency in aging, 49–50
Preadolescence, 37
Pregnancy, disease in, 18
  drug-taking and, 18
  lithium and, 309
  social supports and, 67
Premorbid disabilities, 327, 328
Preoperational period, 21
Preschool years, 24–25. See also specific aspects of this period.
Prevalence, 173
Priest-physician, 6
Projective tests, 109

Protective reaction pattern to stress, 145
Pseudo-epilepsy, 138
Psychedelic-hallucinogens, 227
Psychiatric disorders. See *Disorders, psychiatric.*
Psychiatric emergencies. See *Emergencies, psychiatric.*
Psychiatric terms glossary, 355–357
Psychiatrist, consulting of, 341–343
  legal advice from, 340
  patient assessment by, 339
  patient management by, 339–340
  referral to, 339–343
  role of, 339–340
  seeking of, 340–341
  skills of physician and, 340
Psychoactive drugs, 300
Psychoanalysis, 291–293
  anxiety and, 122
  assumptions of, 291–292
  indications for, 293
  psychoanalytic psychotherapy versus, 293
  technique of, 292–293
Psychoanalytic model, 140
Psychoanalytic theory, anxiety and, 123–124
  of phobias, 126
  of symptom choice, 133
Psychobiologic mechanisms in psychosomatic conditions, 144–145
Psychological development. See *Adolescence, Child,* and *Development.*
Psychological effects. See specific types of drugs or conditions.
Psychological testing. See *Testing, psychological.*
Psychologist, clinical referral to, 110
  testing by, 107
Psychoneurosis, definition of, 118
  oedipal period and, 24
Psychopathologic anxiety, 121–122
Psychopharmacology, 300–318
Psychosis(es), definition of, 118
  of childhood, 262–263. See also *Childhood disorders.*
  of late adolescence, 40
  preoperative, 246
Psychosocial mechanisms, 145
Psychosomatic concepts in initiation of disease, 143–145
Psychosomatic disorders, 138, 149–155. See also specific disorders.
  anorexia nervosa and, 151–152
  asthma, 150
  diabetes mellitus and, 152
  treatment of, 155
  ulcerative colitis and, 153–154
Psychosomatic mechanisms, 143–146
Psychosomatic patterning, 145–146
Psychosomatic-somatopsychic model of illness, 135
Psychotherapy, 289–296
  for aged, 46, 52–53
  for depression, 180
  intensive, 290–291
  major approaches of, 290, 290t
  note taking in, 79
  psychoanalytic, 291–293
    indications for, 293

psychoanalysis versus, 293
  supportive, 285–286
  uncovering, 181
  working relationship in, 77
Psychotropic agents, 300
Pubescence, in boys, 33–34, 34
  in girls, 34, 35
  self-consciousness during, 34–35
Punning, 93
Pygmalionism, 218
Pyrexia, convulsions of, 238
  mental complications of, 238
  symptoms of, 238
  treatment of, 238

Questions, open-ended, 81

Rape pattern, 218
Rapprochement, 22
RAS. See *Reticular activating system.*
"Reactions," 118. See also specific events or crises.
  giving up, 1
  neurotic, 118
Reaction formation, 129
Reality testing, 330
Recall, 72
Recoil phase, 57
Recoil-turmoil phase reactions, 63
Reconstruction, by psychoanalysis, 292
  rehabilitation and, 64
Reconstruction phase reactions, 63–64
Reference, 94
Reflexes, 19
Reformulation, case report of, 115–116
  steps in, 115
Refuge, 66
Regression, at developmental crises, 12
  in crisis, 64
Rehabilitation, 327–331
  accommodations and, 329
  aims of, 327–328
  disabilities treated by, 327–328
  for schizophrenic patient, 327–331
  leisure time and, 329
  reconstruction and, 64
  social environment and, 328–329
  work and, 330
  workshops and, 330
Rejection, 26
Relapses, of depression, 59
  of schizophrenia, 60
Relationships, object, 22. See also specific ones, such as *Mother-child relationship.*
  real, 77
  therapeutic, 77
  transference, 77–78
  transitional, 38–39
Relaxation techniques, 124
Religious denominations as support systems, 67
REM apnea, 168
REM sleep, 163–168
  disorders of, 168
Renal dialysis, 240
Repression, in anxiety, 123
  in conversion disorders, 137, 140
  in dissociative disorders, 133

Reproductive casualty, 18
Respiratory system, 102
Response acquisition procedures, 294
Response decrement procedures, 294
Response increment procedures, 294
Rest-activity cycle, 168
Retardation, mental, 256–257, 345–352
    causal factors in, 347–349, 347t
    criteria for, 345–347, 346t
    educational concerns in, 351–352
    handling of, 257
    harmful genes and, 348
    intelligence test and, 346
    maternal age and, 349
    medical treatment for, 351
    multiple genes and, 348
    parents' reaction to, 257
    physical hazards and, 348
    prevention of, 349–351
    prevention of environmental aspects of, 350–351
    prevention of genetic aspects of, 349
    social issues of, 352
    sterilization and, 350
    subcategories of, 257
    treatment of, 351–352
    vocational training and, 351–352
Reticular activating system, 72–73
    arousal and, 72
    attention and, 72–73
    consciousness and, 72–73
    consciousness disorders and, 73
    habituation, 73
    motor behavior and, 72
    sensory stimuli and, 72
    sleep and, 72
Retinitis pigmentosa, 307
Retirement, 47–48
Rhyming, 93
Rigidity, 50
Risk-taking, 26
Role, impaired, 4
    of patient, 3–4
    of physician, 4–7
"Role stickiness," 63
Role transition, coping skills and, 63
    crisis theory and, 63
Rorschach ink blots, 109

Sadism, 218–219
Schizophrenia, 133. See also Schizophrenic disorders.
    acute, 197–198
        treatment of, 198–199
    affect of, 195
    antipsychotic drugs for, 303–305
    as a lifetime illness, 198–201
    catatonic, 197
        case report of, 93–94
    categories of, 197–198
    chronic, 197–198
        rehabilitation for, 200–201
        signs of, 326
        treatment of, 200–201
    delusions of, 195–196
    diagnosing a first episode of, 193–198, 194t, 195t, 196t

diagnosis of, chief complaint and, 193–194
        history of present illness in, 194, 194t
        family history and, 194
        mental status and, 194–195, 195t, 196t
        past illnesses and, 194
        personal history and, 194
    differential diagnosis of, 196–197
    dopamine and, 74
    dopamine hypothesis of, 192
    drugs and, 60
    electroconvulsive therapy for, 298
    good prognosis, 197
    hallucinations of, 196
    hebephrenic, 197
    insulin coma and, 300
    latent borderline, 207
    life events and, 59–60
    maintenance therapy for, 304–305
    neuroleptics for, 198
    non-paranoid, 197
    paranoid, 197
    placebos and, 60
    poor prognosis, 197
    post-acute, 199–200
    prevention of, 201
    process, 192
    prognosis of, 201
    relapses of, 60
    schizo-affective, 198
    sensorium of, 196
    undifferentiated, 197
Schizophrenic disorders, 189–201. See also Schizophrenia.
    age and, 190
    biochemical theories of, 191–192
    biologic theories of, 190–192
    constitutional theories of, 190
    demographic factors in, 190
    epidemiology of, 189–190
    etiology of, 190–193
    genetic theories of, 190–191
    hospital admission figures, 189
    marital status and, 190
    migrants and, 190
    neurological theories of, 191
    occupation and, 190
    psychosocial theories of, 192–193
    sex of individual and, 190
    social class and, 190
    social factors of, 190
School, achievement in, 26
    adjustment to, 25, 26
    success in, 26
School phobia, 260–261
School refusal, 260–261
Scientist-physician, 5
Scurvy, 244
Secondary gain, from conversion symptom, 138
    of phobia, 126
Sedative drugs, 241
Self versus other, 14–15
Self-concept, in early adolescence, 38
    in hypochondriasis, 141
Self-consciousness, during pubescence, 34–35
    in adolescence, 38

Self-control, 41
　masturbation and, 38
Self-esteem, depression and, 175
　during middle childhood, 26
　in aging, 47
　in retirement, 47
Self-harm, 136
Self-help groups, 67
Semans technique, 215
Semantic skills, 71
Senescence, 43
Sensate focus, 215
Sensorium testing, 95–97
Sensory deprivation, 245–246
Sensory disturbance in conversion disorders, 139
Sensory stimuli, 72
Separation, attachment and, 21
　depression and, 176
　from spouse, 58
　in childhood, 251–252
　irreversible effects of, 21
Separation anxiety, 11
Separation anxiety disorder, 260–261
Separation behavior deviations, 260–261
Separation conflict, 153–154
Serial seven's, 96
Services, emergency. See *Emergency services.*
Sex as adolescent conflict, 36
Sexual activity, 48–49
Sexual behavior, limbic system and, 72
　of aged, 49
Sexual behavior disorders, 211–219
　behavior modification and, 215
Sexual drive, 251
Sexual function impairment by drugs, 213–214
Sexual inadequacy, in men, 211–214
　in women, 214–215
　therapy for, 215–216
Sexual interest, in adolescence, 38
　sexual activity versus, 49
Sexual preferences, anomalous, 216–219
Sexual-response cycle of female, 214
Sexual satisfaction in aged, 49
Sexuality, aging and, 48–50
　oedipal period and, 24
Shock-apathy-depression triad, 57
Side effects. See *Drugs* and types of drugs, such as
　Antidepressants and *Antipsychotic drugs.*
Simmond's disease, 245
SLE, psychological effects of, 240
Sleep, brain wave activity during, 163, *164*
　need for, 164–165, *165*
　reticular activating system and, 72
Sleep apnea, 168
Sleep deprivation, 245
Sleep disorders, 163–168
Sleep phobia, 166
Sleeplessness, 163
Sleepwalking, 167
Smile development, 19
"Social breakdown syndrome," 326
Social class, reproductive casualty and, 18
　school achievement and, 26

Social development in adolescence, 37
Social "drift," 190
Social Readjustment Rating Scale, 59
Social status incongruence, 145
Social supports. See *Supports, social.*
Socialization deviations, 261–262
Society, adolescent relationships to, 36
　aging and, 45
Sodium amytal interview, 140
Somatization, 135–142
　conversion and, 135
　description of, 135
　phenomena of, 135–136
Somatopsychic-psychosomatic model, 61
Somnambulism, 132
　childhood, 133–134
Specialists, 66–67
　techniques for, 286, 286t
Specificity in psychosomatic conditions, 143–144
Speech development, 254
Spouse separation reaction, 58
Stage, critical, 12. See also specific stages of devel-
　opment.
Stagnation, 50
Sterilization of retarded individuals, 350
Stimulants, 242
Stress, 55
　activity in, 65
　as loss, 61
　definition of, 56
　disease and, 144–145
　disorders related to, 61
　"emergency" reaction to, 60
　gastrointestinal disorders and, 61
　gravitational, 60
　grief aspects of, 61
　heart and, 150–151
　in late adolescence, 40
　life events and, 145
　peptic ulcer and, 61
　physical illness and, 1–2
　physical response to, 60–61
　protective reaction pattern to, 145
　ulcers and, 152
Stress-despair-illness sequence, 1
Stressors, 86
"Stripping process," 325–326
Strong Vocational Interest Blank, 109
Studies of physical/emotional disorders, 1–2. See
　also specific disorders.
Stupor, 98–99
Stuttering, 254
Subcortical structures, 71
Sudden death, 151
Suggestion in conversion symptoms, 140
Suicide, 275–279
　alcohol and, 276, 277
　altruistic, 275
　anomic type of, 275
　as cry for help, 276
　attempted, 275–279
　　assessment of, 277–279
　　characteristics of, 276
　　management of, 277–279, 278t
　　method of, 277

Suicide, *cont.*
  characteristics of, 276
  egoistic type of, 275
  fatalistic type of, 275
  in adolescents, 263–264
  life events and, 59
  method of, 277
  potential for, 277t
  prevention of, 278–279, 278t
  psychological theories of, 275–276
  sociological theories of, 275–276
  treatment of, 264–265
  tricyclics and, 313
Support needs, 68
Support network, 66
Support systems, as buffers, 66
  classification of, 66–67
  guidance and, 66
  refuge and, 66
  religions and, 67
Supportive measures, case report of, 284
  general, 284
  medical, 284–285
  of physicians, 283–286, 284t
Supports, social, 66–68
  asthma and, 67
  definition of, 56
  life events and, 67
  pregnancy and, 67
  unemployment and, 67
Suppression, 65
Survivor syndrome, 57
Symbolism, 143
Symptom choice, in conversion disorders, 140. See
      also specific symptoms.
  psychoanalytic theory of, 133
Symptoms in diagnosis, 117. See also specific signs
      and symptoms.
Synchronous emotional response to illness, 146
Syndrome psychiatry, 117
Syphilis, 300
System. See specific name.
"Systems theory," 3
Systemic lupus erythematosus, psychological effects
      of, 240

Target symptom, 199
Teachers, in making psychiatric referrals, 251
  middle aged as, 50
Temperament, 251
  biologic constitution and, 10, 13, 14t
Temperature change, 238
Testing, psychological, 107–111. See also specific
      tests and types of assessment.
  advantages and limitations of, 11
  knowledge about, 108
  referral for, 110
Terrible two's, 22
THC, 227
Thinking, circumstantial, 93
  tangential, 93
Thematic Apperception Test, 109
Theories of child development, 9–13. See also spe-
      cific names and types; and *Development,
      child.*

Therapeutic community, 327
Therapeutic effect, of interview, 82
  of physician-patient relationship, 79–80
Therapeutic milieu, 321, 326–327
Therapeutic nihilism, 46
Therapeutic presence, 53
"Therapeutic window," 314
"Therapeutic zeal," 334
Therapist, 283
Therapy, behavior, 293–296
  conjoint, 290
  family, 290
  group, 290
  individual, 290. See also specific conditions.
  milieu, 321, 326–327
  response to, 333
  techniques of, 283, 285t
Thioridazine, 307
Thought blocking, 93
Thought content disturbances, 94–95
Thought process, 93–94
  associative connections, 93
  case report, 93–94
Thriving, 13
Thyrotoxicosis, anxiety neurosis and, 239
  as psychosomatic disorder, 149
Tics, 256
Toddler years, 21–23
Toilet training conflict, 23
Tolerance to drugs, 75
Torticollis, 306
Toucheurism, 218
Tranquillizers, addiction to, 241
  minor, 315–317
  psychological effects of, 241
Transference, 292
Transition states, 63
Transitional object, 22
Transitional relationships, 38–39
Transsexualism, 217
Transvestism, 217
Trauma, 126
Traumatization, 57
Treatment, adaptation and, 282. See also specific
      types and disorders.
  behavior therapy, 289–296
  by scientific measures, 282
  by supportive techniques, 282
  diagnosis and, 281
  etiological factors and, 281
  family and, 282
  general medical, 281–286
  hospital, 319–324
  individualization of, 281
  of phobias, 126–127
  patient's defenses and, 281
  psychotherapeutic, 289–296
  social-environment, 325–331
  somatic, 297–318
Treatment plan, 99
Tremor, 240
"Triangular conflict," 326
Tricyclics, anticholinergic effects of, 312
  cardiovascular toxicity of, 313
  central nervous system effects of, 312

for depression, 180, 297, 298, 311–313
  incompatibilities and, 313
  interactions and, 313
  maintenance treatment with, 312
  method of treatment by, 311–312
  overdosage of, 313
  side effects of, 312, 313
  suicide and, 313
  toxic reactions of, 312
"Trip," 242
Truancy, 261
Tumors, 235–236
Tunnel vision, 139
Turning points, 63
Type A personality, characteristics of, 61
  heart disease and, 151

Ulcers,
  duodenal, as psychosomatic disorders, 152–153
    dependence conflicts and, 152
    emotions and, 152
  oral needs and, 152
  peptic, as psychosomatic disorder, 149
    stress and, 61
Ultrasonography, 350
Undoing, 128–129
Unemployment, 67

Vaginismus, 214
  treatment of, 216

Vaginitis, 50
Values, 24
Vitamin deficiency, 244
Vocabulary assessment, 97
Vocational assessment tests, 109
Voyeurism, 218

"Wear and tear" aging theory, 44
Wechsler Adult Intelligence Scale, in detecting
        psychotic functioning, 108
  older subjects and, 50
Wechsler Intelligence Scale for Children, 108
Wernicke's encephalopathy, 231
Wilson's disease, 245
Withdrawal, from drugs, 75
  in alcoholism, 225
  to avoid rejection, 26
Wolpe, on desensitization therapy, 216
  on fears, 295
Word salad, 94
Work, in late adolescence, 40
  rehabilitation and, 330
Workshops, 330
Worthiness, maintenance of, in old age, 53

Zoophilia, 218